TEMPOROMANDIBULAR DISORDERS

CLASSIFICATION, DIAGNOSIS, MANAGEMENT

SECOND EDITION

TEMPOROMANDIBULAR DISORDERS

CLASSIFICATION, DIAGNOSIS, MANAGEMENT

Second Edition

Welden E. Bell, D.D.S.

Clinical Professor of Oral and Maxillofacial Surgery
Baylor College of Dentistry

Clinical Professor of Oral Surgery
University of Texas Southwestern Medical School
Dallas, Texas

YEAR BOOK MEDICAL PUBLISHERS, INC.
Chicago • London

0 9 8 7 6 5 4 3 2 1

Library of Congress Cataloging-in-Publication Data

Bell, Welden E.
    Temporomandibular disorders.

    Rev. ed. of: Clinical management of temporomandibular disorders. c1982.
    Includes bibliographies and index.
    1. Temporomandibular joint—Diseases.
2. Temporomandibular joint. I. Bell, Welden E.
Clinical management of temporomandibular disorders.
II. Title. [DNLM: 1. Temporomandibular Joint Diseases.
WU 140 B435t]
RK470.B44 1986   617'.522   85-26292
ISBN 0-8151-0653-X

Sponsoring Editor: Stephany S. Scott
Manager, Copyediting Services: Frances M. Perveiler
Production Project Manager: Sharon W. Pepping
Proofroom Supervisor: Shirley E. Taylor

To honor the memory of
JAMES B. COSTEN
HARRY SICHER
LASZLO L. SCHWARTZ
WILLIAM B. FARRAR

Preface

It has been, and continues to be, my chief objective to develop a book that would serve as both a textbook for students and a practice guide for my colleagues in the dental profession. The first edition was a good start toward that end, being widely used and very well accepted. It is hoped, however, that this updated and thoroughly revised second edition will better accomplish the purpose of the book.

The material has been restructured in a sequence that flows more smoothly from identification of the problem to clinical management. A brief, historical review of the last 50 years of the dental profession's involvement in the correction of temporomandibular disorders should serve to place the entire issue in better perspective. Attention to basic orthopedic principles and a more accurate anatomical understanding of the masticatory structures should help eradicate several serious misconceptions that have spawned confusion in the past. Masticatory physiology is prescribed as the standard by which abnormality may be recognized. A new chapter on etiology has been created, giving special consideration to the roles played by emotional tension, occlusal disharmony, and bruxism. Theories have been omitted in favor of factual evidence. The classification of disorders has been extended to comprise the clinical symptoms usually displayed, by which each such disorder can be identified clinically. The technical matter of examining the patient and the process of arriving at an accurate clinical diagnosis have been refined. Special attention has been given to the different means of confirming the clinical diagnosis. More adequate management guidelines have been suggested as weighed against the currently reported long-term results of therapy.

The most significant improvement, however, lies in documentation. More than 475 new references have been cited as source material from which clinical conclusions have been drawn. Although some revision of the present concepts may be required as new evidence becomes available, the material as presented at this date stands very well authenticated by a mass of research evidence drawn from the published dental and medical literature.

It is again my earnest desire that this effort be found helpful to others in their quest for more rational and effective management of complaints involving the masticatory system.

WELDEN E. BELL, D.D.S.

Contents

1 | A Problem for Clinical Dentistry

Complaints of the masticatory system that involve the temporomandibular joints and masticatory musculature have been troublesome for doctors to manage well. First medical doctors and subsequently dentists have tried to cope with such problems. On the whole, however, clinical results have been less than satisfying. Frequently the patient is disappointed and the doctor is frustrated. But the accumulation of scientific knowledge about the structures and mechanisms involved has been quite satisfactory. It appears, therefore, that the difficulty lies not so much in a lack of basic knowledge as in a failure to apply that information at a clinical level.

DEFINING THE PROBLEM

The clinical management of the dentition comprises the major day-to-day duties of the practicing dentist. Management of the masticatory system, however, does not end with providing the presence, normal structural form, proper alignment, and harmonious occlusion of teeth. The dentition proper represents only the working ends of the apparatus, the tools by which mastication is accomplished, not the system itself.

Prehension, incising, grinding, and swallowing foods are vital body functions. The same is true of respiration and speech, in which the oral structures participate importantly. The mechanisms of oral communication and orofacial expression make social intercourse pleasant and profitable. Chronologically, the oral cavity is the initial organ of sexual expression and throughout life never completely loses this emotional

1

association. The mouth and orofacial structures constitute a region of unusual emotional significance that remains sensitive to threat and responsive to clinical management.

The masticatory system is a complex one indeed. During the many patterns of action required for the preparation of food prior to deglutition, the intricate mechanics involved in the articulation of tooth surfaces (occlusal function) is a study in itself. Mastication calls on an integrated and precisely coordinated biologic system of bones, joints, ligaments, muscles, vessels, nerves, and glands that extends from the lips to the larynx and from the teeth to the esophagus. This system can be affected by disorders and complications without number. It is the purpose of this book to consider in depth one group of disorders of this complex system: the so-called temporomandibular disorders.

More precisely, the objectives of this book are:

1. To consider the anatomical and physiologic factors involved in normal functioning of the masticatory apparatus, other than occlusion per se;
2. To consider departures from normal structural and functional behavior of the masticatory apparatus, other than problems of occlusion per se;
3. The clinical identification of such departures from normal; and
4. To establish guidelines for the clinical management of temporomandibular disorders that constitute such departures from normal.

HISTORICAL BACKGROUND

The historical record of the clinical management of temporomandibular disorders is colorful indeed. Many patients with complaints of this type have found themselves in a medical no-man's-land, in that orthopedists have seemed unable to grasp the full significance of masticatory physiology or cope with its impact on disorders of this type, and dentists who undertake management do so without benefit of adequate training and experience in orthopedic medicine. In retrospect, it appears that this clinical dilemma is really a spinoff from the unfortunate separation of the two professions.

In 1934, the otolaryngologist Costen[1] drew attention to the syndrome that bears his name by concluding that lost vertical dimension in the chewing apparatus was chiefly responsible for the complaints. It was a case of astute observation from which an improper conclusion was drawn. Costen correctly observed that disengagement of the occlusion did benefit many of his patients, just as the restriction of traumatic activity in general is known to ameliorate other types of orthopedic complaints. From this observation, however, he improperly assumed that the disengaging material placed between the teeth yielded benefit *because it opened the bite.* He concluded that the chief cause of the complaint was a "closed bite." As a result, the treatment in vogue for many years was the empirical application of various forms of bite-raising dental procedures.

Although the expected results were disappointing, the belief that occlusion is the key to temporomandibular complaints dominated dental practitioners' thinking until the present. Thus, preoccupied as the dental profession has been with occlusion as the dominant etiologic factor and occlusal therapy as the chief form of treatment, the gap between the professions has widened until the problem has come to rest in the lap of dentistry. Unfortunately, most practicing dentists, untrained in orthopedics and unschooled in diagnostic techniques, have not been able to manage the problem effectively, nor has the dental educational system met the challenge thus presented.

Prior to Costen there was only an occasional article in the dental literature pertaining to this problem. Our basic knowledge of joint structure and function was found in three pages of *Gray's Anatomy.* Most dental articles on the temporomandibular joint (TMJ) referred to such things as spontaneous anterior dislocation, growth disorders, ankylosis, and traumatic injuries. References to the joints and muscles as determinants of masticatory function and dysfunction were rare indeed. Goodfriend[2, 3] contributed to the dental literature in the early 1930s. Costen's real impact on dentistry began in 1937 when he published an article in the *Journal of the American Dental Association.*[4] The same year, Schultz[5] introduced sclerosing therapy as a treatment for joint hypermobility. Schuyler[6] stressed the importance of occlusal disharmony. Dentistry as a profession, however, largely remained unaware of the significance of the TM joint in masticatory complaints.

The decade of the 1940s was a period of confusion and controversy. Untrained in orthopedic medicine, dentists naturally fell back on what they understood—the dentition. With Costen as the dominant authority, reconstructive dentistry was seized upon to treat both temporomandibular and auricular complaints. Bite-raising was the order of the day; the vertical dimension of occlusion took on an undue clinical significance. Occlusionists, however, contended that occlusal disharmony rather than a "closed-bite" was the chief etiologic determinant. As a result, occlusal equilibration became a popular form of treatment.

The contention between occlusionists and bite-raisers was not diminished by Gottlieb's concept of masticatory biofunction as a proper basis for therapy.[7] Thus, more conflicts developed between occlusionists and anatomists.

During the 1950s, the syndrome concept of TMJ disorders had fully flowered. The "Costen's syndrome" or "TM syndrome" was defined in the medical dictionary as a dysfunction of the temporomandibular joint caused by deforming arthritis resulting from mandibular overclosure or displacement. The recognized treatment was occlusal equilibration by "experts," with the alternate therapeutic option resting in the hands of "expert" oral surgeons—meniscectomy,[8-10] corticosteroid therapy,[11, 12] or selective surgery such as the high condylectomy[13] or closed condylotomy.[14] The first book on the subject appeared in 1951, a group of lectures by Sicher, Weinmann, Zimmerman, Brodie, and Thompson, edited by Sarnat.[15]

During this decade the dominant authority was Harry Sicher, whose *Oral Anatomy*[16] had established functional anatomy as a basis upon which to build therapeutic regimens. In 1954 Leonard Rees,[17] the British anatomist, added significantly to Sicher's brilliant work. Gnathology was described by McCollum and Stuart.[18] Electromyographic studies began to bring muscle action into focus.[19-22] Advances were made in radiography, such as the development of arthrography,[23] the refinement of the transcranial technique,[24] TMJ tomography,[25] and cinefluorography.[26] The masticatory musculature also came into its own as a major consideration in the clinical management of masticatory disorders through the efforts of Kraus,[27] Travell,[28] Sicher,[29] and Schwartz.[30] While the "experts" were treating the joints, substantial gains were being achieved in our understanding of masticatory function and dysfunction.

The 1960s found the dental profession ready to accept the challenge. It was ushered in by the appearance of several books on masticatory therapy: Shore,[31] utilizing occlusal equilibration; Schwartz,[32] applying muscle therapy for his temporomandibular pain-dysfunction "syndrome;" and Bell,[33] verbalizing the Sicher concept of biomechanics. Soon other books became available: Freese and Scheman[34] and Sarnat's second edition of *The Temporomandibular Joint*.[35]

The dominant figure during this decade was Schwartz, who in 1956 had introduced the TM pain-dysfunction syndrome,[30] which was considered to be a breakthrough for masticatory therapy. Late in the decade the myofascial pain-dysfunction (MPD) syndrome was named.[36] All the while, serious research was going on, such as investigations into growth and development by Furstman,[37] Moffett,[38] Blackwood,[39] and

DuBrul.[40] Significant advances in neurophysiology were made by Thilander,[41] Kawamura,[42] and Storey,[43] and in psychologic influences by Moulton[44] and Lupton.[45] Also, important advances in occlusal therapy were being made with notable contributions by Ramfjord[46] and Krogh-Poulsen.[47]

The significant change that occurred during the 1960s was a shift of emphasis from biomechanics and the etiologic importance of occlusal factors to the musculature and related emotional and psychologic influences. Definitive occlusal therapy faded in importance and was replaced by temporary splinting methods. Biomechanics and internal derangements were generally ignored; the pain-dysfunction syndrome became dominant as the chief management problem.

In the 1970s, the TMJ bandwagon was in full swing. Continuing education courses and TMJ symposia were offered almost everywhere. "Cookbook" courses and one-disease-one-treatment philosophies of management were rife. Osteopaths and chiropractors offered cranial manipulations and applied kinesiology as therapeutic considerations. Holistic philosophies of therapy became popular. A new organization devoted exclusively to these problems was formed: The American Academy of Craniomandibular Disorders. Specialists in TMJ disorders came on the scene.

An explosion in scientific research took place, especially in growth and development and in masticatory physiology. Noteworthy are the contributions of Carlsson and Oberg[48] in joint remodeling, Ingervall[49] in the form-function relationship of the articular eminence, Enlow[50] in facial growth, and Hansson and Oberg[51] in autopsy studies. Significant also were the research efforts of Hannam, Matthews, and Yemm[52] in the effects of tooth contact, Bessette, Bishop, and Mohl[53] in the electromyographic silent period in elevator muscles, McNamara[54] in the functioning of the two heads of the lateral pterygoid muscle, and Hylander[55] in the effect of masticatory forces. Very important contributions have been made by many clinical occlusionists, including Ash, Dawson, Fox, Funt, Guichet, Haden, Jankelson, Lundeen, McNeill, Nasedkin, Neff, Ramfjord, Rieder, Solberg, Stack, Weinberg, Williams, and Williamson, as well as by nondental researchers, such as Gibbs, Moffett, and Rugh.

The 1970s brought an emphasis on muscle therapy, the MPD syndrome, to which Laskin[36] and Greene[56] contributed importantly. Early in the seventies a courageous new voice was heard—that of Farrar,[57] who challenged the muscle therapy concept and reemphasized the importance of occlusal discrepancies as significant etiologic and therapeutic considerations in the management of temporomandibular disc-interference disorders. As the concept of internal derangements became reestablished, Farrar became the dominant influence of this decade. Mandibular repositioning techniques of occlusal manipulation became popular. As a result of Farrar's influence, arthrography was resurrected and perfected by Wilkes,[58] Farrar and McCarty,[59] and Dolwick et al.[60] There was a conjoint resurgence of surgery, led especially by Wilkes (meniscectomy) and McCarty[61] (plication of the articular disc). The decade ended with a great swing in emphasis from MPD to internal derangements.

The significant change observed during the 1970s was the arrestment of the muscle therapy concept and a restoration of functional biomechanics as the favored clinical approach to the management of TM complaints. There was significant improvement in radiographic and surgical techniques. Occlusionists made peace with anatomists and joined hands in a more rational approach to solving masticatory problems. Clinical management moved into the general practice of dentistry. There were revolutionary new concepts in the mechanisms of pain. Several new books were authored or edited by Gelb,[62] Morgan, Hall, and Vamvas,[63] Dubner, Sessle, and Storey,[64] Sarnat and Laskin,[65] Zarb and Carlsson,[66] and Bell.[67]

With the 1980s the swing of the pendulum focused attention on internal derangements almost to the complete exclusion of the MPD syndrome. Impulsive and sometimes heroic forms of therapy were advocated for otherwise minor masticatory complaints. Every noisy TM joint became a "dislocated disc" and needed a mandibular repositioning appliance or a surgical operation. The American Dental Association awakened and convened a workshop-conference of some 50 workers in this field to consider the etiology, classification, examination, and management of TM disorders.[68] New radiographic techniques were introduced: computed tomographic (CT) scanning[69] and double-contrast arthrography.[70] Significant new textbooks were authored or edited by Irby,[71] Solberg and Clark,[72] Bell,[73] Travell and Simons,[74] Solberg and Clark,[75] and Bell.[76] A new journal dedicated to TMJ problems was introduced, the *Journal of Craniomandibular Practice* (CRANIO).

By viewing the half century since Costen, it can be seen that the dental profession has come a long way—from a state of nearly total unawareness of the significance of temporomandibular disorders to nearly obsessive concern. Through the years, the clinical management of these disorders has swung like a pendulum. There are now indications, however, that empirical mandibular repositioning, overuse of invasive arthrography, and the use of surgical intervention in the absence of diagnostic and therapeutic justification have crested, and the dental profession is looking toward a more rational and moderate approach to therapy. The return of concern for the many muscle disorders is becoming evident. Efforts at better diagnosis are apparent as we realize that rational therapy demands it. No doubt, our progress during the next 50 years depends on it.

LESSONS FROM HISTORY

Temporomandibular therapy since the time of Costen has been largely empirical and oftentimes controversial. Different modalities of treatment have dominated at different times. The profession has witnessed a host of temporarily popular procedures, such as bite-raising, injection of sclerosing solutions into the joints, rehabilitation and reconstruction of the dentition, use of occlusal pivots, surgical removal of the articular disc, occlusal equilibration, use of interocclusal appliances, orthodontics, surgical condylectomy, physiotherapy, injection of cortisone into the joints, muscle relaxant therapy, psychotherapy and tension control, surgical repair of displaced articular discs, and applied kinesiology. Most forms of therapy have concentrated on a particular component of the masticatory apparatus: the dentition, the joints, the musculature. The popularity of any particular treatment modality seemed to bear little relationship to the considerably more orderly accumulation of basic scientific knowledge of the masticatory system. *Important as the dentition is with regard to masticatory function and dysfunction, the passing of time has demonstrated that there is no substitute for a full understanding of the entire masticatory system.* The historical, controversial management of such disorders likely stems from consideration of single components of the masticatory apparatus without regard for the whole system as a functioning unit. History should teach that it is expedient to go back to basics and assimilate at a clinical level the mass of scientific knowledge that has been available for many years, and which should be the basis for the rational diagnosis and effective treatment of temporomandibular disorders.

A better understanding of pain mechanisms and muscle physiology has contributed significantly to the knowledge of masticatory dysfunctions and disorders. The muscular genesis of pain, the secondary effects of deep pain, the modulation of pain impulses, and the discovery of an endogenous antinociceptive system have opened new avenues of thought on masticatory pains. Electromyographic studies have done much to elucidate muscle function, to isolate and identify the action of specific masticatory muscles with the different jaw movements, and to augment the comprehension of what takes place in the process of incising and grinding foods.

More uniform terminology, improved classification of orofacial pain syndromes, more accurate categorization of temporomandibular disorders, and enlightened examining techniques have streamlined the clinical task of identifying disorders of the temporomandibular joints and masticatory musculature. The accumulation of clinical data on etiologic factors, particularly those relevant to abusive habits, bruxism, emotional stress, trauma, and occlusal discrepancies, has given better insight into cause and prevention. Interdisciplinary cooperation in management is doing much to develop guidelines for a rational approach to the whole problem.

There is now a sizable mass of reliable, factual, scientific information available to researchers and clinicians alike. Using this information, unified concepts of normal masticatory function can be formed, criteria for the recognition of masticatory dysfunctions can be established, and effective measures to alleviate temporomandibular complaints can be developed. There is no longer any valid reason for divisive, conflicting, and mutually exclusive concepts of what constitutes normal masticatory function. Purely empirical and trial-and-error therapy are no longer justifiable. Precise differential diagnosis and rational, predictable treatment methods can bring management of most temporomandibular disorders within the grasp of knowledgeable practitioners of dentistry.

RESPONSIBILITY FOR MANAGEMENT

Ordinarily, complaints involving the masticatory system are presented to the dentist directly by the patient or by the referring physician on the assumption that they relate to the dentition. Some complaints are not attended by pain or discomfort, the disorder being wholly that of dysfunction. Such complaints include (1) restrictions of jaw movement that interfere with opening the mouth or with making usual chewing movements, (2) abnormal noises or strange sensations during jaw movements, and (3) sudden alterations in the bite. Some complaints consist of pain only—discomfort with chewing and jaw movements. Most complaints, however, have components of dysfunction and pain in myriad combinations. The management of all such complaints involves diagnosis and treatment.

Diagnosis

It is a serious mistake to assume that the presenting symptoms automatically indicate the proper category into which the particular complaint should fall. Nor do they signify the seriousness of the problem or responsiveness to treatment. It is the responsibility of the examining dentist to make a diagnosis prior to undertaking definitive treatment. An accurate diagnosis is the first step in the treatment of any disorder, and the process cannot be abridged.

The diagnosis of disorders of the masticatory system requires the services of a dentist knowledgeable in pain and oriented toward masticatory function. Only he has the training and expertise to trace pain sources and judge masticatory function. It is the professional obligation of every dentist who undertakes the management of such disorders to make himself proficient in these areas.

A diagnosis should (1) identify and classify the disorder properly, (2) establish the reason for dysfunction and the source of pain, (3) determine the etiology, if at all possible, and (4) provide a basis for prognosis in the light of effective therapy.

Treatment

Although the dentist is responsible for the diagnosis, subsequent treatment may or may not rest in his hands. If etiologic factors in the case are exclusively related to conditions amenable to dental treatment, then the responsibility for therapy should remain the dentist's. Interdisciplinary dental cooperative effort, however, may be needed to ensure a successful outcome. Some temporomandibular disorders are associated with conditions that are not responsive to dental treatment measures. Management of these conditions should be done by an appropriate medical practitioner or by a cooperative interdisciplinary team.

Preliminary consultations prior to definitive therapy may do much to smooth the clinical course and ensure the outcome of complex masticatory conditions.

TEMPOROMANDIBULAR KINEMATICS

Like all synovial joints, the temporomandibular joints are under the control of the musculature with respect to proprioceptive and sensory guidance, habit patterns, and volition. Afferent monitoring input provides the central nervous system (CNS) with a continuous inflow of signals arising from the oral mucosa, the mucogingival tissues, the muscular structures of the mouth, the periodontal ligaments, and the capsular and articular ligaments of the temporomandibular joints, as well as from the masticatory muscles themselves. This mass of sensory input helps guide the disc-condyle complex through the translatory cycles, the chewing movements being altered as needed by the particular demands of function at any particular moment. Deeply ingrained habit patterns become established so that chewing becomes unconscious and nearly automatic, unless volition is used to override habitual and muscle-guided movements.

When the teeth are out of contact, nondental sensory and proprioceptive signals dominate guidance of chewing movements. The periodontal receptors come into play as the teeth are stimulated by the contact of food and each other, thus modifying guidance by periodontal sensory input. It is important to understand, however, that another form of guidance that is not controlled by afferent input from any source or by volition becomes dominant as maximum intercuspation takes place. This is the effect of structural tooth form—the meshing of inclined planes of teeth—a force that is irresistible as the final determinant of joint position at the end of a chewing stroke or clenching the teeth. This force, which completely dominates the positioning of the condyle, occurs suddenly and every time the teeth are firmly occluded and disappears just as suddenly when the occluding effort is released.

Joint position is determined by muscle action (regardless of the factors of guidance and control) until the moment of maximum intercuspation, when a new and irresistible force suddenly determines that position. This new force lasts only as long as the teeth remain fully occluded. Unless strict harmony exists between these two factors that determine joint position, disruption of normal joint function may result. The tooth-dictated position must be harmonious with that determined by muscle action.

During maximum intercuspation, the fully occluded posterior teeth absorb most of the force exerted by the elevator muscles, thus relieving the joints and musculature of maintaining adequate stability. This may be witnessed by observing that the articular disc space does not collapse when the teeth are occluded in the absence of an interposed disc between condyle and articular eminence (Fig 1–1).

Temporomandibular joint kinematics, therefore, require strict harmony between the dentition and muscle action for normal functioning of the masticatory apparatus to take place. This is why temporomandibular disorders are a problem for clinical dentistry.

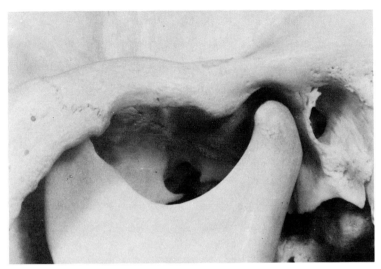

FIGURE 1-1 Photograph of dry skull showing relationship of mandibular condyle to articular eminence with teeth in normal occlusion. No intervening articular disc is present. Note that occlusion of teeth prevents collapse of articular disc space.

REFERENCES

1. Costen J.B.: Syndrome of ear and sinus symptoms dependent upon disturbed function of the temporomandibular joint. *Ann. Otol. Rhinol. Laryngol.* 43:1, 1934.
2. Goodfriend D.J.: Dysarthrosis and subarthrosis of the mandibular articulation. *Dent. Cosmos* 74:523, 1932.
3. Goodfriend D.J.: Symptomology and treatment of abnormalities of the mandibular articulation. *Dent. Cosmos* 75:844, 947, 1106, 1933.
4. Costen J.B.: Some features of the mandibular articulation as it pertains to medical diagnosis, especially otolaryngology. *J. Am. Dent. Assoc.* 24:1507, 1937.
5. Schultz L.W.: A curative treatment for subluxation of the temporomandibular joint or of any joint. *J. Am. Dent. Assoc.* 24:1947, 1937.
6. Schuyler C.H.: Fundamental principles in the correction of occlusal disharmony, natural and artificial. *J. Am. Dent. Assoc.* 22:1193, 1935.
7. Gottlieb B.: Traumatic occlusion and the rest position of the mandible. *J. Periodontol.* 7:21, 1947.
8. Ireland V.E.: The problem of the clicking jaw. *Proc. R. Soc. Lond.* 44:363, 1951.
9. Dingman R.O., Moorman W.C.: Meniscectomy in the treatment of lesions of the temporomandibular joint. *J. Oral Surg.* 9:214, 1951.
10. Kiehn C.L.: Meniscectomy for internal derangement of temporomandibular joint. *Am. J. Surg.* 83:364, 1952.

11. Horton C.P.: Treatment of arthritic temporomandibular joints by intra-articular injection of hydrocortisone. *Oral Surg.* 6:826, 1953.

12. Henny F.A.: Intra-articular injection of hydrocortisone into the temporomandibular joint. *J. Oral Surg.* 12:314, 1954.

13. Henny F.A., Baldridge O.L.: Condylectomy for the persistently painful temporomandibular joint. *J. Oral Surg.* 15:24, 1957.

14. Ward T.G., Smith D.G., Sommars M.: Condylotomy for mandibular joint arthrosis. *Br. Dent. J.* 103:147, 1957.

15. Sarnat B.G. (ed.): *The Temporomandibular Joint.* Springfield, Ill., Charles C Thomas, Publisher, 1951.

16. Sicher H.: *Oral Anatomy.* St. Louis, C.V. Mosby Co., 1949.

17. Rees L.A.: The structure and function of the mandibular joint. *Br. Dent. J.* 96:125, 1954.

18. McCollum B.B., Stuart C.E.: *A Research Report.* South Pasadena, Cal., Scientific Press, 1955.

19. Moyers R.E.: An electromyographic analysis of certain muscles involved in temporomandibular movement. *Am. J. Orthod.* 36:481, 1950.

20. Prozansky S.: The application of electromyography in dental research. *J. Am. Dent. Assoc.* 44:49, 1952.

21. MacDougall J.D.B., Andrew B.L.: An electromyographic study of the temporalis and masseter muscles. *J. Anat.* 87:37, 1953.

22. Perry H.T.: Implications of myographic research. *Angle Orthod.* 25:179, 1955.

23. Norgaard F.: Temporomandibular Arthography. Copenhagen, Munksgaard, 1947.

24. Updegrave W.J.: Temporomandibular articulation: X-ray examination. *Dent. Radiogr. Photogr.* 26:41, 1953.

25. Ricketts R.M.: Laminography in the diagnosis of temporomandibular disorders. *J. Am. Dent. Assoc.* 46:620, 1953.

26. Berry H.M. Jr., Hoffman F.A.: Cinefluorography with image intensification for observing temporomandibular joint movements. *J. Am. Dent. Assoc.* 53:517, 1956.

27. Kraus H.: *Principles and Practice of Therapeutic Exercises.* Springfield, Ill., Charles C Thomas, Publisher, 1950.

28. Travell J., Rinzler S.H.: The myofascial genesis of pain. *Postgrad. Med.* 11:425, 1952.

29. Sicher H.: Problems of pain in dentistry. *Oral Surg.* 7:149, 1954.

30. Schwartz L.L.: A temporomandibular pain-dysfunction syndrome. *J. Chronic Dis.* 3:284, 1956.

31. Shore N.A.: *Occlusal Equilibration and Temporomandibular Joint Dysfunction.* Philadelphia, J. B. Lippincott Co., 1959.

32. Schwartz L. (ed.): *Diseases of the Temporomandibular Joint.* Philadelphia, W.B. Saunders Co., 1959.

33. Bell W.E.: *Temporomandibular Joint Disease.* Dallas, Egan Press, 1960.

34. Freese A.J., Scheman P.: *Management of Temporomandibular Joint Problems.* St. Louis, C.V. Mosby Co., 1962.

35. Sarnat B.G. (ed.): *The Temporomandibular Joint,* ed. 2. Springfield, Ill., Charles C Thomas, Publisher, 1964.
36. Laskin D.M.: Etiology of the pain-dysfunction syndrome. *J. Am. Dent. Assoc.* 79:147, 1969.
37. Furstman L.: The early development of the human temporomandibular joint. *Am. J. Orthod.* 49:672, 1963.
38. Moffett B.C., Johnson L.C., McCabe J.B., et al.: Articular remodeling in the adult human temporomandibular joint. *Am. J. Anat.* 115:119–130, 1964.
39. Blackwood H.J.J.: Cellular remodeling in articular tissue. *J. Dent. Res.* 45:480, 1966.
40. DuBrul E.L.: Development of the hominid oral apparatus, in Schumacher G. (ed.): *Morphology of the Maxillomandibular Apparatus.* Leipsig, VEB George Thieme, 1967.
41. Thilander B.: Innervation of the temporomandibular joint capsule in man. *Trans. R. School Dent.* 7:1, 1961.
42. Kawamura Y., Majima T.: Temporomandibular joint's sensory mechanisms controlling activities of the jaw muscles. *J. Dent. Res.* 43:150, 1964.
43. Storey A.T.: Sensory functions of the temporomandibular joint. *Can. Dent. Assoc. J.* 34:294, 1968.
44. Moulton R.E.: Emotional factors in nonorganic temporomandibular pain. *Dent. Clin. North Am.* Nov. 1966, p. 609.
45. Lupton D.E.: Psychological aspects of temporomandibular joint dysfunction. *J. Am. Dent. Assoc.* 79:131, 1969.
46. Ramfjord S.P.: Dysfunctional temporomandibular joint and muscle pain. *J. Prosthet. Dent.* 11:353, 1961.
47. Krogh-Poulsen W.G., Olsson A.: Occlusal disharmonies and dysfunction of the stomatognathic system. *Dent. Clin. North Am.* Nov. 1966, p. 627.
48. Carlsson G.E., Oberg T.: Remodeling of the temporomandibular joint. *Oral Sci. Rev.* 7:58, 1974.
49. Ingervall B.: Relation between height of the articular eminence of the temporomandibular joint and facial morphology. *Angle Orthod.* 44:15, 1974.
50. Enlow D.H.: *Handbook of Facial Growth.* Philadelphia, W.B. Saunders Co., 1975.
51. Hansson T., Oberg T.: Arthrosis and deviation in form in the temporomandibular joint: A macroscopic study on a human autopsy material. *Acta Odontol. Scand.* 35:167, 1977.
52. Hannam A.G., Matthews B., Yemm R.: Changes in the activity of the masseter muscle following tooth contact in man. *Arch. Oral Biol.* 14:1401, 1969.
53. Bessette R., Bishop B., Mohl N.: Duration of masseteric silent period in patients with TMJ syndrome. *J. Appl. Physiol.* 30:864, 1971.
54. McNamara J.A. Jr.: The independent functions of the two heads of the lateral pterygoid muscle. *Am. J. Anat.* 138:197, 1973.

55. Hylander W.L.: The human mandible: Lever or link? *Am. J. Phys. Anthropol.* 43:227, 1975.

56. Greene C.S.: Myofascial pain-dysfunction syndrome: The evolution of concepts, in Sarnat B.G., Laskin D.M. (eds.): *The Temporomandibular Joint,* ed. 3. Springfield, Ill., Charles C Thomas, Publisher, 1979, pp. 277–288.

57. Farrar W.B.: Diagnosis and treatment of anterior dislocation of the articular disc. *N.Y. J. Dent.* 41:348, 1971.

58. Wilkes C.H.: Arthrography of the temporomandibular joint. *Minn. Med.* 61:645, 1978.

59. Farrar W.B., McCarty W.L., Jr.: Inferior joint space arthrography and characteristics of condylar paths in internal derangements of the TMJ. *J. Prosthet. Dent.* 41:5, 1979.

60. Dolwick M.F., Katzberg R.W., Helms C.A., et al.: Arthrotomographic evaluation of the temporomandibular joint. *J. Oral Surg.* 37:793–799, 1979.

61. McCarty W.L., Farrar W.B.: Surgery for internal derangements of the temporomandibular joint. *J. Prosthet. Dent.* 42:2, 1979.

62. Gelb H. (ed.): *Clinical Management of Head, Neck and TMJ Pain and Dysfunction.* Philadelphia, W.B. Saunders Co., 1977.

63. Morgan D.H., Hall W.P., Vamvas S.J. (eds.): *Diseases of the Temporomandibular Apparatus.* St. Louis, C.V. Mosby Co., 1977.

64. Dubner R., Sessle B.J., Storey A.T.: *The Neural Basis of Oral and Facial Function.* New York, Plenum Publishing Corp., 1978.

65. Sarnat B.G., Laskin D.M. (eds.): *The Temporomandibular Joint,* ed. 3. Springfield, Ill., Charles C Thomas, Publisher, 1979.

66. Zarb G.A., Carlsson G.E. (eds.): *Temporomandibular Joint Function and Dysfunction.* Copenhagen, Munksgaard, 1979.

67. Bell W.E.: *Orofacial Pains, Differential Diagnosis,* ed. 2. Chicago, Year Book Medical Publishers, 1979.

68. Laskin D., Greenfield W., Gale E., et al.: *The President's Conference on the Examination, Diagnosis and Management of Temporomandibular Disorders.* Chicago, American Dental Association, 1983.

69. Helms C.A., Katzberg R.W., Manzione J.V.: Computed tomography, in Helms C.A., Katzberg R.W., Dolwick M.F. (eds.): *Internal Derangements of the Temporomandibular Joint.* San Francisco, University of California, 1983.

70. Moffett B.C. (ed.): *Diagnosis of Temporomandibular Joint Internal Derangements: Double Contrast Arthrography and Clinical Correction.* Seattle, University of Washington, 1984.

71. Irby W.B. (ed.): *Current Advances in Oral Surgery,* Vol. III. St. Louis, C.V. Mosby Co., 1980.

72. Solberg W.K., Clark G.T. (eds.): *Temporomandibular Joint Problems.* Chicago, Quintessence Publishing Co., 1980.

73. Bell W.E.: *Clinical Management of Temporomandibular Disorders.* Chicago, Year Book Medical Publishers, 1982.

74. Travell J.G., Simons D.G.: *Myofascial Pain and Dysfunction.* Baltimore, Williams & Wilkins Co., 1983.
75. Solberg W.K., Clark G.T. (eds.): *Abnormal Jaw Mechanics.* Chicago, Quintessence Publishing Co., 1984.
76. Bell W.E.: *Orofacial Pains,* ed. 3. Chicago, Year Book Medical Publishers, 1985.

2

Orthopedic Principles

Although dentistry is concerned with functioning teeth, each tooth being attached to the alveolar bone by a *true fibrous joint,* and although the masticatory system involves the craniomandibular articulation which is the *most complex synovial system of the body,* dental education usually is quite deficient in providing adequate instruction in orthopedic medicine. A good understanding of the basic principles of orthopedics should be fundamental to everyday dental practice. It is prerequisite to the rational management of temporomandibular disorders.

JOINTS

The word *articulation,* meaning the place of junction between two discrete objects, is used in orthopedic nomenclature to designate the place of union or junction between two or more bones of the skeleton. Such articulations are commonly called *joints.* Joints are classified as *synarthrodial* or *diarthrodial.*

In *synarthrodial or fibrous joints,* the parts are united by fibrous tissue. When the intervening fibrous tissue is continuous, the joint is referred to as a *suture.* Some common sutures are those of the cranial bones. When the bones are connected by ligaments only, the joint is referred to as *syndesmosis;* an example is the tibiofibular articulation. When the fibrous joint is composed of a conical process inserted into a socket-like portion, it is referred to as *gomphosis.* The teeth in the alveolar process form such a joint.

Diarthrodial joints are discontinuous articulations that permit greater freedom of movement between the united parts. The articulating surfaces are composed of a tissue able to sustain compression and movement simultaneously, a condition that precludes the presence of blood vessels and nerve receptors in the pressure-bearing areas. Metabolic and nutritional requirements of such nonvascularized tissue are provided by surface contact of joint fluid, called *synovial fluid*. The presence of synovial fluid requires that the articular surfaces be encapsulated to confine it. The inner surface of the capsule is composed of a specialized connective tissue that secretes the synovial fluid, the *synovial membrane*. Because of this structural arrangement imposed on movable joints by the demands of simultaneous compression and movement, diarthrodial joints are referred to as *synovial joints*. These joints facilitate locomotion in the musculoskeletal system. Synovial joints may be classified as *simple* or *compound*.

Simple synovial joints involve only two articular surfaces. They may be structured for flexion and extension only—hinge movement. Hinge joints *(ginglymoid)* have articular surfaces contoured to permit movement in a single plane and are supported by closely placed collateral ligaments that resist movement in other planes. The phalangeal joints are of this type. More flexible condyloid joints *(condyloarthrosis)* permit movement in more than a single plane—flexion, extension, abduction (turning outward or laterally), and adduction (turning inward or medially). Such joints present a contouring and ligamentous arrangement compatible with movement in different planes. The metacarpophalangeal articulation of the index finger is of this type. A still more flexible simple joint is the carpometacarpal joint of the thumb. Some synovial joints are structured to permit linear sliding movement between the united parts *(arthrodial)*, the surfaces being flat or slightly curved and unrestrained by closely placed ligaments. Some joints have a ball-and-socket arrangement *(enarthrosis)*, such as the hip joint.

Compound synovial joints involve three or more articular surfaces. When the sliding movement is quite limited, the term *amphiarthrosis* applies. This movement is seen in intercarpal, carpometacarpal, and intermetacarpal joints. Pivotal movement is termed *trochoid* and is seen in the elbow during pronation and supination of the forearm. Compound joints may be structured chiefly for hinge movement, such as the knee joint. Others have extensive freedom of movement, such as the elbow joint, in which flexion, extension, abduction, adduction, and trochoid movement are possible.

The type and distribution of joints are determined by functional requirements. When movement is limited and the forces across the joint are tractive, the union of the moving parts is by means of collagenous fibers to form a *fibrous joint*. When movement is very limited, the bones remain in close proximity, and the fibrous content is quite dense, as seen in cranial sutures and tooth attachments. Growth forces at such joints are also tractile in nature. When the requirement for movement ceases, such joints may undergo a degree of calcification, as seen in some cranial sutures after skeletal maturation. When the need for movement is greater, the bones are separated, and the ligamentous attachment is more flexible, as seen in the tibiofibular articulation. Compressive force may be converted into traction by the arrangement of the collagenous fibers that constitute the interbony ligament. This is demonstrated by the fibers that attach the teeth to the alveolar bone. The fibers of the periodontal ligament (a true articular ligament) are arranged in such a way as to convert compressive lateral and axial stresses upon the tooth into tractive forces on the bone. Movement between tooth and bone, though quite limited, is none the less a normal functional capability of the gomphosis joint. Such movement is needed for normal functioning, growth changes, and remodeling requirements of a healthy, functioning masticatory system. Calcification of the articular ligament (dental ankylosis) arrests such movement and removes the tooth from normal masticatory function.

When movement is limited and compressive forces are present, *cartilaginous joints* are required. The articulations between the ribs and the sternum are of this type. It should be noted that cartilage is required when growth occurs in the presence of compressive stress. Cartilage is the only tissue designed for this purpose. Endochondral bone growth is indicative of such stresses, as is seen at epiphyseal junctions in long bones and in the condylar development of the mandible. Under the impact of tractive force, osseous development is interstitial or appositional intramembranous growth which occurs in conjunction with osseous remodeling activity.[1]

When functional demands require controlled movement, the articulating bones must be completely disconnected and yet held firmly in place. This requires a different type of joint. The pressure that holds the parts together would cause undesirable sensory effects if the surfaces were innervated and would cause an inflammatory reaction if they were vascularized. The articulating surfaces therefore are composed of a tissue that is neither innervated nor vascularized. In the absence of neural structures, the articular tissues are incapable of sensation of any kind. In the absence of blood vessels, nutritional and metabolic activities must be provided for by way of a special joint fluid that is supplied by vessels free from interarticular pressure. Encapsulation is required to contain the joint fluid. This arrangement constitutes diarthrosis—a *synovial joint*.

The disconnected bones of a synovial joint are supported by two mechanisms: (1) a system of ligamentous structures that *passively* limit the amount of separation permitted by the articular surfaces and that restrain the degree and control the direction of joint movement, and (2) a system of skeletal muscles that *actively* hold the parts in sharp contact during all functional activities and that furnish power for working movements. The muscles therefore are no less functional components of a synovial joint than the ligaments. Since muscle action requires anchorage (Newton's third law), the joint musculature must be attached to a stable base, thus requiring a feedback mechanism that will provide a high degree of muscular coordination. Therefore, a controlling proprioceptive reflex mechanism is also an important component of synovial joint function. The articulating surfaces, of course, have no proprioceptors; the proprioceptors in the ligaments are chiefly inhibitory in action while those of the musculature are both excitatory and inhibitory.

SYNOVIAL JOINTS

The structural features of diarthrodial joints should be understood and appreciated. Although, like all other joints, the craniomandibular articulation has special features peculiar to the demands of specialized function, the general structural characteristics and behavior are typical of all synovial joints. Hence, an understanding of basic orthopedic principles is needed.

Encapsulation

The fibrous capsule is attached near the periphery of the articular surfaces. One can usually identify this attachment area on the dry bone, the surface thus enclosed being the nonvascularized pressure-bearing portion and indicative of the articular surface.

The capsule is well vascularized and innervated. The vessels supply the tissue fluid, which has free metabolic interchange with the synovial fluid within the joint cavity. The synovial membrane that secretes the synovial fluid lines the inner surface of the fibrous capsule and may overlie slightly the articular surfaces peripherally, especially if the articular body is convex. The synovial fluid supplies the nutritional and metabolic requirements of the nonvascularized tissues within the capsule. It also serves as joint lubricant and furnishes phagocytic capability. It fills the joint cavity. The capsule is innervated by sensory receptors for proprioceptive monitoring and conscious sensibility. Although the capsule is innervated with nociceptors, they have a moderately high threshold, so that pain is usually not felt unless the strain, distortion, or distention is considerable. Such discomfort is intermittent. If the capsule becomes inflamed, however, the pain threshold is lowered, discomfort may become evident especially when movement puts it under strain, and tenderness to manual palpation increases. Inflammatory pain may become continuous and thus induce secondary referred pain or myospastic activity. The fibrous capsule is lined with synovial membrane which is a specialized tissue consisting of a superficial layer three or four cells thick over a bed of loose connective tissue rich in blood vessels. It supplies the synovial fluid that fills the joint cavity.

Articular Tissues

The noninnervated, nonvascularizied articular tissue in most synovial joints is hyaline cartilage. As such, it is referred to as *articular cartilage.* This tissue is structured to resist compressive forces and shearing movements. It is to be distinguished from *growth cartilage,* which has quite a different purpose, that of endochondral osseous development. Although the attached side of articular cartilage receives some nourishment from the subarticular tissue, the free functioning surface is dependent upon the synovial fluid for nutrients, metabolic exchange, phagocytosis, and lubrication. Hyaluronic acid, a mucopolysaccharide, in the synovial fluid has lubricative qualities essential to normal joint functioning.

DuBrul[2] identified two types of lubrication in synovial joints: (1) weeping lubrication and (2) boundary lubrication. Except when the articulating surfaces are under compressive force, the articular tissue freely soaks up synovial fluid from the reservoir. Under compressive force, this fluid exudes onto the surface in tiny droplets and forms a layer of liquid that acts as a lubricating film. Thus, the articulating surfaces may be moved under pressure without sustaining damage. This weeping lubricating effect makes extensive joint movement, even under considerable pressure, entirely harmless to the joint. There is a limit, however. When all the fluid is expelled, further movement is without adequate lubrication, and the resultant friction is potentially damaging to the articular surfaces. Three determinants are important: (1) the length of time; (2) the degree of pressure; and (3) the extent of movement. Momentary high pressure even with extensive movement is harmless, as is limited sustained pressure without movement. But sustained pressure with movement can exhaust the limit of available absorbed synovial fluid contained in the articular tissue. When the limit of weeping lubrication is exceeded, frictional movement becomes the source of possible damage to the joint.

Boundary lubrication pertains to the reservoir of synovial fluid in the joint cavity which lubricates the articular tissues by surface contact and is the means of replenishing that which enters into the weeping lubricating mechanism. Conditions that alter the composition and consistency of synovial fluid may profoundly influence this normal lubrication system. Synovitis, which usually produces effusion within the synovial sac, is such a condition. When the synovial fluid becomes too viscid, its lubricating qualities are seriously impaired, a condition clinically referred to as *gelation.*

Joint Stability

The stability of completely disconnected articular surfaces depends upon continuous sharp contact of those surfaces at all times and under all conditions of function.[3, 4] By definition, *dislocation* is the separation of articular surfaces. Joint stability therefore is the means of preventing dislocation of the articulating parts.

Sharp contact of articular surfaces is maintained, not by ligaments, but by muscle action.[4] Resting muscle tonus in those that cross the joint maintains the minimal level of *passive* interarticular pressure. This pressure is increased by positive gravitational force in weight-bearing joints. In hanging joints, negative gravitational force is countered by the myotatic reflex. As the muscle spindles are elongated by the weight of the part, a reflex contraction of the muscle takes place to maintain a constant length of the spindles. This increased contraction of the muscle exactly offsets the effect of gravity, and a constancy of passive interarticular pressure on the joint surfaces is maintained. The resting posture of the part therefore depends on muscle tonus, which is due to the myotatic-reflex-controlled contraction of the muscles plus the inherent elasticity of the muscle tissue itself. It should be noted that in the cadaver (and to a large extent in locally anesthetized structures also), only the effect of muscle tissue elasticity remains; there is a lack of muscle contraction. It should also be understood that in examining joint movements, so-called cadaver function (or operating-table function) may be misleading to the observer, for what he witnesses is not the effect of muscle action on the skeleton, but rather the effect of skeletal movement on the denervated soft tissue structures. Cadaver function can appear almost the opposite of vital function. Nor can joint function be accurately judged by static viewing, such as by microscopic sections or radiographic films. Even fluoroscopic examination may be misleading, because only the subarticular osseous structures can be visualized, not the vital, functioning soft tissue parts. Actually, joint function can only be visualized in the mind by conceptualization.

Loading

Loading of the joint is due to muscle action as affected by resistance during working movements. Thus, *active* interarticular pressure on the joint surfaces occurs. If continued loading takes place slowly, some deformation of the articular tissue occurs as the synovial fluid is squeezed out. Movement tends to offset this deforming action.[5] The distribution of compressive stress is important. Joint surfaces do not fit together exactly. According to DuBrul,[2] the "closed-packed position" of the joint is when broad areas of the opposing articular surfaces fit most closely. This occurs when the greatest pressure is transmitted and therefore tends to minimize the deforming action of such pressure by distributing the stress more widely. Most heavy pressure on joints during normal functioning is of momentary duration and may be sustained without tissue damage.

The presence and distribution of proteoglycans found in the collagen matrix of superficial layers of articular tissue is a measure of the resilience of that tissue, which in turn is indicative of the location and degree of compressive loading.[6] This can be taken as a means of identifying within joints the areas that bear the burden of functional stress. Joints are able to manage ordinary loading. If overloading occurs at a tolerable rate of change, tissue remodeling may take place in the deeper layers of the articular tissue, thus changing its morphology while permitting the articular surface to remain intact.[7] If the demand for change exceeds the capability of the tissue to remodel, degenerative effects may occur.[8] Intolerable loading relates to the degree of load, to the duration, or to both. Keeping functional demands within tolerable limits therefore is important in maintaining the integrity of the articular structures in synovial joints.

Articular Ligaments

The type, direction, and extent of movement of a joint during normal functioning is restricted by several factors:

1. The shape and structural relationship of the articular facets
2. The size and structure of the articular capsule

3. The location, length, and structure of collateral ligaments and other articular ligaments
4. The stretching length of the muscles that power the joint
5. The presence of other restraints, such as the surrounding structures

Articular ligaments should be understood and appreciated. Although the term *ligament* may be used rather loosely in the literature because it is used to designate different types of anatomical structures, when applied to joints, it should have a specific meaning. An articular ligament is composed of nonelastic, noncontractile collagenous connective tissue. Depending on its structural strength, on its location relative to the articular surfaces, and on its length, a ligament restricts, restrains, and limits the functional movements of the joint. Its action is wholly passive; ligaments do not enter actively into joint function. Ligaments limit the extent to which articular surfaces can be separated or distracted without incurring tissue damage. They do not keep the articular surfaces in contact, however; nor do they maintain joint stability. When abused, a ligament may be damaged by strain, laceration, or detachment. Continued microtraumas may induce elongation (looseness) or other degenerative change. Since a ligament is nonelastic, it does not stretch and return again to its original length, as other elastic structures do (such as muscle tissue). Elongated or degenerated ligaments remain so. They also lose much of their normal innervation, thus contributing less proprioceptive control and pain.

Some joint capsules are ligamentous, some are elastic, some serve little more than to support the synovial membrane. Collateral ligaments are paired to hinge joints. They are usually short, strong, and closely placed at the sides of the joint so as to permit freedom of movement in the intended plane but prevent movements of the joint in other planes. The strength, placement, and length of other articular ligaments restrict the functional activities of the joint. The size and shape of the articular facets and the array of ligaments passively set the limits of joint functional capability. The actual functioning, however, is the result of muscle action.

Ligaments are innervated by both proprioceptors and nociceptors. The nociceptors are high threshold unless they are inflamed. Abusive strain induces a momentary painful response that is readily associated with the force involved. Inflammation may induce more continuous tenderness, soreness, or severe pain depending on the phase and extent of the inflammatory process and the demands of function.

Proprioceptors in ligaments provide a continuous inflow of information to the CNS that monitors joint position and function. Together with proprioceptive input from the related musculature, such monitoring information supplies the afferent signals for the efferent feedback mechanism that controls joint movements.[9] The stimulation of ligament proprioceptors induces an inhibitory response in the muscles and as such serves a protective function.

Interarticular Pressure

All synovial joints bear pressure. The passive interarticular pressure induced by muscle tonus and by positive gravitational force provides for continuous sharp contact of the articulating surfaces in the resting joint and during nonstressed movements. Since muscle tonus varies, passive interarticular pressure also varies, but within fairly narrow limits. Muscle tonus varies with emotional tension, illness, fatigue, time of day, activities, and age. The effect of gravitational force varies with posture.

Active interarticular pressure results from the contraction of muscles as opposed by resistance—the stresses and forces of skeletal activity. It is extremely variable and may extend all the way from negative pressure to high compressive force, according to the demands of function.

Meniscus

A meniscus (from the Greek *meniskos,* meaning crescent) is a wedge-shaped crescent of fibrocartilage or dense fibrous tissue, one side of which forms a marginal attachment at the articular capsule, and the other two sides extend into the joint cavity and end in a free edge. The structure does not divide the joint cavity into separate compartments, nor does it restrict or confine the synovial fluid. It facilitates movements of the bony parts but does not act as a true articular surface, in that it is not a determinant of that movement. Two such structures are found in the knee joint: the medial meniscus, attaching to the medial margin of the superior articular surface of the tibia, and the lateral meniscus, attaching to the lateral margin of the superior articular surface of the tibia.

SPECIAL FEATURES OF CRANIOMANDIBULAR ARTICULATION

The craniomandibular articulation consists of two synovial (true diarthrodial) joints, a right and a left temporomandibular joint. These joints have characteristics that are not shared by all other synovial joints. It is essential that these special features be recognized and appreciated.

Phylogenetic Heritage

Costen's syndrome included several symptoms, some clearly auricular, some temporomandibular.[10] His therapy, which was unmistakably masticatory, seemed also to alleviate the auricular component of the complaint. Anatomists, however, insisted that the joint and ear symptoms be delineated, thus dividing the syndrome into two parts. Treatment of the ear portion remained to otolaryngologists, while treatment of the masticatory portion was allotted to dentists. It is interesting to note, however, that in due time researchers established an intimate structural relationship between the ear and the joint.

The mandibular joint of lower animal life has undergone considerable change, especially from the amphibia through the mammal-like reptiles (Fig 2–1).[11] In the mammal, the primitive jaw articulation of the lower vertebrates is located in the middle ear as the articulation between the malleus and incus bones. The temporomandibular joint is phylogenically recent and peculiar to mammals. It also is the last joint to develop in the human embryo.[12]

In the important development of the craniomandibular articulation over eons of time, certain structures of the ear and temporomandibular joint became intimately related.[11] The tensor tympani muscle, which flexes the tympanic membrane (arising from the cartilaginous portion of the eustachian tube and inserting into the malleus bone), is innervated by the mandibular division of the trigeminal nerve, which also innervates the masticatory muscles. Likewise, the tensor palati muscle, which elevates the palate and opens the eustachian tube by straightening it (arising from the sphenoid bone and wall of the eustachian tube and, after passing around the hamular process of the pterygoid bone, inserting into the aponeurosis of the soft palate), also is innervated by the mandibular division of the trigeminal nerve. Thus, the eustachian tube, which connects the cavity of the middle ear with the nasopharynx for the purpose of maintaining equalized air pressure on the ear drum, is under the control of muscles innervated by nerves that subserve mastication. During deglutition, the palate is elevated to valve off the nasopharynx and the eustachian tubes are simultaneously opened. Rood and Doyle[13] have reported that the dilator muscle of the eustachian tube (the dilator tubae) is also innervated by the trigeminal nerve. Thus, normal auditory function is intimately related to masticatory

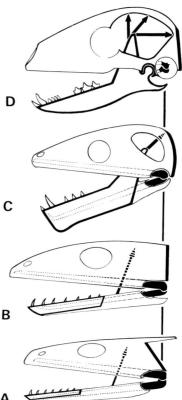

FIGURE 2–1   Evolution of mammalian jaw joint. Back of skull and dentary bone in *heavy outline. Arrows* indicate muscle vectors. *A,* amphibian. Note notch on rear skull margin and muscle attached on undersurface of skull roof. *B,* reptile. Note increase in dentary bone and straight rear skull margin. *C,* mammal-like reptile. Note great increase in dentary bone with coronoid process and opening in skull roof (temporal fossa). *D,* mammal. Note dentary bone now contacts skull, forming the dentary-squamosal (temporomandibular) joint—an entirely new jaw joint. The primitive jaw articulation now forms the malleolar-incus joint of the ear ossicles. (From Du Brul E.L., in Sarnat B.G., Laskin D.M. (eds.): *The Temporomandibular Joint,* ed. 3. Springfield, Ill. Charles C Thomas, Publisher, 1979. Reproduced with permission.)

function. At the same time, the tensor tympani muscles also flex the ear drums, the sound of which may be heard accompanying the act of swallowing.

Another interesting structural relationship between the joint and the ear was brought to light by Pinto's discovery in 1962 of the mandibular-malleolar ligament.[14] This structure connects the temporomandibular capsule with the malleus bone, which in turn attaches to the tympanic membrane. Thus, when the condyle is translated forward, the ear drum is flexed. The sound of flexion can be heard by protruding the mandible or moving it laterally from side to side.

This structure was initially referred to by Rees,[15] who described fibroelastic tissue of the superior retrodiscal lamina that appeared to represent the discomalleolar band of fetal life which connects the lateral pterygoid tendon to the malleus bone through the squamotympanic fissure. Coleman[16] determined that the so-called Pinto ligament was composed of retrodiscal fibers in connection with the anterior mal-leolar ligament. These fibers were tightly attached to the walls of the fissure through which they passed, so that traction applied to the ret-rodiscal tissue did not move the malleus bone. Marshall[17] agreed with this observation. Mohl[18] did not place much importance on the liga-ment. Although the clinical significance of the mandibulomalleolar lig-ament is debatable, it does indicate a structural relationship between the temporomandibular joint and the middle ear. This relationship is intimate indeed, and symptoms in common should present no surprise or problem to dentists or otolaryngologists.

Bilaterality of the Craniomandibular Articulation

The craniomandibular articulation is bilateral, being composed of two joints, a left and a right temporomandibular joint, which form a func-tioning unit. They cannot function separately. What affects one joint must also influence the other.

Each of the two joints is compound and is classified as a ginglymo-arthrodial (hinge-sliding) joint. By definition, a compound joint in-volves three or more articular surfaces. In the temporomandibular joint, the articular disc supplies true articular surfaces above and below. Actually, the temporomandibular joint is a double joint composed of a lower ginglymoid and an upper arthrodial joint. Sicher described it as a hinge joint with a movable socket.[19] The usual concept that the con-dyle articulates with the fossa-eminence, with an interposed meniscus, is not accurate. More correctly, the condyle articulates with the articu-lar disc to form the disc-condyle complex, which in turn articulates with the temporal bone.

Chronological Changes in the Joint

The temporomandibular joint undergoes significant developmental change from infancy to skeletal maturity. These changes correspond to edentulousness at birth, the eruption and articulation of the deciduous dentition, the eruption and articulation of the permanent dentition, and the skeletal maturation of the maxillary bones.

Although the joint at birth displays the structural components of the adult joint (Fig 2–2),[20] it lies in line with the occlusal plane rather than an inch or more superior to it, as in the adult jaw (Fig 2–3). The articular eminence is low, the fossa is relatively flat, and hinge move-ment is the normal type of action. Throughout fetal life, the fibrous articular surfaces and disc are vascularized and innervated. This state

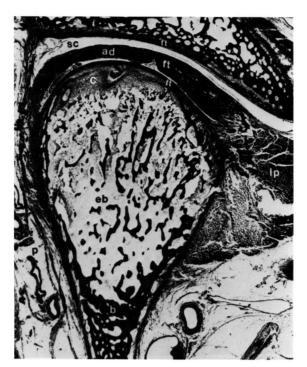

FIGURE 2–2   The human temporomandibular joint at term. Note temporal bone *(t),* superior compartment *(sc)* of the joint, the articular disc *(ad),* cartilaginous area *(c)* of the condyle, endochondral bone *(eb)* formation, parotid gland *(p),* and the lateral pterygoid muscle *(lp).* The outer surfaces of the condyle and temporal portion of the joint cavity are covered with dense fibrous connective tissue *(ft).* The articular disc is also composed of dense fibrous connective tissue. (From Furstman L., in Sarnat B.G., Laskin D.M. (eds.): *The Temporomandibular Joint,* ed. 3. Springfield, Ill., Charles C Thomas, Publisher, 1979. Reproduced with permission.)

disappears as function induces the compression of the disc between the condyle and temporal bone.[21] The growth changes that take place from birth to maturity are great.

The growth process is complex indeed and not completely understood. As the mandible moves forward and downward, its size increases in the opposite superior and posterior directions. This involves not only condylar growth, but also widespread remodeling of the entire bone, as resorptive and depository activity takes place. As the ramus grows posteriorly, the condyle simultaneously grows posteriorly and superiorly by active endochondral osseous proliferation. Intramembranous growth processes likewise take place throughout the osseous structures.[22]

During the growth process, accommodation occurs first for the totally edentulous mouth, followed by the eruption and final alignment of a complete deciduous dentition, the spacing and shedding of deciduous teeth for succedaneous ones to follow, the eruption and alignment of a complete adult dentition, and, finally, the skeletal maturation and cessation of active developmental growth. Clinically, structural considerations of the temporomandibular joint at any particular time during the developmental years must take into account the state of development of the dentition at that time. The shape and size of the condyle relative to the depth of the articular fossa and elevation of the eminence should remain compatible as transition occurs from edentulous babyhood, through the relatively flat, end-to-end deciduous dentition, to the adult permanent dentition with its considerable interlocking of occlusal surfaces. During certain transitional periods, change may be quite rapid. The articular eminence is usually formed by age 7 or 8 years.

It should be noted that even after skeletal maturation and cessation of development, the process of osseous remodeling normally continues so that satisfactory accommodation in osseous structure can meet changing functional demands.

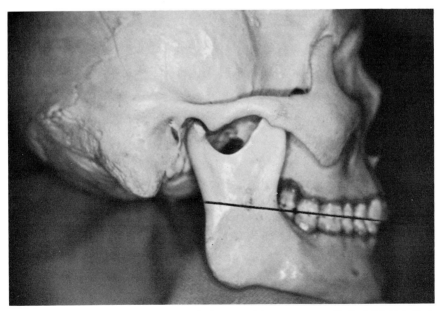

FIGURE 2–3   Relationship of occlusal plane to adult temporomandibular joint. Note that mandibular condyle is an inch or more superior to plane of occlusion. At birth, it normally lies in line with plane of occlusion.

Condylar Cartilage

Condylar cartilage is not articular cartilage. This distinction is important in the understanding of mandibular growth as well as of joint function. The condylar cartilage pertains to the process of endochondral bone formation. It is *growth cartilage*. In long bones the epiphyseal and articular cartilages are never confused because they are separated by bone tissue. In the mandibular condyle, however, the growth cartilage is on the surface of the bone just beneath the fibrous articular surface. Its location, no doubt, is the reason why it has so often been confused with articular cartilage.

Condylar cartilage does not enter into the problems of joint function—that is, sustaining compression and movement. Rather, it has to do with bone formation in the growth and development of the mandibular condyle. Deformity results when its function in growth is interfered with.

It is known that bone growth is intramembranous in tensile relationships and endochondral in compression relationships. The concept that endochondral growth pushes the bones apart has been questioned seriously. Presently, it is thought that displacement of osseous structures due to the expansive effect of developing muscles and other soft tissues exerts tension on the tissues where the bones tend to move apart, thus triggering proliferation of bone and enlargement. Perhaps it is the location of compressive influence due to functional requirements (as with the mandibular condyle) that accounts for the presence of endochondrosis. It seems to be generally agreed that active remodeling at the articulation and, indeed, throughout the individual bone, is an integral part of the process of growth and development.[22]

The growth cartilage of the mandibular condyle is different from the epiphyseal cartilage of long bones, which is subject to the genetic controls of growth. The condylar cartilage is secondary cartilage that arises ectopically rather than from primary cephalic cartilage. It has no inherent genetic controls and serves only to meet the developmental demands of function.[1] It quickly undergoes atrophic change in the absence of function but regains its endochondral capability when functional demands are reestablished.[23, 24]

Articular Surfaces

The articular surfaces of the temporomandibular joints are different from other synovial joints (except those of the clavicles) in that they are not composed of hyaline cartilage. Rather, these surfaces are composed of nonvascularized and noninnervated *dense fibrous tissue* which functions like cartilage insofar as it is suited to the demands of movement and compression simultaneously.[25]

This difference becomes important in the matter of regenerative capabilities of the joint. It is known that hyaline cartilage has a low propensity in this regard when damaged or lost. The temporomandibular joints, however, enjoy a considerably greater potentiality—a feature of real importance in treatment planning.[26] It is also known that degenerative arthritis is a primary disease of articular hyaline cartilage. The temporomandibular joints do not have articular cartilage—an important departure from usual synovial joint structure.

Remodeling

Remodeling involves morphologic changes in bone as an adaptive response to altered environmental demands. Structural adaptation of the articular surfaces of the temporomandibular joint is necessary for the normal development of the craniofacial skeleton and for the changing demands of function of the masticatory system throughout life.

Remodeling is said to be *progressive* when proliferation of tissue occurs and *regressive* when osteoclastic resorption is evident. The extraosseous surface of the mandibular condyle is composed of three layers (Fig 2–4): a layer of nonvascularized dense fibrous tissue which consti-

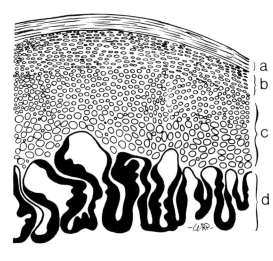

FIGURE 2–4 The condylar cartilage has a fibrous covering *(a)* that overlies a region of rapidly proliferating prechondroblasts *(b)*. In area *c*, the cells have become chondrocytes that "mature" in the deeper part of the zone. Each cell undergoes hypertrophy, and a limited deposition of intercellular matrix occurs. Near zone *d*, the matrix calcifies, and cartilage resorption with subsequent bone deposition begins along the posterosuperior moving interface between *c* and *d*. (From Enlow D.H.: *Handbook of Facial Growth.* Philadelphia, W.B. Saunders Co., 1975. Reproduced with permission.)

tutes the articular surface, a deeper zone of proliferative cells that can produce either a cartilaginous or an osseous matrix, and a still deeper layer of hyaline cartilage next to the bone. Remodeling is evidenced by increased activity in the proliferative zone.[22] Early remodeling changes appear to be largely progressive, with thickening of the articular soft tissue taking place along with osseous change. Such change occurs more in the condylar than the temporal surface, and little or none occurs in the articular disc.[27]

The degree of compressive stress seems to significantly influence changes within the stress-bearing portions of the joint. Moderate loading appears to facilitate normal remodeling. Excessive loading appears to arrest remodeling and may induce metaplasia of a hyaline cartilage-like tissue, not only in the articular surface of the condyle, but in the articular disc and upper articular surface as well. If compressive force is sufficently great, localized resorption results.[28]

All such remodeling changes embrace an element of time. It takes time for the biomechanical adaptations to occur. Adaptive changes, therefore, may be expected *if time permits*. If the demands for change are too rapid, however, degenerative breakdown may take place instead.

The temporomandibular joint is not a rigid, static, unchanging structure. Rather, like all other joints, it is adaptable to the demands of function, providing (1) the forces applied are not destructively excessive (such as movement of articular surfaces under sufficient pressure to induce frictional abuse), (2) the demands for change are not excessively rapid (such as acute trauma, too rapid orthodontic movement, or sudden changes due to natural or iatrogenic causes), and (3) the host conditions are not unsatisfactory for normal responsive behavior (such as advanced age, illness, diabetes, and rheumatoid disease). It should be noted that the adaptive capability of the dentition far exceeds that of the joints. *Therefore, if therapeutic change is contemplated, it is better to attempt adaptation of the dentition to the joints rather than vice versa.*

Age should be considered in the biomechanical adaptive process of the joints. Clinically, the adaptive processes appear to be quite adequate during the developmental period and to remain so well into adult life. In later years, however, the obvious decrease in response suggests a serious decline in the adaptive and regenerative capability. This has a bearing on treatment planning and prognosis.

Structural Requirements Imposed by Translatory Movement

The temporomandibular joint is the most complex of all synovial joints. The double-joint arrangement enables movements that are utter extremes. Hinge action in the lower joint is purely rotatory. Sliding action in the upper joint can take place in all directions, even pivotally. The extensive translatory movement of the disc-condyle complex gives the joint its great range of motion. This remarkable movement, which reaches a zenith in the higher primates, imposes, however, a number of structural requirements that should be well understood.

Provision for Stability. Adequate stability during translation is necessary. Since the craniomandibular articulation functions bilaterally, the disc-condyle complexes are suspended bilaterally by two temporomandibular ligaments, one situated in the lateral portion of the articular capsule in each joint. These ligaments prevent dislocation inferiorly during the translatory cycle. They also limit posterior movement of the condyles, thus preventing posterior dislocation, especially at the end of a power stroke—even when edentulous.

Stability during the translatory cycle is maintained by firm contact between the disc-condyle complex and the eminence. This is accomplished by muscle action involving the posterior temporalis in combination with the inferior head of the lateral pterygoid muscle. During power strokes that force the teeth against a bolus of food, stability is ensured by the action of the superior head of the lateral pterygoid muscle in two ways: (1) a holding action applied to the condylar neck, thus permitting the return movement of the translatory cycle to be controlled until intercuspation takes place, and (2) a firm anterior rotatory traction applied to the articular disc, thus rotating a thicker portion of disc firmly into the widened articular disc space created by torquing of the mandible.

During maximum intercuspation, stability is provided by the occlusion of the teeth. This permits muscle action to drop back to the resting state as the dentition also assumes an attitude of physiologic rest.

Capsular Attachment. The temporomandibular articular capsule is attached to the condyle, disc, and temporal bone in such a manner as to create two separate joint cavities (with the help of the retrodiscal tissue), but not to interfere with or restrain the function of the condyle to translate anteriorly the full extent of the temporal articular surface. It attaches rather closely, therefore, in all but the posterior region of the joint, where it forms loose folds. This permits the full translatory cycle to take place wtihout capsular restraint as the folds open up.

Retrodiscal Tissue. *It is necessary that the two joint cavities be isolated so as to retain their separate portions of synovial fluid.* This separation is accomplished only partially by the disc. It is completed by the presence of a mass of loose connective tissue attached to the posterior edge of the articular disc and extending to the posterior capsule. This tissue is well vascularized and innervated. Its upper and lower surface structures or laminae enter importantly into the functioning of the disc-condyle complex, as will be seen later. These surfaces are covered with synovial membrane. Therefore, the retrodiscal tissue is an important source of synovial fluid in both joint cavities.

As translation takes place, the loose, flexible retrodiscal tissue follows the disc-condyle complex. Thus, translatory movements are accomplished without compromising the integrity of the two joint cavities or the vascular structures that are the source of synovial fluid. This structural arrangement is unique and of great importance in the normal functioning of the joint.

Intracapsular Vascularity

Most synovial joints do not have blood vessels within the confines of the articular capsule. Therefore, the clinical identification of intracapsular inflammation is usually taken as being symptomatic of inflammatory arthritis. The temporomandibular joint is different in that it is really two joints within a single capsule, and the retrodiscal tissue which helps separate the upper and lower joint cavities lies within the confines of the articular capsule. Since this tissue is vascularized and subject to injury by the mandibular condyle, intracapsular inflammation of the temporomandibular joint may stem from causes other than inflammatory arthritis. An understanding of this peculiarity has considerable diagnostic importance.

Articular Disc Damage

The TM articular disc is a unique structure and is subject to unique functional conditions, some of which may result in damage. Articular *remodeling* is normal—a nonpathologic adaptation in which the cells respond to the stimuli of whatever mechanical forces are acting on the joint—while *degeneration* is the destruction of articular tissue that begins whenever the contours of a joint have not adapted successfully to the functional or other forces imposed upon it.[29] Cellular activity is involved in both conditions. Since the TM articular disc does not have the capacity to undergo cellular remodeling,[30] the use of the term *degeneration* is not appropriate to describe deteriorative conditions of the disc.

Changes in the articular disc that result from trauma or from abusive mechanical loading and/or frictional movement include deformation, deterioration, perforation, fracture, displacement, and dislocation.

Deformation is a change in configuration that occurs passively in response to compressive loading.

Deterioration is a change in configuration that occurs actively in response to frictional movement.

Perforation or *fracture* may result from extensive deformation or deterioration.

Displacement is the alteration of the normal disc-condyle relationship due to the loss of disc contour.

Dislocation is the gross displacement of the disc from between the condyle and articular eminence, which results in the collapse of the articular disc space and entrapment of the disc.

The term *derangement* refers to the lack of normal functional behavior from any cause. It describes a dysfunction, not a structural change. Disc-interference disorders may be described as internal derangements of the TM joint. More precisely, disc-interference disorders include those internal derangements that specifically result from impaired disc-condyle complex function. They do not include internal derangements due to inflammatory conditions of the joint such as inflammatory degenerative, traumatic, or rheumatoid arthritis.

REFERENCES

1. Enlow D.H.: Role of the TMJ in facial growth and development, in *The President's Conference on the Examination, Diagnosis and Management of Temporomandibular Disorders*. Chicago, American Dental Association, 1983, pp. 13–16.
2. DuBrul E.L.: The biomechanics of the oral apparatus. Chapter 3. Structural analysis, in DuBrul E.L., Menekratis A.: *The Physiology of Oral Reconstruction*. Chicago, Quintessence Publishing Co., 1981, pp. 21–38.
3. Sicher H.: Functional anatomy of the temporomandibular joint, in Sarnat B.G. (ed.): *The Temporomandibular Joint*, ed. 2. Springfield, Ill., Charles C Thomas, Publisher, 1964, pp. 28–58.
4. DuBrul E.L.: The biomechanics of the oral apparatus. Chapter 4. Posture and movement, in DuBrul E.L., Menekratis A.: *The Physiology of Oral Reconstruction*. Chicago, Quintessence Publishing Co., 1981, pp. 39–53.
5. Frankel V.H., Nordin M.: *Basic Biomechanics of the Skeletal System*. Philadelphia, Lea & Febiger, 1980.
6. Kopp S.: Topographical distribution of sulphated glycosaminoglycans in the surface layers of the human temporomandibular joint. *J. Oral Pathol.* 7:283, 1978.

7. Blackwood H.J.J.: Pathology of the temporomandibular joint. *J. Am. Dent. Assoc.* 79:118, 1969.
8. Mongini F.: Abnormalities in condylar and occlusal positions, in Solberg W.K., Clark G.T. (eds.): *Abnormal Jaw Mechanics*. Chicago, Quintessence Publishing Co., 1984, pp. 23–50.
9. Sicher H.: Positions and movements of the mandible. *J. Am. Dent. Assoc.* 48:620, 1954.
10. Costen J.B.: Syndrome of ear and sinus symptoms dependent upon disturbed function of the temporomandibular joint. *Ann. Otol. Rhinol. Laryngol.* 43:1, 1934.
11. DuBrul E.L.: Evolution of the temporomandibular joint, in Sarnat B.G. (ed.): *The Temporomandibular Joint*, ed. 2. Springfield, Ill., Charles C Thomas, Publisher, 1964, pp. 3–27.
12. Moffett B.C.: The morphogenesis of the temporomandibular joint. *Am. J. Orthod.* 52:410, 1966.
13. Rood S.R., Doyle W.J.: Morphology of the tensor veli palatini, tensor tympani, and dilator tubae muscles. *Ann. Otol. Rhinol. Laryngol.* 87:202–210, 1978.
14. Pinto O.F.: A new structure related to the TM joint and middle ear. *J. Prosthet. Dent.* 12:95, 1962.
15. Rees L.A.: The structure and function of the temporomandibular joint. *Br. Dent. J.* 96:125, 1954.
16. Coleman R.D.: Temporomandibular joint: Relationship of the retrodiskal zone to Meckel's cartilage and lateral pterygoid muscle. *J. Dent. Res.* 49:626, 1970.
17. Marshall W.G.: The relationship between the meniscus of the TMJ and the anterior ligament of the malleus. *J. Dent. Res.* 54:649 (abs. No. 26), 1975.
18. Mohl N.D.: Functional anatomy of the temporomandibular joint, in *The President's Conference on the Examination, Diagnosis and Management of Temporomandibular Disorders*. Chicago, American Dental Association, 1983, pp. 3–12.
19. Sicher H.: *Oral Anatomy*. St. Louis, C.V. Mosby Co., 1949.
20. Furstman L.: Embryology, in Sarnat B.G., Laskin D.M. (eds.): *The Temporomandibular Joint*, ed. 3. Springfield, Ill., Charles C Thomas, Publisher, 1979, pp. 53–69.
21. Levy B.M.: Embryological development of the temporomandibular joint, in Sarnat B.G. (ed.): *The Temporomandibular Joint*, ed. 2. Springfield, Ill., Charles C Thomas, Publisher, 1964, pp. 59–70.
22. Enlow D.H.: *Handbook of Facial Growth*, ed. 2. Philadelphia, W.B. Saunders Co., 1982.
23. Glineburg R.W., Laskin D.M., Blaustein D.I.: The effects of immobilization on the primate temporomandibular joint. *J. Oral Maxillofac. Surg.* 40:3, 1982.
24. Lydiatt D.D., Davis L.F.: The effects of immobilization on the rabbit temporomandibular joint. *J. Oral Maxillofac. Surg.* 43:188–193, 1985.

25. DuBrul E.L.: *Sicher's Oral Anatomy,* ed. 7. St. Louis, C.V. Mosby Co., 1980.
26. Toller P.A.: Temporomandibular arthropathy. *Proc. R. Soc. Lond.* 67:153, 1974.
27. Hansson T.: Temporomandibular joint changes related to dental occlusion, in Solberg W.K., Clark G.T. (eds.): *Temporomandibular Joint Problems.* Chicago, Quintessence Publishing Co., 1980, pp. 129–143.
28. Meikle M.C.: Remodeling, in Sarnat B.G., Laskin D.M. (eds.): *The Temporomandibular Joint,* ed. 3. Springfield, Ill., Charles C Thomas, Publisher, 1979, pp. 205–226.
29. Moffett B.: Definitions of temporomandibular joint derangements, in Moffett B.C. (ed.): *Diagnosis of Internal Derangements of the Temporomandibular Joint.* Vol. 1. Seattle, University of Washington, 1984, pp. 5–8.
30. Moffett B.: Histologic aspects of temporomandibular joint derangements, in Moffett B.C. (ed.): *Diagnosis of Internal Derangements of the Temporomandibular Joint,* Vol. 1. Seattle, University of Washington, 1984, pp. 47–49.

3 | Structural Components

A good understanding of the functional anatomy of the craniomandibular articulation is an absolute prerequisite for accurate diagnosis and effective treatment of temporomandibular disorders, and necessarily is the basis for judging when departures from normal occur.

ERRONEOUS ANATOMICAL CONCEPTS

Unfortunately, the dental profession has been plagued by several erroneous notions about TM joint structure and function. The continuation of such errors is not justified. No doubt, much of the confusion that has pervaded this field in the past was due in part to an improper understanding of joint structure and function.

Meniscus Concept

A meniscus is a passive anatomical structure that facilitates joint movements without becoming a determinant of those movements. The articulating surfaces are not capsule-enclosed and, as such, are not true articular facets. The removal of a meniscus therefore does not seriously alter the functional behavior of a joint.

The TM articular disc is different. It is not a passive structure that just facilitates joint movement. Rather, it is an active component of the joint. It is completely encapsulated and has true articular facets on both the superior and inferior surfaces. It has its own power system and therefore is capable of functioning quite independently of either condyle or articular eminence. It is a determinant of joint function in that it is the structure that converts an otherwise simple joint into a compound one. Furthermore, the disc is essential to normal joint functioning in that it is the means of providing the continuous sharp contact of the articulating structures of the joint under all conditions. The TM articular disc is a unique structure in the body. Its removal converts the TM into a simple joint. A TM joint without its disc, or with a seriously malfunctioning one, loses the means of maintaining stability during translatory cycles, especially during power strokes. It can never again function normally.

Simple-Joint Concept

A serious misunderstanding of anatomy is the idea that the mandibular condyle articulates with the articular eminence with an interposed "meniscus"—as it seems to appear radiographically. By orthopedic definition, this arrangement makes the TM a *simple joint* with only two articulating surfaces. The correct anatomical concept, as described by Sicher[1] in 1949, is that the mandibular condyle articulates with the articular disc to form a separate simple joint, the disc-condyle complex; this complex, in turn, articulates with the temporal bone. Thus, the TM is a *true compound joint,* having four articular surfaces, with articular facets on the condyle, on the lower surface of the disc, on the upper surface of the disc, and on the temporal fossa-eminence. The simple-joint concept centers attention on the osseous components which are seen radiographically, rather than on the much more important functioning of the articular disc which is radiographically invisible.

Articular Cartilage

In spite of frequent references in the literature to the contrary, there is no articular cartilage in the TM joint.[1-6] The condylar cartilage, which is often mistaken for articular cartilage, is different; it is *growth cartilage* that is utilized in endochondral osseous development. Excellent research on the condylar cartilage (even though sometimes mistaken for articular cartilage) has been reported in the dental literature.[7, 8] Instead of hyaline cartilage, the articular surfaces of the TM joint are composed of dense fibrous tissue.[1, 2, 9] This difference is significantly important both diagnostically and therapeutically.

Clicking Due to Condyle Slipping Over Disc

Since the 1950s, there has been a prevailing notion that linear sliding in the lower joint compartment permits the condyle to slip over various "bands" of the articular disc during translatory movements, thus causing the clicking noise that frequently occurs in TM disorders. This concept appears to have originated as the result of a serious misinterpretation of Rees' brilliant description of TM joint structure and function in 1954.[2] Rees lost his life in an accident prior to the publication of his work and therefore could not put the record straight. Schwartz[10] used Rees as his authority for the notion that during translatory movements the disc remained stationary against the mandibular fossa while the condyle moved over it. According to him, when the condyle slipped over a different "band" of the disc, a clicking noise resulted. This notion of the condyle sliding linearly over different "bands" of the disc as the cause of clicking has persisted with some modification down to the present.[11-14] Anatomists,[1, 9] including Rees,[2] agree, however, that the movement between condyle and disc in the normal TM joint is a *rotatory* sliding movement around a horizontal axis that passes through the medial and lateral poles of the condyle and is not a *linear* sliding movement at all. Toller[15] reported that, in arthrographically examining 19 patients with clinical disc noise complaints, none showed the condyle riding over either the anterior or the posterior border of the articular disc. A recent study of 115 cadaver joints showed that it is highly improbable that anterior disc displacement should occur when the condyle slips behind the articular disc and pushes it forward.[16] The important issue in Schwartz's concept of the cause of disc noise is that it is wholly impossible in *normal* joints. When such interference does take place, significant damage to the joint must have occurred first.

Nonpressure-Bearing Joint

In the past there have been notions that the TM was not a pressure-bearing joint. This was based on a theory that the mandible functioned as a "reflexly controlled nonlever."[17] Such a theory of course had no anatomical foundation and even violated the orthopedic definition of a synovial joint. It is still occasionally heard, however.[18]

Disc Adaptability

There is a rather prevalent notion that the TM disc equalizes the incongruity of the condylar and temporal articular surfaces of the joint by altering its shape during translatory movements.[19, 20] Actually, the dense, nonvascularized, fibrous structure of a normal disc precludes such a degree of adaptability. It has resiliency and flexibility, the qualities needed to maintain continuous surface contact with the articular eminence during the translatory cycle.[21] It can be deformed by static overloading or by condylar pressure when it is dislocated anteriorly, but it does not change its shape to any appreciable degree during translatory cycles.

Synovial Membrane on Articular Surfaces

An old notion that synovial membrane completely lines the synovial cavities, including the articular surfaces, occasionally is encountered.[19, 20] This, of course, is not true, except at the periphery of the articular tissue.[9] Actually, the ongrowth of such vascularized tissue onto articular surfaces constitutes the chief pathologic manifestation of rheumatoid arthritis.

Lateral Pterygoid Incoordination

A very prevalent notion is that the two heads of the lateral pterygoid muscle conjointly draw the condyle and disc forward during translatory movements.[19, 22] It is assumed therefore that strict coordination between these heads is essential to normal joint functioning and that incoordination, with resulting myospastic activity, may be both a cause and a result of disc interference disorders.[22, 23] McNamara[24] and others[25, 26] have shown, however, that these two heads function as different muscles, even nearly in a reciprocal manner. While the inferior head protracts the condyle, the superior head normally remains *inactive throughout the entire translatory cycle* unless a power stroke is made. Rather than being coordinated with the inferior head, the superior head functions in conjunction with the elevator masticatory muscles. So, with whatever problems that occur relative to the superior and inferior lateral pterygoid muscles, at least functional incoordination is not one of them.

Posterior Ligament Holds Disc on Condyle

A fairly common belief is that the elastic retrodiscal tissue—sometimes mistakenly called a posterior "ligament"—holds the articular disc on the condyle during the closed, resting position of the joint.[27, 28] It is therefore assumed that if this "ligament" becomes too loose due to condylar encroachment, the disc can slip off the condyle in an anterior direction, thus constituting an anterior dislocation. It is true that the superior retrodiscal lamina has a high content of elastic fibers, and it does exert tractive force on the disc in a posterior direction. But, this does not occur in the closed, resting position of the joint. At that time, this tissue is relaxed and exerts no elastic traction on the disc. It is only when the condyle translates forward that the effect of elasticity of this tissue takes place. In the resting joint, the predominant force on the disc is that of muscle tonus in the superior lateral pterygoid muscle anteriorly. *It is the contour of the disc and not the retrodiscal tissue that prevents displacement forward.*

As Sherlock Holmes would have said, "Remove the impossibles and what remains may likely be the truth." So, if we can eliminate the "impossibles" from this field, we should be in excellent position to understand what is really true.

Currently, much of what is known about masticatory disorders is backed up by sound documentation. Unfortunately, such cannot be cited for all problems of TM function and dysfunction. It is necessary therefore to extrapolate information from other sources and *presume* that it does in fact apply to the masticatory system. It is necessary to utilize principles of physics and biomechanics as well as biology, to apply logic and common sense, and to use as best we can the lessons of clinical experience until genuine documentation becomes available. However, many years ago Sicher[29] sounded a warning: "Clinical success does not prove anything but the acceptability of the method employed; any attempt to prove an anatomical concept by clinical success is merely a rationalization and certainly is not to be regarded as truly scientific evidence."

CHEWING UNIT

The process of mastication requires a complete functioning unit, structurally interrelated and biologically integrated. Chewing is a mechanical process in which physical laws cannot be ignored. Laws governing movement, force, resistance, friction, and noise must be given due consideration. Like locomotion, mastication involves structures of the musculoskeletal system that behave according to certain principles of biomechanics.

The chief working component of the mouth proper, relative to mastication, is the dentition—teeth functioning in such a way as to hold, incise, tear, and grind foods. The lips, cheeks, tongue, and palate position and control the foods in the mouth. These structures are muscle-activated and neurologically guided by central direction, reflex activities, and feedback mechanisms. The teeth are anchored in bony frameworks that are bilaterally connected by the craniomandibular articulation, which is composed of two separate but functionally related temporomandibular joints. Skeletal muscles power the mandibular frame. They are activated and guided by impulses from the CNS in response to preconditioned habit patterns, reflex activity, feedback mechanisms, and volition. Swallowing invokes activity of the tongue, palate, pharynx, epiglottis, and esophagus. Saliva is an essential factor in mastication; it softens and binds food particles, initiates the digestive process, lubricates the oral structures, and facilitates swallowing. Salivation is a glandular activity under control of the visceral nervous system and responsive to systemic factors. To all this is added an effective sensory system for detecting and selectively choosing proper foods. Influencing the whole process are the factors of systemic relationships, emotional situations, and volition.

Mastication involves many structures—bones, joints, muscles, teeth, glands, nerves of different types, blood vessels—and systemic and central nervous system processes. Any attempt to examine one part in isolation from the rest is futile. Since the objective of this book is to consider particularly temporomandibular disorders, only the craniomandibular articulation and its activating musculature will be taken into account. This is not to imply that other structures of the chewing unit, particularly the occlusion of teeth, are any less important. Each is essential in its own way to the normal functioning of the whole system.

In man, the articulation of a one-piece mandible with the cranium is a bilateral structure joining the mandibular condyles with articular facets on the temporal bones. All movements of the mandible affect both joints. Functionally, they cannot be considered as isolated structures.

These joints are compression-movement articulations, which require that the pressure-bearing articular surfaces be nonvascularized and noninnervated. As such, they are classified as diarthrodial or synovial joints.

Each temporomandibular joint is capable of two distinct movements, rotating and sliding. Rotation is confined strictly to the condyle-articular disc portion of the joint, while linear sliding movement is confined strictly to the articular disc-temporal bone portion.

The temporomandibular is a double joint, one above the other. It is a lower hinge joint and an upper sliding joint, all in a single capsule. As such, it is classified as a ginglymo-arthrodial joint.

The two joints that constitute the temporomandibular joint have several structures in common, namely:

1. The *articular disc together with the retrodiscal tissue,* which divides it into two separate joints

2. The *capsular ligament,* which encapsulates each of the two joints, thus confining the synovial fluid to separate compartments or synovial cavities
3. The *musculature,* which provides for stability and movement in both joints

CAPSULAR LIGAMENT

The capsular ligament is composed of fibrous connective tissue. It attaches to the periphery of the articular facets on the temporal bone above and the mandibular condyle below. The sides of the capsule anteriorly are little more than loose connective tissue supporting the synovial membrane. The temporomandibular ligament strongly reinforces the lateral wall of the capsule. Anteriorly, the capsule fuses with the articular disc. Posteriorly, it attaches to the retrodiscal tissue in loose folds that permit freedom of movement of the disc-condyle complex anteriorly.

The capsule offers little restraint on mandibular movements except in the outer ranges. Rather, it appears to relate more to the dynamics of synovial fluid. In the closed position, the fluid in both upper and lower joint cavities appears to be distributed evenly anterior and posterior to the disc. In forward translation, much of the fluid is located posteriorly, the synovial fluid conforming to the shape of the capsule. This suggests that the functioning of the capsule is an important factor in lubricating and nourishing the articular surfaces, the fluid being swished back and forth between the articulating surfaces as translatory movements take place.

The fibrous capsule is well vascularized and innervated. It is lined with synovial membrane which secretes the synovial fluid into the joint cavities. The vascular supply is chiefly from the superficial temporal artery. The anterior tympanic artery supplies the retrodiscal tissue.

Afferent nerve fibers for proprioception and nociception are branches of the auriculotemporal, masseteric, and posterior deep temporal nerves.[30] Fibers of the auriculotemporal innervate the posterior capsule and retrodiscal tissue; those of the masseteric and temporal nerves innervate the anterior part of the capsular ligament. These nerves terminate in the periphery of the articular disc. Free nerve endings, generally conceded to mediate pain sensation, are abundant throughout the capsule, thus giving it the propensity to sense pain. Ruffini's corpuscles, Golgi tendon organs, and Pacinian corpuscles are found in the capsular ligament, especially in the lateral and posterolateral parts, thus proprioceptively monitoring condylar position and movement. Visceral fibers, accompanying somatic fibers of the auriculotemporal nerve, supply the blood vessels of the capsule.[31]

Griffin and Harris[32] identified mechanoreceptors in the fascia of the lateral and medial ligaments of the articular disc. Although a great deal seems to be known about the neurophysiology of the craniomandibular articulation by extrapolation from other body structures, Storey[33] pointed out that actually much of it is only presumed.

LOWER JOINT

The articulation of the mandibular condyle with the articular disc forms a simple hinge joint (ginglymoid), which henceforth will be referred to as the *disc-condyle complex.*

Articular Surfaces

The articular facet of the mandibular condyle is small compared with that of the temporal bone (Fig 3–1). It is rounded mediolaterally and quite convex anteroposteriorly. The posterior margin of the articular surface extends a considerable distance, permitting more extensive ro-

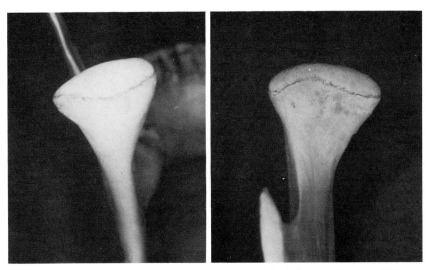

FIGURE 3–1 Subarticular bone of mandibular condyle. *Left,* posterior view. *Right,* anterior view. Attachment of capsular ligament outlined with pencil. Note that articular facet is more extensive posteriorly.

tation of the disc posteriorly than anteriorly. The articular surface is composed of dense, nonvascularized, noninnervated fibrous tissue rather than cartilage. This tissue is quite thin over most of the articular facet but thickens appreciably in the anterosuperior aspect, indicating the area best suited to sustain maximum pressure.

Immediately beneath the dense fibrous articular surface is the *proliferative zone*. Deeper to the proliferative zone and adjacent to the osseous structure of the condyle is the *condylar cartilage* (see Fig 2–4). It should be understood that this pertains to endochondral growth. It is distinctively different structurally and functionally from articular cartilage of other synovial joints and should not be confused with it.

The inferior surface of the articular disc forms the other facet that articulates with the condyle to make up the disc-condyle complex. This surface is slightly concave mediolaterally and boldly concave anteroposteriorly, making it compatible with the condylar surface for flexion-extension movement in the sagittal plane.

Articular Disc.   The articular disc is composed of dense fibrous tissue that is nonvascularized and noninnervated except in the peripheral, nonpressure-bearing areas. A few cartilaginous cells may be present. The size and shape of the disc are determined by the shape of the condylar and eminence articular surfaces. The lower articular surface of the disc is contoured in both dimensions to fit the condylar facet so as to permit uninterrupted rotatory sliding movement around a horizontal axis. These compatible surfaces form the arc of a circle, the radius of which extends to the hinge axis that passes through the medial and lateral poles of the condyle. The upper articular surface of the disc is shaped in both dimensions to fit the temporal articular facet. These compatible surfaces permit linear sliding movement in all directions, even pivoting.

The anteroposterior profile of the disc is thinner in the central portion. The anterior and posterior margins are considerably thicker. The greater the steepness of the articular eminence, the greater the thickness of the disc posteriorly. The disc is composed of rather homogeneous dense fibrous tissue and does not present the appearance of well-demarcated "bands" as is commonly believed.

The disc contour is important and should be well understood. As the interarticular pressure from the osseous components of the joint narrows the articular disc space and bears on the disc, the contour of the disc causes an automatic biomechanical self-centering effect, a rotatory movement of the disc to bring a thinner portion between the bones. Conversely, when pressure between the bony parts is decreased and the disc space widens, the disc is free to rotate a thicker portion to fill the space. If disc contour is lost, it loses also this self-centering capability.[34]

Disc contour is important in another way: it prevents linear sliding movement between disc and condyle without inhibiting rotatory sliding movement. It is the thicker posterior margin of the disc that prevents linear displacement of the disc anteriorly. It is the thicker anterior margin of the disc that prevents linear displacement of the disc posteriorly. *It is the disc contour therefore that causes the disc and condyle to translate together without displacement.* Linear displacement of the disc is impossible unless there is first some appreciable loss of contour due to applied force, either immediately, as from acute trauma, or gradually, as from functional abuse.

The articular disc is normally too dense to permit compression great enough to be radiographically apparent. It has flexibility, however, to maintain surface contact satisfactorily with the articular eminence during translatory movements. A normal disc cannot appreciably alter its contour during movements.

The medial portion of the articular disc forms as a condensation in the tendon of the superior lateral pterygoid muscle. Thus, an unusually strong bond is formed between disc and muscle. Actually, the disc may be considered as a continuation of the superior lateral pterygoid muscle.[34, 35]

Synovial Sac

The synovial cavity of the lower joint is formed anteriorly by the inferior segment of the anterior wall of the joint capsule, laterally and medially by the lateral walls of the capsule, and posteriorly by the inferior retrodiscal lamina. All of these structures are ligamentous, even though the capsular parts are not strong. Synovial membrane lines these structures. The passive volume of synovial fluid in the lower joint averages about 0.9 ml.[15] Synovial fluid cannot be aspirated from the TM joint.[36]

Collateral Discal Ligaments

Collateral ligaments attaching the articular disc to the medial and lateral poles of the condyle were described by Krogh-Poulsen and Moelhave in 1957.[37] These nonelastic structures, like other true ligaments, are composed of collagenous connective tissue fibers. *They do not stretch appreciably.* If subjected to abusive and repeated strain, they may elongate, thus impairing their efficiency to passively restrain discal movement.[38] Like all collateral ligaments, these ligaments serve to restrict the movements of the joint to hinge action in a single plane. Being short and closely placed to the articulating surfaces, the ligaments limit gross movement between the articular disc and mandibular condyle to rotation. They are not so rigidly attached, however, as to prevent slight shifting movements of the disc laterally. The discal ligaments attach the articular disc to the condyle in such a manner as to cause it to passively follow the condyle wherever it moves.[9] They resist displacement between disc and condyle. *The disc may rotate forward on the condyle, but it cannot be bodily displaced anteriorly or posteriorly as long as these ligaments are intact and functonal.*

The discal ligaments are vascularized and innervated. When strained, they may sense pain. When injured, they may become inflamed. They proprioceptively monitor position and movement.

Like all hinge joints, the disc-condyle complex has an anatomical axis of rotation. It passes mediolaterally through the attachments of the articular disc to the condyle: that is, through the medial and lateral condylar poles. If projected onto the face, this axis terminates at a point near the center of the mandibular condyle. If projected medially, it crosses its fellow of the opposite side near the anterior margin of the foramen magnum. Since the disc-condyle complex moves anteroposteriorly during translatory movements, the intercondylar hinge axis also moves. To be a useful point of orientation on the face, the intercondylar hinge axis registration should be accomplished by using rotatory movement of the condyle only. The degree to which translation is permitted, therefore, represents technical error.

The arc of rotation of the disc-condyle complex is the arc of a circle, the radius of which extends from the anatomical rotatory axis of the condyle. If this radius is projected to the mandibular incisor area, a circle is described, a segment of which represents the arc of rotation at the incisor area. It should be noted that normal translatory opening follows a path that terminates anterior to this arc of rotation (Fig 3–2).

Retrodiscal Tissue

The retrodiscal tissue attaches to the posterior edge of the articular disc. It extends posteriorly to and fuses with the posterior wall of the articular capsule. Its *superior lamina* attaches to the tympanic plate. Composed of connective tissue containing many elastic fibers, this lamina has the quality of elasticity[39, 40] which counters the forward traction of the superior lateral pterygoid muscle on the articular disc. Except

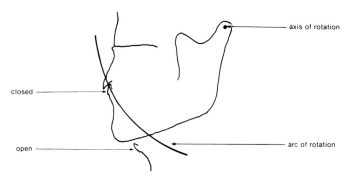

FIGURE 3–2 Tracing from lateral radiographs of face in *closed* and *open* positions. Condylar *axis of rotation* is indicated at about center of condyle. An arc from axis of rotation drawn through the incisal edge of mandibular incisor in closed position describes the *arc of rotation*. Note that in normal translatory opening the position of mandibular incisor is anterior to arc of rotation.

during forward translation, when this superior lamina is stretched, the effect of muscle tonus in the superior lateral pterygoid muscle is dominant and exceeds the elastic traction of the retrodiscal tissue. *At rest, the articular disc normally occupies the most forward rotated position on the condyle that is permitted by the width of the articular disc space.*

The elasticity of the superior lamina does not hold the articular disc on the condyle in the closed joint position, as is sometimes believed. In the closed relationship this lamina is relaxed and exerts no traction on the disc. It exerts an appreciable posterior tractive force on the disc during the forward phase of the translatory cycle only.

The *inferior retrodiscal lamina* attaches anteriorly to the articular disc and posteriorly just below the posterior margin of the condylar articular facet. It is different from the superior lamina in that it is composed chiefly of collagenous fibers, making it nonelastic. This lamina serves as a check ligament that passively limits forward rotation of the disc on the condyle. Like all ligaments, it does not enter actively into disc functioning.

The *body of retrodiscal tissue* consists of loose connective tissue that is highly vascularized and innervated. Synovial membrane covers both the superior and inferior laminae. Thus, the retrodiscal tissue is a major contributor to synovial fluid metabolism, which is essential to the normal functioning of a synovial joint. It ensures free metabolic exchange, nutrition, and lubrication of the articulating surfaces in both upper and lower joints, whether at rest or during translatory movement.

UPPER JOINT

The upper part of the compound temporomandibular joint consists of the disc-condyle complex articulating with the articular facet of the temporal bone in a manner that permits freedom of sliding (arthrodial) movement. This requires flattened articular surfaces that are not restrained by ligamentous structures.

Articular Surfaces

The temporal articular facet that accommodates the disc-condyle complex occupies the anterolateral part of the glenoid fossa and the whole of the articular eminence (Fig 3–3). As indicated by evidence of attachment of the capsular ligament on the dry bone, the articular surface falls safely clear of adjacent bony structures. Laterally, the articular surface ends several millimeters short of the outer margin of the inferior surface of the supra-articular crest.

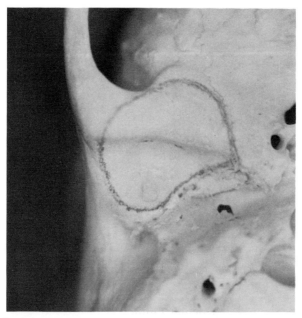

FIGURE 3–3 Subarticular bone of temporal articular facet. Attachment of capsular ligament is outlined with pencil. Articular surface is narrow posteriorly, widest at articular eminence. Structures medial and posterior are not included within capsular attachment. Note forward extent of articular surface.

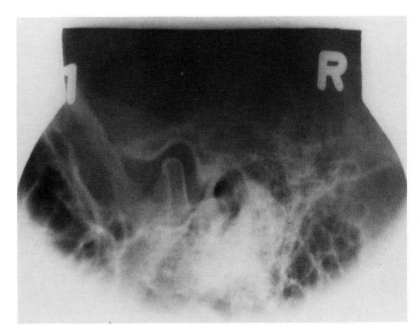

FIGURE 3–4 Transparietal flat-plate radiograph of temporomandibular joint. Note that what appears to be subarticular osseous structure is actually the more dense outer margin of the joint; what appears to be articular eminence is articular tubercle. The anterior slope of articular eminence is obscured by the zygomatic arch.

Since lateral flat-plate radiographs of the temporomandibular joint cause this outer margin to obscure the true subarticular surface of the temporal bone, what appears as the upper osseous surface is obviously an artifact (Fig 3–4). This discrepancy increases proportionately in the eminence region as the distance of the articular facet from the edge of the supra-articular crest becomes greater. The true osseous surface, which lies slightly medially and superiorly, is visualized radiographically only by the tomographic method. *Thus, the inclination of the articular eminence is not as steep as it appears to be on flat-plate radiography, and the true articular disc space is wider than is radiographically apparent.*

The supra-articular crest anterior to the articular eminence bows out to form the zygomatic arch, thus obscuring the osseous joint surface anterior to the eminence. The shape of the articular surface anterior to the crest of the articular eminence is a gentle slope superiorly, being nearly flat in many joints (Fig 3–5). It does not follow the dramatic upward sweep of the lateral margin of the articular tubercle, as visualized radiographically.

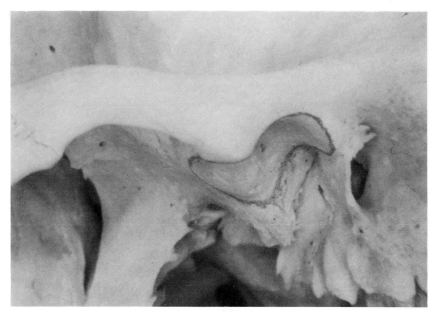

FIGURE 3–5 Lateral view of dry skull showing temporal articular facet. Attachment of capsular ligament is outlined with pencil. Note that anterior slope of articular eminence is only moderately inclined superiorly compared with the posterior slope.

Mediolaterally, the temporal articular facet is gently concave throughout its full anteroposterior sweep. It conforms to the slight mediolateral convexity of the articular facet of the mandibular condyle. Thus, the articular disc is of fairly uniform thickness mediolaterally, being gently concave below and convex above.

The extreme anterior and posterior borders of the temporal articular surface lie nearly parallel to the Frankfort horizontal plane (Fig 3–6). Between these extremities, the upward concavity of the fossa just about equals the downward convexity in the eminence area. Since the shadow of the *superior margin* of the supra-articular crest is visible radiographically, and since this structure *in the eminence area* is nearly parallel to the Frankfort plane, a useful means of estimating the inclination of the articular eminence is radiographically available (Fig 3–7). It should be noted, however, that the actual osseous surface is a few degrees flatter than this would indicate.

The articular surface proper of the temporal facet, like the condylar facet below, is composed of a thin layer of nonvascularized, noninnervated, dense fibrous tissue. Over the posterior surface of the articular eminence, this tissue thickens perceptibly, indicating the area best suited to sustain maximum pressure. Anatomically, the direction of greatest pressure from the mandible to the temporal bone is upward and forward. It projects from the anteriorly inclined mandibular condyle, through the thin central portion of disc, and into the body of the articular eminence, which is well braced.

Beneath the fibrous articular surface is a proliferative zone of cells that function in the same manner as in the condyle. The occasional presence of a hyaline cartilage-like proliferation in the temporal articular surface only demonstrates the potential of the cells of the proliferative zone to differentiate into a cartilaginous matrix.

The disc-condyle complex articulates with the temporal bone to form the upper sliding portion of the temporomandibular joint. The superior surface of the articular disc is the lower articular surface of this sliding joint. The surface is shaped to be compatible with the fossa-eminence articular facet. Mediolaterally, it is slightly convex. Anteroposteriorly, it is slightly concave. The contour of this surface correlates with the prominence of the articular eminence. The flatness and compatibility of the articular surfaces, the absence of collateral ligaments,

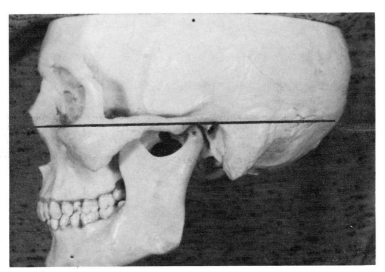

FIGURE 3–6   Dry skull with Frankfort horizontal indicated. Note that superior surface of supra-articular crest in the area of the articular eminence is nearly parallel to the Frankfort plane. Since the supra-articular crest is clearly visible on a flat-plate radiograph of the temporomandibular joint, it serves as an accurate means of estimating the angle of inclination of the articular eminence.

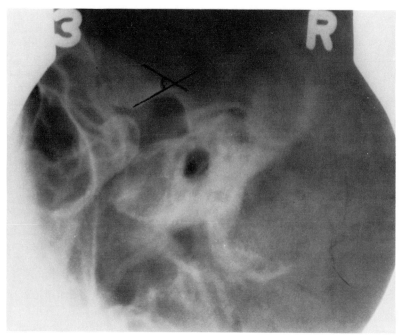

FIGURE 3–7   Transparietal radiograph of temporomandibular joint. Observe shadow of supra-articular crest. Angle formed by supra-articular crest and posterior slope of articular eminence indicates the approximate angle of inclination of the eminence in degrees. Average inclination is 30 to 60 degrees. This eminence is about 57 degrees.

and the loose attachment of the capsular ligament ensure freedom of sliding movement in all directions. The slight mediolateral convexity of the disc, with compatible concavity of the temporal facet, strongly favors sliding movement in the sagittal plane.

Synovial Sac

The synovial cavity of the upper joint is formed anteriorly by the superior segment of the anterior wall of the capsule, laterally and medially by the lateral walls of the capsule, and posteriorly by the elastic superior retrodiscal lamina. Synovial membrane lines these surfaces. It is rather deeply folded in the retrodiscal lamina area to permit freedom of forward translation of the disc-condyle complex without injury to the membrane. The passive volume of synovial fluid in the upper joint averages about 1.2 ml.[15]

Temporomandibular Ligament

The mandible is suspended from the craniofacial skeleton by two strong *lateral ligaments,* currently referred to by anatomists under the older terminology, *the temporomandibular ligaments.*[9] Although bilateral, as related to the whole craniomandibular articulation, these ligaments do not function as collateral ligaments. They are the suspensory mechanism of the mandible that resists downward and posterior displacement. As such, they protect the individual temporomandibular joint against gross disarticulation inferiorly and posteriorly.

The temporomandibular ligament is composed of two parts: an *outer oblique portion,* arising from the outer surface of the articular tubercle and extending down and back to insert into the outer surface of the condylar neck, and an *inner horizontal portion,* arising from the same area and running horizontally backward to insert into the lateral pole of the condyle and posterior part of the articular disc (Fig 3–8).[9]

The outer oblique portion of the temporomandibular ligament limits the amount that the condyle can be distracted inferiorly in the closed joint position as well as during the translatory cycle. It does not determine the resting position of the mandible; that is a function of

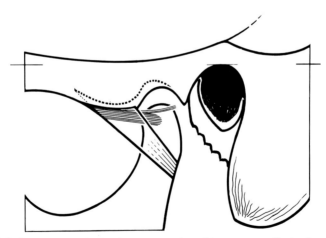

FIGURE 3–8 Diagram of adaptive construction of temporomandibular ligament. Condyle is pulled out of position and disc is omitted for clarity. Outline of articular eminence (surface) is represented by heavy interrupted line. Outer, oblique band runs from articular tubercle to condylar neck. Inner, horizontal band *(hatched)* runs from the articular tubercle to the lateral condylar pole and back of disc. (From Du Brul E.L.: *Sicher's Oral Anatomy,* ed. 7. St. Louis, C.V. Mosby Co., 1980. Reproduced with permission.)

muscle action. It does determine the condylar position when muscle action is entirely absent (paralysis, motor denervation, anesthesia, cadaver studies).

The inner horizontal portion limits how far the disc-condyle complex can go posteriorly. Normally this limit is not reached because intercuspation of teeth at the end of a power stroke firmly anchors the condylar position. In posterior edentulousness, however, the final determinant of condylar position depends on the holding action of the lateral pterygoid muscle, with the limit to posterior movement being established by the temporomandibular ligament. A serious consequence of inadequate posterior dental support is sequential elongation of this ligament until it no longer restrains the condyle from damaging the retrodiscal tissue.

The inner horizontal portion of the temporomandibular ligament has a special restraining function: it arrests posterior condylar movement during pivoting of the working joint when lateral excursions are made. It serves two important purposes: (1) it prevents encroachment of the pivoting lateral pole of the condyle on structures posterior to it; and (2) it holds the condyle and disc in their normal relationship during the pivoting movement, thus reducing strain on the discal ligaments.[41] It is this restraining influence on the lateral pole of the condyle that alters mandibular movement and causes the condyle to rotate vertically around the lateral pole rather than around the anatomical vertical axis.

The temporomandibular ligament is in close structural relationship with the lateral aspect of the capsular ligament, which it strongly reinforces. Its attachments are in intimate structural relationship with the lateral discal ligament. The intimate arrangement of these important structures has special significance in some traumatic conditions of the TM joint. For example, a torn capsule could seriously disrupt normal disc-condyle complex functioning by detaching the lateral discal ligament. Or it could alter the protective suspensory mechanism by rupturing one or both portions of the temporomandibular ligament. Such a trauma could have major consequences. Likewise, surgical opening of the articular capsule cannot be done with impunity, since it is fraught with similar possible consequences.

It should be understood that these important ligamentous structures (discal ligaments, capsular ligament, and temporomandibular ligament) are innervated for proprioceptive monitoring of movement and position. Under strain, various effects may tend to disrupt normal muscle action. These ligaments also are innervated for pain detection and are vascularized. Thus, inflammatory processes may develop if injury is sustained.

JOINT MOVEMENTS

The joint is structured to deliver rotatory movement in the lower joint and linear sliding movement in the upper compartment. Hinge-axis rotation is the normal functional movement of the disc-condyle complex. Translatory movement is a combination of sliding in the upper joint and rotation in the lower. Most jaw movements entail such a combination.

Empty-mouth movements constitute the bulk of temporomandibular function. Such movements include all activities except those which involve the special contraction of elevator muscles, such as chewing movements or special use of the jaws for holding objects. Empty-mouth functioning goes on 24 hours a day, as with swallowing.

During empty-mouth translatory cycles, continuous sharp contact of the articulating parts is accomplished by muscle tonus as affected by gravity. The weight of the mandible represents negative gravitational force that stimulates the muscle spindles in elevator masticatory muscles, thereby initiating the myotatic or stretch reflex and automatically increasing tonicity in those muscles. The posterior fibers of the temporalis and the inferior head of the lateral pterygoid muscle are of particular importance in maintaining continuous sharp contact during translatory movements.

Chewing brings into play power strokes, which impose a special burden on the musculature to maintain adequate stability. Such strokes have a marked effect on interarticular pressure in both the chewing side and the opposite joint.

Interarticular Pressure

Interarticular pressure may be passive or active. Passive interarticular pressure is due to muscle tonus and varies as muscle tonus varies. Active interarticular pressure is due to the contraction of elevator muscles and varies with the demands of function.

Limitation of Movement

The gross extent of mouth opening is limited by extra-articular factors such as the stretching length of the elevator muscles and the size of the orifice of the mouth. The capsule offers little resistance to opening. The posterior wall of the capsule limits the forward movement of the disc-condyle complex, but that does not preclude further opening of the mouth.

Within the joint, rotatory movement of the disc on the condyle is limited anteriorly by the inferior retrodiscal lamina and posteriorly by the anterior capsular ligament. Violation of hinge movement and separation between disc and condyle are resisted by the discal collateral ligaments. Gross distraction of the condyle inferiorly or displacement of the condyle posteriorly is resisted by the temporomandibular ligament.

Activators of Movement

The masticatory muscles constitute the source of power for movement of the mandible. The mouth is opened by the depressor action of the digastric and mylohyoid muscles in conjunction with contraction of the inferior head of the lateral pterygoid muscles. This activity is best demonstrated when the mouth is opened against resistance. When there is no resistance to opening, very little active muscle contraction is required to overcome the effect of muscle tonus in the elevator muscles. Closing the mouth is accomplished by contraction of the elevator muscles. Empty-mouth closure requires minimal muscular effort. Power strokes require strong contraction of elevator muscles, controlled by a holding action exerted by depressor and superior lateral pterygoid muscles. Protrusion and lateral excursion are executed by contraction of the inferior lateral pterygoid muscles bilaterally and unilaterally, respectively. Retrusion of the mandible from the forward translated position is accomplished by contraction of posterior fibers of the temporalis and deep portion of the masseter in conjunction with the mylohyoid and digastric muscles. With all such movements, the activators are resisted by antagonists that exert holding and controlling effects. Active movement, therefore, invokes muscle activity in antagonist muscles as well.

Mandibular movements are accomplished by the complex interaction of many muscles, the usefulness of which requires a high degree of muscular coordination. Jaw movements are learned over a considerable period of time. Unconscious mandibular activity is guided largely by preconditioned habit patterns that become deeply ingrained and tend to resist change. Volitional movements, however, easily override such habitual muscle action. The product of conscious voluntary mandibular movement may or may not conform to habitual chewing movements and, therefore, may or may not be compatible with normal joint functioning. The immediate guidance of muscle action on an automatic level is the product of afferent input from oral tissues, periodontal ligaments, articular ligaments, and the muscles themselves.

The final determinant of joint position is tooth form, the result of intercuspation of teeth. Normal functioning depends on a high degree of harmony between the forces imposed by the action of muscles and those of the occluded dentition.

Translatory Cycle

The translatory cycle utilizes both rotatory and translatory movement. It begins from a rest position that is determined by muscle tonus. The forward phase of the cycle consists of the disc-condyle complex moving downward and forward along the posterior slope of the articular eminence. It rounds the crest of the eminence and then moves forward along the articular plane that forms the anterior surface of the articular eminence. The return phase of the translatory cycle is a retracing of the disc-condyle complex back to rest position. The translatory cycle is similar, whether it occurs with protrusion, lateral excursion, or opening. The difference lies in the degree of rotation mixed with translation, and whether the cycle is bilateral or unilateral. When the translatory cycle is unilateral (as in the nonworking joint during a lateral excursion), the disc-condyle complex moves medially as it descends the articular eminence. This displaces the complex slightly in an inferior direction as the outer limit of lateral excursion is reached. Simultaneously, the opposite (working side) disc-condyle complex pivots until the inner horizontal portion of the temporomandibular ligament arrests further posterior movement of the lateral pole. From that point on, the disc-condyle complex rotates around a vertical axis that passes through the lateral pole rather than the center of the condyle. Ordinarily, the forces of tooth form initiated by intercuspation of teeth do not appreciably influence the translatory cycle during empty-mouth movements.

Power strokes alter the translatory cycle considerably in the return phase. Such cycle begins from rest position. It goes through the forward phase and begins the return phase, as described, until the bolus of food is encountered. As power is brought to bear on the food object, torquing of the mandible may take place. This alters the interarticular pressure in both joints. It continues to exert influence until the teeth penetrate the food object and come into full occlusion. Afferent input guidance changes during the power stroke as periodontal receptors are stimulated. The power stroke may end with maximum intercuspation, followed by relaxation of the musculature to the rest position. This brings into play the dominant positioning force of tooth form as maximum intercuspation is achieved. The dominating influence of tooth form ceases as biting is released and the muscles relax. The final determinant of joint position exerted by firmly occluded inclined planes of the teeth may or may not be compatible with the position established by muscle action alone.

It should be evident that the effect of the dentition on the translatory cycle occurs with power strokes. This stimulates the periodontal receptors, thus influencing muscle guidance. It initiates the element of tooth form—the final determinant of joint position as maximum intercuspation begins and ends. It should also be noted that empty-mouth clenching of teeth (bruxism), with or without movement, brings similar forces into play that have considerable influence on the temporomandibular joints and the musculature.

REFERENCES

1. Sicher H.: *Oral Anatomy*. St. Louis, C.V. Mosby Co., 1949.
2. Rees L.A.: The structure and function of the mandibular joint. *Br. Dent. J.* 96:125, 1954.
3. Blackwood H.J.J.: Pathology of the temporomandibular joint. *J. Am. Dent. Assoc.* 79:118, 1969.
4. Toller P.A.: Temporomandibular arthropathy. *Proc. R. Soc. Lond.* 67:153, 1974.
5. Furstman L.: Embryology, in Sarnat B.G., Laskin D.M. (eds.): *The Temporomandibular Joint*, ed. 3. Springfield, Ill., Charles C Thomas, Publisher, 1979, pp. 52–69.
6. Enlow D.H.: *Handbook of Facial Growth*, ed. 2. Philadelphia, W.B. Saunders Co., 1982.
7. Glineburg R.W., Laskin D.M., Blaustein D.I.: The effects of immobilization on the primate temporomandibular joint. *J. Oral Maxillofac. Surg.* 40:3, 1982.
8. DeBont L.G.M., Boering G., Havinga P., et al.: Spatial arrangement of collagen fibrils in the articular cartilage of the mandibular condyle: A light microscopic and scanning electron microscopic study. *J. Oral Maxillofac. Surg.* 42:306, 1984.
9. DuBrul E.L.: *Sicher's Oral Surgery*, ed. 7. St. Louis, C.V. Mosby Co., 1980.
10. Schwartz L. (ed.): *Diseases of the Temporomandibular Joint*. Philadelphia, W.B. Saunders Co., 1959.
11. Shore N.A.: *Occlusal Equilibration and Temporomandibular Joint Dysfunction*. Philadelphia, J.B. Lippincott, Co., 1959.
12. Farrar W.B.: Diagnosis and treatment of anterior dislocation of the articular disc. *New York Dent. J.* 41:348, 1971.
13. Gelb H. (ed.): *Clinical Management of Head, Neck, and TMJ Pain and Dysfunction*. Philadelphia, W.B. Saunders Co., 1977.

14. Dolwick M.F.: The temporomandibular joint, in Helms C.A., Katzberg R.W., Dolwick M.F. (eds.): *Internal Derangements of the Temporomandibular Joint.* San Francisco, University of California Press, 1983, pp. 1–14.
15. Toller P.A.: Opaque arthrography of the temporomandibular joint. *Int. J. Oral Surg.* 3:17, 1974.
16. Hellsing G., Holmlund A.: Development of anterior disk displacement in the temporomandibular joint: An autopsy study. *J. Prosthet. Dent.* 53:397–401, 1985.
17. Robinson M.: Temporomandibular joint: Theory of reflex controlled nonlever action of the mandible. *J. Am. Dent. Assoc.* 33:1260, 1946.
18. Garry J.F.: Early iatrogenic orofacial muscle, skeletal, and TMJ dysfunction, in Morgan D.H., House L.R., Hall W.P., et al. (eds.): *Diseases of the Temporomandibular Apparatus*, ed. 2. St. Louis, C.V. Mosby Co., 1982, pp. 35–69.
19. Miller C.W.: The temporomandibular joint. *J. Am. Dent. Assoc.* 44:386, 1952.
20. Ermshar C.B.: Anatomy and neurology, in Morgan D.H., House L.R., Hall W.P., et al. (eds.): *Diseases of the Temporomandibular Apparatus*, ed. 2. St. Louis, C.V. Mosby Co., 1982, pp. 8–25.
21. Mohl N.D.: Functional anatomy of the temporomandibular joint, in *The President's Conference on the Examination, Diagnosis and Management of Temporomandibular Disorders.* Chicago, American Dental Association, 1983, pp. 3–12.
22. Vamvas S.J.: Differential diagnosis of TMJ disease, in Morgan D.H., House L.R., Hall W.P., et al. (eds.): *Diseases of the Temporomandibular Apparatus*, ed. 2. St. Louis, C.V. Mosby Co., 1982, pp. 211–223.
23. Koole P., Beenhakker F., Brongersma T.J., et al.: Electromyography before and after treatment of TMJ dysfunction. *J. Craniomand. Pract.* 2:326, 1984.
24. McNamara J.A., Jr.: The independent function of the two heads of the lateral pterygoid muscle. *Am. J. Anat.* 138:197, 1973.
25. Mahan P.E., Wilkinson T.M., Gibbs C.H., et al.: Superior and inferior bellies of the lateral pterygoid muscle: EMG activity at basic jaw positions. *J. Prosthet. Dent.* 50:710, 1983.
26. Gibbs C.H., Mahan P.E., Wilkinson T.M., et al.: EMG activity of the superior belly of the lateral pterygoid muscle in relation to other jaw muscles. *J. Prosthet. Dent.* 51:691, 1984.
27. Guichet N.E.: Clinical management of occlusally related orofacial pain and TMJ dysfunction. *J. Craniomand. Pract.* 1(4):60, 1983.
28. Travell J.G., Simons D.G.: *Myofascial Pain and Dysfunction.* Baltimore, Williams & Wilkins Co., 1983.
29. Sicher H.: Positions and movements of the mandible. *J. Am. Dent. Assoc.* 48:620, 1954.
30. Thilander B.: Innervation of the temporomandibular joint capsule in man. *Trans. R. School Dent.* 7:1, 1961.

31. Kawamura Y.: Neurophysiology, in Sarnat B.G., Laskin D.M. (eds.): *The Temporomandibular Joint*, ed. 3. Springfield, Ill., Charles C Thomas, Publisher, 1979, pp. 114–126.

32. Griffin C.J., Harris R.: Innervation of the temporomandibular joint. *Aust. Dent. J.* 20:78, 1973.

33. Storey A.T.: Neurophysiological aspects of TM disorders, in *The President's Conference on the Examination, Diagnosis and Management of Temporomandibular Disorders*. Chicago, American Dental Association, 1983, pp. 17–23.

34. Moffett B.: Histologic aspects of temporomandibular joint derangements, in Moffett B.C. (ed.): *Diagnosis of Internal Derangements of the Temporomandibular Joint*, Vol. 1. Seattle, University of Washington, 1984, pp. 47–49.

35. Perry H.T., Xu Y., Forbes D.P.: The embryology of the temporomandibular joint. *J. Craniomand. Pract.* 3:126–132, 1985.

36. Mahan P.E.: The temporomandibular joint in function and pathofunction, in Solberg W.K., Clark G.T. (eds.): *Temporomandibular Joint Problems*. Chicago, Quintessence Publishing Co., 1980, pp. 33–47.

37. Krogh-Poulsen A.W., Moelhave A.: Om discus articularis temporomandibularis. *Tondlaegebladt* 61:265, 1957.

38. Moffett B.: Questions and answers, Session 2, in Moffett B.C. (ed.): *Diagnosis of Internal Derangements of the Temporomandibular Joint*, Vol. 1. Seattle, University of Washington, 1984, pp. 51–57.

39. Griffin C.J., Sharpe C.J.: The structure of the adult human temporomandibular meniscus. *Aust. Dent. J.* 5:190, 1960.

40. DuBrul E.L.: The biomechanics of the oral apparatus. Chapter 3. Structural analysis, in DuBrul E.L., Menekratis A.: *The Physiology of Oral Reconstruction*. Chicago, Quintessence Publishing Co., 1981, pp. 21–38.

41. DuBrul E.L.: The biomechanics of the oral apparatus. Chapter 4. Postures and movement, in DuBrul E.L., Menekratis A.: *The Physiology of Oral Reconstruction*. Chicago, Quintessence Publishing Co., 1981, pp. 39–53.

4
Masticatory Physiology

A good understanding of the normal functioning of the masticatory system is necessary for interpreting conditions that are abnormal and potentially symptomatic. Since mastication is a musculoskeletal activity, considerations of biology alone will not suffice. Mechanics are involved to which physical laws apply: force, resistance, movement, friction, pressure, torque, noise, gravity. Such mechanics involve biologic structures—biomechanics.

The biomechanics of mastication entail the forces of muscle action as affected by skeletal enertia and working resistance. Although the muscular and skeletal components of biomechanical action cannot be separated, for the sake of discussion, an arbitrary division of various factors of function is necessary.

Like other musculoskeletal systems, the masticatory apparatus must have the capability of remarkably varied function. From the inactive, resting state through nonstressed movements to biting against a resistant bolus of food, marked differences in biomechanical forces are encountered. A wide latitude of what constitutes normal response should moderate our concept of masticatory function. Rigidity in this respect may cause us to define as abnormal many borderline functions and thus create management problems that are not justified.

It should be understood that this system may be subject to momentary strains and abuses—excessive force, movement, or resistance—and in turn display momentary symptoms of dysfunction without there being any real damage to the structures or need for therapy. Examples of this are momentary pain, muscular incoordination, noise, or arrested movement as single, isolated symptoms when sudden, strained, or excessive functional demands are placed on the chewing apparatus.

One should be prepared to accept such isolated instances of dysfunction as falling within the range of normal. It is when such symptoms become repetitive or continuous, and particularly when symptoms occur in combinations, that investigative action is justified.

MUSCLE STRUCTURE AND FUNCTION

Muscle contraction is the source of power for all musculoskeletal functioning. The basic structure and innervation of muscles are established genetically; they are resistant to change.[1]

Stability, position, and movement are determined by the skeletal musculature, which is coordinated by efferent neural impulses from the CNS. Incoming information is supplied by a continuous inflow of monitoring afferent neural impulses from muscles and other peripheral structures. Understanding masticatory function requires some knowledge of muscle structure and behavior.

Muscles do not act singly. Useful muscle action is concerted and purposeful. Agonist muscles cooperate to perform an action; antagonist muscles act in opposition to agonist muscles and produce the control and graduated action necessary for useful movements. No specific function can be assigned to a single muscle without due consideration for the cooperative and opposing actions of other muscles.

Skeletal muscles are composed of many bundles (fasciculi) of fibers, each bundle containing a number of parallel fibers. A muscle fiber consists of sarcoplasm, which is composed of alternate light and dark portions that account for its striated appearance. Each fiber is made up of myofibrils.

The thicker myofibrils are composed chiefly of myosin, a protein (globin) that has enzymatic properties, acting as an adenosine triphosphatase. The thinner myofibrils contain actin. Together, these proteins are responsible for the contraction and relaxation of muscle tissue. Each fiber is surrounded by a delicate elastic sheath, called sarcolemma, which gives muscle tissue its elasticity.

The basic unit of the neuromuscular system is the *motor unit*, which consists of a single α motor neuron and a group of muscle fibers. The number of fibers contained within a motor unit relates to the complexity of the action involved: the more precise the movement required, the fewer the fibers per motor neuron.

Muscle fibers are classified as Type I and Type II. The Type I fibers contract slowly and resist fatigue. Type II fibers contract rapidly and are of two categories: Type IIA are fatigue resistant, while Type

IIB fibers fatigue quickly. Type I corresponds to the slow-oxidative (SO) fibers identified by histochemical analysis. Type IIA corresponds to the fast-oxidative glycolytic (FOG) fibers. Type IIB corresponds to the fast-contracting glycolytic (FG) fibers.[2] All the muscle fibers in a motor unit are of the same histochemical fiber type, but the distribution of these fibers may be scattered over a considerable volume of muscle tissue.[3] Motor units differ from each other not only in size but also in the biochemical and physiologic properties of their muscle fibers.

Masticatory muscles contain all three fiber types. The human masseter muscle consists of 50% to 60% FG fibers.[4-6] As such, it is capable of strong rapid contractions but tends to fatigue. The lateral pterygoid muscle consists of about 70% Type I slow-twitch fibers throughout.[7] As such, it tends to resist fatigue and, presumably, myospasticity as well.

Skeletal muscles that are capable of powerful contractive force, but fatigue readily, appear to contain a high percentage of fast-twitch fibers, while "holding muscles" display a high percentage of slow-twitch fibers.[2] Type I slow-twitch fibers are more sensitive to atrophic change.[6]

MUSCLE CONTRACTION

When stimulated by activity in the motor neuron, the fibers of a motor unit contract. When the stimulation ceases, the fibers relax. This operates on an all-or-none principle. Contractile activity results from active groups of muscle fibers intermingled with inactive groups throughout the muscle. The activity shifts from group to group so that alternating periods of activity and rest preclude the fatiguing of any particular group. The degree of contractile activity of a muscle depends on the relative number of muscle fibers active at a given time. Muscle fatigue results when the demand for contractile activity exceeds the capability of group interchange within the muscle.

Contractile activity may shorten the muscle under constant loading, thus inducing skeletal movement. Such contraction is termed *isotonic*. Contractile activity may increase tension within the muscle while maintaining a constant muscle length, thus producing a holding action. Such contraction is termed *isometric*. Both types of contractile activity may occur in the same muscle, giving it great versatility. Coordinated muscle action consists of various combinations of such contractile activity in agonist and antagonist muscle groups.

Contractile activity may occur reflexly in automatic response to stimulation of receptors within the muscle and its tendinous attachments. Such reflex activity is somewhat self-regulatory and subject to the influence of other sensory input and to stimulation from the CNS. Contractile activity may follow preconditioned habit patterns, some of which may be so deeply ingrained as to induce nearly automatic and unconscious behavior. Contractile activity may occur in response to volition, which usually is capable of overriding habitual muscular activity.

Muscle Tonus

Muscle tonus may be defined as the resistance of the muscle to elongation or stretch. *Hypertonicity* refers to a relative increase in passive resistance to stretching the muscle; *hypotonicity* refers to a decreased passive resistance to stretch. Muscle tonus is based primarily on the myotatic or stretch reflex, as far as active contraction of muscle fibers is concerned. The sum total of muscle tonus includes the effect of the elastic properties of muscle tissue itself.

Muscle tonus is somewhat self-regulatory, through the positive action of elongated muscle spindles that reflexly cause the muscle to contract. This relieves the tension on those spindles. It is subject to the adjusting effect of fusimotor activity, which increases spindle sensitivity to stretch by its shortening effect on the spindles. Muscle tonus is influenced by afferent input from other sensory receptors, such as those of the skin and mucosa, as well as by action of the CNS relative to systemic factors, both psychic and somatic. Such extraneous influence may be excitatory or inhibitory. Emotional tension increases muscle tonus.[8]

Muscle tonus serves two purposes: (1) it furnishes the muscular activity needed to maintain sharp contact of the articulating parts in joints when at rest or under negative interarticular pressure imposed by the effect of gravity; and (2) it maintains the muscles in an optimum state of readiness for contraction. The tonus of skeletal muscle is functionally adaptive to conditions that alter its resting length. Thus, an optimum resting length is maintained. Muscles are most efficient at generating force when they are at their physiologic resting length.[9] It has been shown that a marked increase in the vertical dimension of occlusion which would necessitate an increase in the resting length of the masticatory elevator muscles is readily adapted to. Thus, a new physiologic resting length for those muscles is established.[10]

Protective Muscle Splinting

When a muscle or other component of the musculoskeletal system is injured or threatened, as perceived by proprioceptive and sensory input from those and adjacent structures, protective muscle splinting may occur. This consists of increased tonicity of the musculature that has to do with movement of the threatened part, as if to stabilize it in space. Hypertonicity induces discomfort when the involved muscles are actively contracted, the resulting pain acting as an effective deterrent or inhibitory influence on such contractile efforts. This effect frequently is accompanied by a sensation of muscular weakness (pseudoparalysis), which reinforces the inhibitory influence on movement of the injured part. But no structural muscular dysfunction occurs.

Muscle splinting is considered to be a protective mechanism within the physiologic range of normal skeletal muscle behavior. It is induced involuntarily and is thought to be a response to altered environmental sensory and proprioceptive input. It is influenced by the reaction of the higher centers to painful stimuli and feelings of change, danger, or threat. The condition usually returns to normal as soon as the injury or threat disappears. Protracted muscle splinting may terminate as muscle spasm.

Involuntary Muscle Spasm

Muscle spasm is the involuntary contraction of a muscle or group of muscles that are functionally related. It is attended by interference with function and is manifested by involuntary rigidity, distortion, or movement. Clonic muscle spasm is of momentary duration; tonic spasm persists for a period of time. Cycling muscle spasm is protracted tonic spastic activity that becomes self-perpetuating. Isometric spasm causes muscular rigidity with marked resistance to stretch; isotonic spasm causes shortening of the muscle, which produces distortion or skeletal movement.

Clinical Significance

At a clinical level, masticatory muscle contractions may be divided into involuntary responses and working movements. Involuntary responses include (1) *muscle tonus,* which is the continued but variable degree of contraction of resting muscles that furnishes stability to the craniomandibular articulation as well as a position of physiologic rest for the mandible; (2) *muscle splinting,* which is a temporary state of hypertonicity induced as a protective mechanism to stabilize the threatened part in space and deter movement by pain inhibition and a feeling of weakness but which does not otherwise induce structural muscular dysfunction; and (3) *cycling muscle spasm,* which is a protracted self-perpetuating state of involuntary tonic contraction attended by structural muscular dysfunction, expressed as rigidity or shortening of the muscle. It should be noted that these clinical effects differ largely in the degree of involuntary contraction of the muscles and, therefore, may not be differentiated with precision.[11] But, since treatment differs considerably, they should be identified *if possible*.

The working contractions of masticatory muscles provide for (1) voluntary conscious mandibular movements, and (2) semiautomatic habitual chewing movements based on central patterns and influenced by proprioceptive and sensory feedback from the muscles, joints, periodontal ligaments, and soft oral tissues.

INNERVATION

Neural pathways subserving the masticatory musculature have to do with motor function. Each of the masticatory muscles receives branches from the mandibular division of the trigeminal nerve. The masseter is innervated by the masseteric nerve, the temporalis by three temporal nerves, the medial pterygoid by the medial pterygoid nerve, the lateral pterygoid by the lateral pterygoid nerve, the mylohyoid by the mylohyoid nerve, and the anterior belly of the digastric muscle by a branch from the mylohyoid nerve. It should be noted that sensory pathways are not described.

Several considerations relative to the sensory innervation of the musculature should be kept in mind. It has been known for a long time that noxious stimulation of spinal ventral roots causes pain felt diffusely in the muscles innervated by those fibers.[12] It has been established that about 27% of the nerve fiber population contained within the spinal ventral (motor) roots consists of very fine nonmyelinated nerves.[13] It is known that at least some sensory fibers are contained within the motor nerves, since some sensory innervation to the temporomandibular capsule is by way of the masseteric and temporal (motor) nerves.[14] It also is known that the nerve cell bodies of proprioceptive fibers of the trigeminal nerve are not located with those of other sensory fibers in the dorsal root (gasserian) ganglion but rather are found in the mesencephalic nucleus located in the midbrain.[15] This would indicate that the afferent fibers relaying trigeminal proprioception need not pass through the dorsal sensory root. It is known that these[16] and other sensory fibers[17] are contained within the motor root. Taken together, this evidence justifies the assumption that sensory innervation to the masticatory muscles is by way of motor nerves to those muscles and that at least some of that sensory input is conducted to the CNS by way of the trigeminal motor, rather than sensory, root. Thus, the sensibility of the masticatory musculature may remain even though the trigeminal dorsal root is interrupted.

REFLEX ACTIVITY

Some muscle activity occurs automatically through reflex acton. Other activity occurs in response to a proprioceptive and sensory feedback mechanism. Mandibular movements actively involve the muscle proprioceptors along with the inhibitory influences of stimulated mechanoreceptors of the TM joint ligaments and periodontal ligaments as well as of sensory receptors in the oral mucogingival tissues.

Myotatic (Stretch) Reflex

When a muscle is stretched, it automatically contracts. The receptors for this reflex mechanism are the *muscle spindles,* which are mechanoreceptors arranged in parallel with the muscle fibers. They respond to *passive stretch* of the muscle. They cease to discharge if the muscle contracts isotonically, the spindles signaling muscle length. The neural relay is a monosynaptic circuit composed of two neurons, an afferent arm synapsing directly with a motoneuron that connects back to motor endplates of the muscle where the spindles are located. There is a reciprocal neural circuitry by which other muscles are simultaneously affected, namely, stimulation of agonist muscles and inhibitory influence on antagonist muscles. The muscle spindles are sensitive not only to the structural length of muscle fibers but also to the rate of change of elongation as well. The sensitivity of the spindles to change is regulated by a biasing mechanism that establishes control over the effectiveness of myotatic reflex activity. Thus, one function of the muscle spindles is unconscious automatic control of muscular contractions during working movements and holding actions, according to the demands of function. They also serve to maintain stability of the parts at rest as an antigravity mechanism.

The myotatic reflex automatically operates when muscle stretch elongates the muscle spindles. This effect maintains sufficient muscle tonus to ensure continuous surface contact in synovial joints when the negative effect of gravity tends to separate them. With masticatory muscles, it is by the myotatic reflex that the weight of the mandible is overcome when the jaw is at rest. The stretching of elevator muscles due to mandibular weight would tend to separate the articulating parts of the temporomandibular joints. As the relaxed muscles stretch, the muscle spindles are elongated. As a result, the muscles contract until the tension of the spindles is equalized. The resulting increased tonicity in the elevator muscles maintains sharp contact of the articulating parts in the joints.

According to Kubota and Masegi,[18] the mandibular elevator muscles have significantly more muscle spindles than any other body muscle. The myotatic reflex not only maintains the passive interarticular pressure in the TM joints, but also is an important determinant of the mandibular rest position as it relates to the effect of weight of the part.

The myotatic reflex also influences muscle behavior during functional activities. This mechanism no doubt accounts for the *jaw-jerk reflex,* in which contraction of elevator muscles may be activated by downward tapping on the chin or the mandibular incisors or by tapping the point of insertion of the masseter muscle. It appears that such reflex activity may be influenced by associated sensory input from cutaneous, mucosal, and periodontal receptors.

It is important to know that myotatic reflex activity is absent in the lateral pterygoid and anterior digastric muscles. Presumably this is due to the dearth of spindles in those muscles.[19] It should be obvious that such activity would disrupt masticatory movements. Such activity would be greatest when the lateral pterygoid muscles are stretched in the act of achieving maximum intercuspation of the teeth—a critical moment in the chewing stroke when the smooth holding action of those muscles is of paramount importance. Reflex contraction of the muscle at that time would create conflictory forces completely disruptive to full occlusion of the teeth.

Nociceptive (Flexion) Reflex

When sudden, unexpected, *painful* stimulation of a part occurs, the muscles automatically react to cause withdrawal from the source of noxious input. This is called the nociceptive reflex. It is considered to be a protective mechanism to minimize injury. As related to the masticatory musculature, it accounts for the *jaw-opening reflex.* This is seen especially when one bites oneself or unexpectedly bites down hard on a rock; the jaws literally fly apart.

This reflex activity involves groups of muscles and is polysynaptic, the relay involving interneurons. In the jaw-opening reflex, active contraction of depressor and protractor muscles takes place with simultaneous relaxation of antagonist elevator muscles.

Since the nociceptive reflex is activated by painful stimulation, the receptor organs that initiate it no doubt are pain receptors. To what extent the receptors of the periodontal ligaments and the proprioceptors of the musculature and joints are involved is largely conjectural. It should be noted that this reflex is initiated by pain. For example, striking a hard object in chewing does not in itself induce a withdrawal jaw-opening reflex.[20] If pain occurs, the reflex takes place.

Inverse Stretch Reflex

When a muscle is stretched its full resting length, contraction ceases and the muscle relaxes fully. This response to *strong stretch* is known as the inverse stretch reflex. The receptors that initiate this activity are thought to be Golgi tendon organs, mechanoreceptors found in tendons of skeletal muscles arranged in series with the muscles. They are sensitive to mechanical distortion. Thus, they signal muscle tension and have inhibitory influence on muscle contraction.

The Golgi tendon organs likely play an important role in muscular activity as an inhibitory influence that helps to regulate contractile efforts of all types. Their activity influences, and is influenced by, the myotatic reflex mechanism. They no doubt have a role in coordinated muscle activity, as they are dominated not only by proprioceptive and sensory feedback mechanisms but by habitual and voluntary muscle action as well. Their protective effect to prevent injury as a result of hard muscular contraction is recognized. *The importance of this reflex in maintaining the normal resting length of skeletal muscles should be understood.*

Contracture of Elevator Muscles. The inverse stretch reflex causes a muscle to relax when it is elongated or stretched to its full length. If this normal physiologic maneuver is not permitted to take place occasionally, the muscle gradually shortens as its resting length decreases. The resulting contracture is called *myostatic contracture.*[21]

An occasional yawn activates such a mechanism in the elevator muscles and is needed to prevent their contracture, which would reduce mouth-opening capability. If some condition is imposed on the elevator muscles that prevents normal action of the inverse stretch reflex, the extent to which the mouth can be opened is jeopardized. This can occur as the result of such structural conditions as intraoral adhesions, periarticular restraint of opening, intracapsular adhesions, protracted locking of the articular disc, or other arthropathy that restricts mouth opening. It may result from the inhibitory effects of protracted pain, habitual voluntary restraint of opening, or unduly protracted intermaxillary fixation.

Anterior Drift of Edentulous Mandible.   Another instance of inverse stretch reflex has to do with the lateral pterygoid muscles. An inverse stretch mechanism in those muscles is stimulated when they are fully stretched. This occurs with maximum intercuspation of the teeth. Just as an occasional yawn is necessary to maintain the full resting length of elevator muscles and, therefore, prevent loss of the ability to open the mouth normally, so also is an occasional clenching of the teeth necessary to maintain the full resting length of the lateral pterygoid muscles. This ensures the physiologic rest position of the mandible. Clenching the teeth occasionally is not only a normal physiologic activity of the masticatory muscles, it is a necessary one.

It should be noted that the effectiveness of activating the inverse stretch reflex to maintain the resting length of the lateral pterygoid muscles depends on the presence of teeth that can be fully occluded. Edentulousness eliminates the stretching of these muscles, and the reflex mechanism cannot be activated in this condition. A denture does not necessarily reestablish the reflex mechanism because the stretching force may be dissipated by the resilience of the supporting soft tissues or by actual movement of the denture on its supporting base. This is particularly true when the alveolar ridges are atrophic. Thus, edentulousness may predispose to myostatic contracture of the lateral pterygoid muscles. Clinically this is recognized as a gradual progressive anterior drift of the mandible.

Palatal (Swallow) Reflex

Swallowing reflexly occurs when the palate is stimulated. This is known as the palatal or palatine reflex and occurs periodically under empty-mouth conditions as well as with eating. It may be induced voluntarily. This reflex is accompanied by closing the mouth, the so-called *jaw-closing reflex,* which can be induced independently by lightly stroking the tongue. These reflex activities appear to depend on superficial sensory receptors more than on muscle proprioceptors.

Pharyngeal (Gag) Reflex

Light touch or mild stimulation of the back of the pharynx may initiate a more or less convulsive contraction of the constrictor muscle of the pharynx. This is known as the pharyngeal reflex. It may also be induced by light stimulation of the palate, tongue, and other soft tissues in the posterior part of the mouth. Psychic stimuli may initiate the reflex, as well. These reflex activities appear to depend largely on sensory receptors. The masticatory musculature participates considerably in this reflex activity.

Inhibitory Effect of Periodontal Stimulation

The mechanoreceptors of periodontal ligaments, like proprioceptors in other joint ligaments, are inhibitory on the muscles that cross the joint—the mandibular elevators.[22] Stimulation of these receptors by tooth contact reflexly decreases elevator muscle action.[23, 24] This periodontal reflex is thought to be a protective mechanism to decrease impact damage to teeth during masticatory functon.[25]

Electromyographic (EMG) silent periods may be induced by pain and other oral sensations,[26] by tooth contact,[23] and during normal masticatory functioning.[27] An artificial masseteric EMG silent period can be induced by tapping the chin when the teeth are occluded. The duration of this masseteric EMG silent period is inversely related to the magnitude of biting force.[28] The wider the distribution of occlusal stress, the shorter the period. This is observed especially with occlusal splinting therapy for acute muscle disorders. Such splinting reduces the masseteric EMG silent period in masticatory pain-dysfunction patients, who reportedly have longer-than-normal such periods.[29, 30] It has been found to be shortened significantly when the number of biting contacts is increased.[31] This has been noticed following occlusal equilibration therapy. Conversely, the silent period was significantly increased in duration by experimental bruxism.[32]

Some effort has been made to utilize the masseteric EMG silent period as a diagnostic and monitoring aid in the management of patients with pain-dysfunction symptoms. It varies, however, from time to time and from patient to patient so that it has been difficult to arrive at a "normal" value.[28] Its clinical usefulness therefore has yet to be demonstrated.[33]

MANDIBULAR REST POSITION

The resting position of the mandible is determined by muscle tonus of the elevator muscles which, in turn, is determined by the myotatic reflex as it is affected by the weight of the mandible.[34] The EMG activity of the elevator muscles at rest represents the degree of contraction required to overcome gravity and maintain the sharp contact of the articulating surfaces of the TM joints. Ordinarily, rest position provides 1.3 to 3.0 mm of interocclusal clearance (freeway space).[35] The rest position is not coincident with the position of minimal EMG activity, which ranges from 4.5 to 12.6 mm of separation of the teeth.[35]

The mandibular rest position is not constant, as has been thought by many in the past. There exists no single, constant resting position of the mandible.[36] The notion that such a position persists as a reliable criterion for determining the proper vertical dimension of occlusion in edentulous mouths is not accurate.[37] The rest position changes with both head posture and muscle tonus. As the head posture shifts forward, the interocclusal clearance decreases.[38] It varies therefore with head position, total body posture, functional activities, fatigue, anticipation, time of day, age, and especially emotional tension.[39]

It has been thought by many that closure from rest position to occlusal position was a pure hinge movement, and therefore rest position was reliable as a means of obtaining the proper occlusal position by executing a simple hinge movement from it. Many years ago, Nevakari[40] demonstrated conclusively that the closing path was normally a continuation of translatory movement in most subjects, and rest position therefore was not reliable for finding the proper occlusal position. As the head posture shifts posteriorly, the anterior movement of the mandible through interocclusal clearance decreases.[38]

VERTICAL DIMENSION OF OCCLUSION

It has been thought that increasing the vertical dimension of occlusion (VDO) would cause increased activity in the elevator muscles, with pain and dysfunction resulting. It has been determined, however, that increasing VDO actually induces relaxation in most subjects.[37] This usually is evident with occlusal splinting therapy. Akagawa et al.[41] determined that increased VDO within interocclusal clearance displayed only transient acute inflammation in the deep and superficial masseter muscles, but no degenerative change. Increased VDO in excess of interocclusal clearance displayed a sequence of early acute inflammation to muscle fiber regeneration in the deep masseter, with a lesser degree occurring in the superficial masseter and anterior temporal muscles. No significant changes occurred in other masticatory muscles, except noninflammatory atrophy in the lateral pterygoid muscle. These effects have been interpreted as evidence of the inherent adaptability of the musculature to a new resting posture. Carlsson et al.[42] determined that

VDO can be altered considerably by using bite planes without seemingly affecting the resting muscle tonus of the mandibular muscles. Ramfjord and Blankenship[43] increased VDO in adult monkeys for periods ranging from 3 to 36 months, with the following results: (1) No pathologic changes in the TM joints occurred, (2) the teeth beneath the splint were intruded while the nonoccluding teeth were extruded, and (3) VDO gradually returned toward the pretreatment values. Manns et al.[44, 45] reported that elongation of the elevator muscles to near their point of least EMG activity (4+ mm) was effective in producing neuromuscular relaxation.

MANDIBULAR MOVEMENTS

Many years ago, anatomists, by employing principles of biomechanics, were able to discern the necessary actions of the various muscles that execute chewing movements. It is significant that all muscles that enter actively into mandibular functioning are innervated by the trigeminal nerve, the proprioceptors of which have their nerve cell bodies located in the mesencephalic nucleus of the midbrain, rather than in the gasserian ganglion, where the nerve cell bodies of other trigeminal sensory afferents are located. Although the principles of biomechanics have afforded considerable insight into the action of various muscles during mandibular movements, it remained for electromyographic studies to confirm and refine understanding in this respect.

As summarized by Hylander,[46] electromyographic studies have contributed much to the knowledge of masticatory muscle action during chewing strokes. It has become evident that the masseter and medial pterygoid muscles serve primarily as sources of power, while the temporalis and lateral pterygoid muscles are important for stability and control. At rest and during empty-mouth translatory cycles, sharp contact of the articulating parts of the temporomandibular joints is maintained by the posterior fibers of the temporalis muscles, which exert vertical traction on the condyles to press them firmly against the posterior slope of the articular eminences. As the mouth opens and the condyles slide forward, these fibers swing forward to an oblique angle, thus holding the condyles up against the slope of the eminences. As this effect diminishes, contraction of the inferior lateral pterygoid muscles continues to maintain sharp stabilizing contact of the articulating parts during the forward phase of the translatory cycle.[47]

Electromyographic studies have shown that during the forward phase of a translatory cycle for opening the mouth, activity occurs first in the mylohyoids and then the digastrics, as the mandible is moved inferiorly. Next, activity occurs in the inferior lateral pterygoid muscles, as the condyles are moved anteriorly. *The superior lateral pterygoid muscles remain inactive throughout the forward phase of the cycle and do not show appreciable activity unless a power stroke is exercised.* If the translatory cycle is for a unilateral chewing stroke (lateral excursion), the activity in the inferior lateral pterygoid muscle on the chewing side slightly precedes that of the opposite side, presumably to reinforce its vital function of maintaining adequate stability in the chewing joint preparatory to the power stroke that is to follow. Then activity occurs in the inferior lateral pterygoid on the nonworking side to move that condyle forward to accomplish a unilateral translatory cyclic movement.[46]

In the absence of a power stroke, the return phase of the translatory cycle is initiated by activity in the medial pterygoid muscles, followed by the masseters. There is little increased activity in the temporalis and lateral pterygoid muscles, which continue their function of maintaining joint stability.

If resistance is met during the return phase and a power stroke ensues, marked activity occurs in the medial pterygoid and masseter muscles as they execute strong elevator force on the mandible. This is accompanied by marked activity in the *superior* lateral pterygoid muscles as a holding action on the mandibular condyles. They simultaneously provide strong anterior traction on the articular discs. If the power stroke is for bilateral incising of a food object held in the hand and assisted by the hand pulling anteriorly on the object, considerable activity of the posterior and middle temporalis fibers in conjunction with medial pterygoid and masseter activity takes place, presumably to counter the extrinsic anterior pulling force on the mandible exerted by the hand. If the power stroke is for unilateral chewing, the return phase of the translatory cycle is initiated by activity in the medial pterygoid muscles while the mandible still is being moved ipsilaterally. Next, activity increases in the temporalis on the chewing side, presumably to reinforce stability preparatory to the power stroke to follow. Then, activity is increased in the elevator muscles bilaterally, with only minor activity in the lateral pterygoids. As the power stroke begins, marked activity occurs in the temporalis on the chewing side, followed immediately by maximum activity in the other elevator muscles bilaterally. This is accompanied by marked activity in the superior lateral pterygoid muscles, the activity being greater on the chewing side.[46]

The action of the lateral pterygoid muscle during masticatory movements should be well understood. It has been shown that the upper and lower heads function independently.[48, 49] Mahan et al.[50]

showed that the inferior lateral pterygoid muscle was electromyographically active during opening, protrusion, and contralateral (nonworking) excursion, especially against resistance, but remained only minimally active when clenching the teeth. The superior lateral pterygoid muscle was minimally active during protrusion, even against resistance, but strongly active during elevation of the mandible, return from lateral excursion, and especially with clenching. Gibbs et al.[51] pointed out that simultaneous isometric and isotonic muscle contraction commonly occurs in basic jaw movements to provide fine control, mandibular stability, and protection to the masticatory apparatus especially during rapid movements. DuBrul[39] stressed the need for maintaining firm contact between the articulating parts at all times by the musculature. All condylar excursions were guided exclusively by neuromuscular mechanisms. Bony contours, ligaments, and tooth contacts limited, rather than guided, the mandibular movements. Even the condylar position dictated by the occluded dentition when the teeth are firmly clenched is a mechanically imposed restriction of movement, not a form of guidance.

Clinical Significance

Most of the information gained from electromyographic studies only confirms what had previously been discerned as the necessary functioning of the masticatory muscles. It graphically indicates the marked difference between power strokes and empty-mouth movements. It shows the effect of prehensile incising and of unilateral chewing movements. The most significant information has to do with lateral pterygoid muscle action. The inferior heads, in conjunction with posterior temporalis fibers, furnish continuing stability to the craniomandibular articulation.[52] The inferior head protrudes the mandible and has much to do with executing the forward phase of the translatory cycle. The superior head furnishes anterior traction on the articular disc. This is accomplished by muscle tonus only, for this head shows no increased activity during the anterior movement of the condyle. It does not draw the disc forward along with the condyle during translatory movement. Rather, it functions in such a way as to permit quite separate action of the articular disc and condyle. It becomes active only during power strokes.

Active contraction of the superior lateral pterygoid muscle serves two functions: (1) it exerts strong holding action on the mandibular condyle, thus exercising control over the return movement of the disc-condyle complex during the power stroke;[50] and (2) it exerts strong anterior traction on the articular disc. This action takes place during the critical period when the width of the disc space is altered by the forces of the power stroke.

When the teeth are fully occluded, either at the completion of a power stroke or with empty-mouth clenching, strong positive anterior rotatory traction on the articular disc is present. This effect occurs in conjunction with elevator muscle action. At this time, the width of the articular disc space is minimal, and the articular disc is centered on the condyle with the thinnest portion interposed between condyle and articular eminence.

Following maximum intercuspation, the superior lateral pterygoid and elevator muscles relax. As the interarticular pressure decreases, the articular disc space widens slightly. The traction force on the disc returns to that of muscle tonus in the superior lateral pterygoid muscle as opposed by the relaxed (nonstretched) superior retrodiscal lamina. Thus, the predominant muscle effect rotates the articular disc anteriorly.

It should be appreciated that this precisely coordinated action, which takes place every time the teeth are firmly occluded, can be severely interfered with by such factors as incoordinated muscle action, spasticity of muscles that interferes with normal activity, occlusal disharmony that sets up conflictory forces, and edentulousness.

ARTICULAR DISC MOVEMENTS

Muscle action influences articular disc movements. During gross mandibular movements, rotation of the condyles in the discs (to separate the jaws) and rotation of the discs on the condyles (to maintain surface-to-surface contact between the discs and articular eminences during translatory movements) result from muscle action as affected by disc contour. It is also by muscle action that the articular disc spaces are kept filled as the width changes owing to fluctuation in interarticular pressure.

The superior lateral pterygoid muscle attaches anteromedially to the articular disc. The effect of muscle tonus exerts sufficient rotatory force to keep the disc in the most anterior position permitted by the width of the articular disc space. This force is opposed by the superior retrodiscal lamina, the effect of which exceeds that of muscle tonus through the forward phase of the translatory cycle and rotates the disc posteriorly. In this way, the disc is protected against spontaneous anterior dislocation at the critical time when the translatory cycle shifts to the return phase.

During power strokes, a change in the width of the articular disc space occurs as a result of altered interarticular pressure. As the elevator muscles contract to execute the biting stroke, simultaneous contraction of the superior lateral pterygoid muscle takes place. This rotates the disc anteriorly, thus keeping the disc space filled, regardless of its width. This effect continues throughout the power stroke and maximum intercuspation.

The effect of muscle action on articular disc function may be summarized as follows:

1. During rest and empty-mouth translatory cycles, it maintains constant anterior traction on the articular disc as countered by the posterior tractive force of the superior retrodiscal lamina. This action of muscle tonus ensures the forward rotatory position of the disc in the resting posture of the joint without interfering with the necessary posterior tractive force of the superior retrodiscal lamina during the forward movement of the condyle.

2. During power strokes and maximum intercuspation, it provides strong anterior traction on the articular disc to overcome the posterior tractive force of the stretched superior retrodiscal lamina, thus maintaining satisfactory joint stability when the disc space varies in width due to the changing interarticular pressures induced by the forces of mastication.

BIOMECHANICS

The biomechanics of the TM joint are determined by the morphology and structural arrangement of its parts (Fig 4–1) as they relate to the demands of function. The craniomandibular articulation should be visualized as two hinge joints suspended by strong temporomandibular ligaments. Each of the hinge joints is capable of a linear sliding movement down and around the articular eminence. This can take place symmetrically, as with protrusion and mouth opening, or asymmetrically, as with lateral excursions. Since the articular discs take part in both rotatory and translatory movements, they play the dominant role. The discs are the key to stability in this articulation.[53]

INTERARTICULAR PRESSURE

The interarticular pressure in the TM joint, as in other synovial joints, varies considerably during the normal functioning of the mandible.

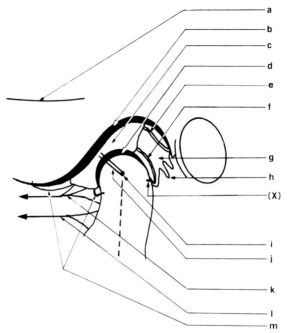

FIGURE 4–1   Schematic drawing illustrates essential structures that constitute the functioning temporomandibular joint; *a,* supra-articular crest; *b,* temporal articular surface, composed of nonvascular fibrous tissue; *c,* articular disc; *d,* condylar articular surface, composed of nonvascular fibrous tissue; *e,* superior retrodiscal lamina (elastic); *f,* inferior retrodiscal lamina (collagenous); *g,* retrodiscal loose connective tissue; *h,* posterior capsular ligament (collagenous); *i,* condylar axis of rotation; *j,* discal collateral ligament (collagenous); *k,* superior lateral pterygoid muscle; *l,* inferior lateral pterygoid muscle; *m,* anterior capsular ligament (collagenous); *x,* posterior margin of condylar articular facet. Note that the inclination of the articular eminence is about 52 degrees from the horizontal supra-articular crest.

The pressure remains relatively constant during nonstressed, empty-mouth movements. The width of the articular disc space, being related to interarticular pressure, also remains relatively constant. But, the demands of function bring on wide fluctuations in interarticular pressure, and with it variations also in the width of the disc space. Such variation seriously threatens joint stability by permitting separation of the articulating parts. This is in addition to the already very unstable condition produced by the extensive forward translatory movements of the disc-condyle complexes.

Biting against resistance during a power stroke, which occurs during the forward unstable phase of translation, induces a variety of torque forces in the mandible that are transmitted to the TM joints. This alters the active interarticular pressure in the joints. The pressure in the chewing-side joint decreases, at times even becoming negative with perceptible widening of the disc space, while pressure in the non-working joint increases (Fig 4–2).[46] Walker[54] has shown that the mandible functions as a loaded beam during asymmetric biting. The axis of the beam runs obliquely between the occlusal bite point on the working

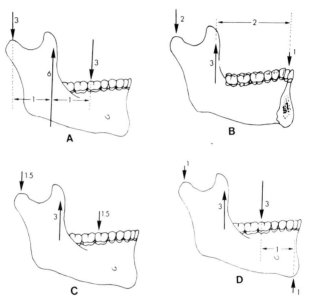

FIGURE 4–2 Biomechanics of the mandible in the lateral projection. *A,* no distinction is made between forces on the ipsilateral and contralateral sides. The perpendicular distance between the resultant muscle force and the bite force is 1 unit. The perpendicular distance between the resultant muscle force and the condylar reaction force is also 1 unit. Six units of muscle force yield 3 units of both bite force and condylar force. *B,* forces acting on the contralateral side of the mandible. The muscle force on the contralateral side is divided into condylar reaction force and a force that is transmitted to the ipsilateral side through the mandibular symphysis. The distance between the contralateral resultant muscle force and the symphysis is 2 units. Three units of muscle force yield 2 units of condylar reaction force and 1 unit of force transmitted through the symphysis. *C,* forces acting on the ipsilateral side without consideration of the force being transmitted through the symphysis from the contralateral side. The 3 units of resultant muscle force are divided equally between the bite force and the condylar reaction force. *D,* forces acting on the ipsilateral side. The distance between the force acting through the symphysis and the bite force is 1 unit. The 3 units of muscle force on the ipsilateral side and the 1 unit of force acting through the symphysis yield 1 unit of reaction force and 3 units of bite force. (From Hylander W.L., in Sarnat B.G., Laskin D.M. (eds.): *The Temporomandibular Joint,* ed. 3. Springfield, Ill., Charles C Thomas, Publisher, 1979. Reproduced with permission.)

side and the opposite nonworking condyle. If the muscle action vectors are posterior to this axis, the working condyle remains somewhat loaded. But, if the muscle action vectors lie anterior to it, the working condyle becomes completely unloaded. Thus, when unilateral biting takes place on the third molar tooth, an extremely unstable and threatening condition in the joint is induced at the moment when joint stability is needed most. Without adequate provision for this biomechanical crisis, dislocation would be imminent.[53] The widening of the disc space under these conditions has been observed radiographically.[55]

Unilateral biting forward to the third molar does not completely unload the working joint, but torque forces reduce the interarticular pressure in the working joint, and greater pressure is sustained by the nonworking joint.[46] This unequal distribution of stress alters disc-space width accordingly and produces a serious instability problem. Hylander[56] has shown that the working condyle becomes unloaded when unilateral biting is on the third molar while it remains loaded when occlusal force is generated on the first two molars or bicuspids.

Gibbs et al.[57] have measured the interdental clenching force at from 55 to 280 lbs, of which about 36% is utilized as chewing force while as much as 41% may be used with swallowing solid foods. Forces developed in eccentric contact of the teeth were relatively low. Denture wearers were able to exert only about 15% of the force delivered by dentate patients.[58] Considerably more biting force occurs in the posterior mouth than anteriorly because of the shorter resistance arm; the graded decrease in the size of the occlusal surfaces anteriorly compensates for the lengthening resistance arm.[59]

The direct and torquing forces that affect the TM joints during mastication are great and highly variable, which make for instability. To this is added the inherent instability entailed in the extensive translatory movement during which most chewing is done. The need for the continuing sharp contact of the articulating surfaces is extremely high and critical to prevent joint dislocation. The TM joints have a unique arrangement for providing the necessary stability with the articular discs playing the key role. This mechanism should be well understood.[53]

EMPTY-MOUTH MOVEMENTS

Most functioning of the craniomandibular articulation occurs with minimal muscular activity. Consequently, interarticular pressure remains constant. Active contraction of the various muscles is limited to that required for mandibular movement in the absence of resistance and stress. Power strokes and maximum intercuspation do not enter the picture. Such functioning is referred to as *empty-mouth movements.*

The dentition has little, if any, influence on such movements under normal circumstances because the teeth are not occluded firmly. Any contact of the teeth is very light and does not tend to alter the positioning force of muscle action. Unless solid food is being ingested, swallowing usually does not bring into play the effect of firmly articulated inclined planes of teeth.[60] Only empty-mouth clenching of the teeth initiates the determinant positioning force exerted by tooth form. Although occasional clenching of the teeth is normal, just as is occasional yawning, clenching in excess of that needed to maintain the resting length of the lateral pterygoid muscles constitutes bruxism.

Since empty-mouth functioning involves neither power strokes nor maximum intercuspation, articular disc movement is needed chiefly to facilitate two biomechanical functions, namely, separation of the jaws and translation of the condyle.

To Separate the Jaws

Separation of the chewing frames that support the teeth is accomplished by rotation of the condyles *in the articular discs.* The relative movement in the disc-condyle complex is that of rotation of the disc posteriorly on the condyle (Fig 4–3). The limit of such rotation is the posterior border of the condylar articular facet—a limit that seldom is reached in the absence of translation of the condyle. Pure rotatory

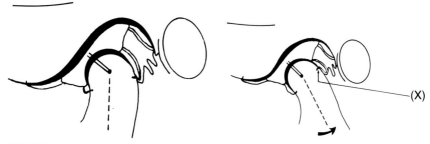

FIGURE 4–3   Effect of separating the jaws on movement within the disc-condyle complex. *Left,* resting closed position of the joint. *Right,* rotation of the condyle in the articular disc to separate the jaws. Note that the relationship between disc and eminence does not change. Rotation of the condyle moves the posterior margin of the condylar articular facet *(x)* closer to the posterior edge of the articular disc. This amounts to posterior rotatory movement in the disc-condyle complex.

opening does not occur frequently, unless volition is involved. It has been established that some degree of translation almost invariably occurs when the jaws are separated.[40]

To Translate the Condyle

Most movements of the mandible involve part of the translatory cycle in addition to separation of the jaws. Normal functioning is a combination of both factors. The translatory cycle movements within the joint are much the same whether due to opening, protrusion, or lateral excursion. Straight-line opening and straight-line protrusion produce nearly identical and bilaterally symmetric translatory cyclic movements in the joint. Deviated or deflected movements produce compensatory asymmetry of movement. Lateral excursion produces maximum asymmetry: the disc-condyle complex on the working side pivots, while that on the nonworking side translates. The translating disc-condyle complex during lateral excursion moves slightly medially as it descends the articular eminence. This difference is not grossly significant except that it restrains somewhat the extent of anterior movement in the forward phase of the translatory cycle. This observation is readily apparent radiographically; the normal extent of forward movement of the condyle in lateral excursion is invariably *less* than in opening or protrusion (Fig 4–4).

As the forward phase of the cycle takes place, the upper surface of the articular disc slides down the articular eminence, rounds the crest, and moves forward along its anterior plane. During the return phase

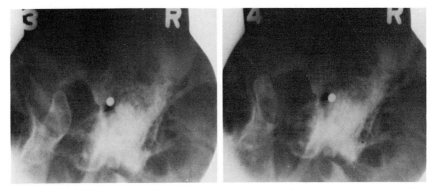

FIGURE 4–4 Transparietal radiographs of temporomandibular joint in lateral position *(left)* and open position *(right)*. Note that in lateral position the condyle moves to the crest of the articular eminence. In open position it moves well beyond the crest, a considerably greater distance than in lateral position. This is a normal movement pattern.

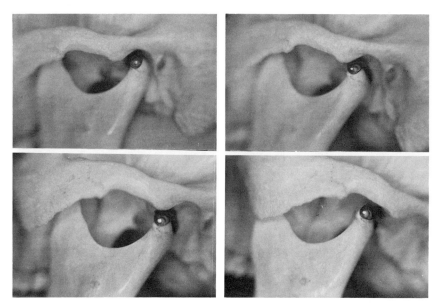

FIGURE 4–5 Photographs of dry skull with a simulated articular disc hinged on condyle to illustrate posterior rotation of the articular disc on the condyle during forward translatory movement of the disc-condyle complex (opening movement). *Top left,* joint in resting closed position. *Top right,* condyle moved halfway toward crest of eminence. *Bottom left,* condyle at crest of articular eminence. *Bottom right,* condyle at full forward translatory position. Note that as condyle moves anteriorly, the articular disc rotates posteriorly on the condyle. Owing to this rotatory movement, during forward translation the articular disc moves a shorter distance than the condyle.

of the cycle, the upper surface of the disc retraces the sliding movement back to the resting or lightly occluded position.

If the upper articular facet were entirely flat, so that sliding between the disc-condyle complex and temporal bone were straight, the sliding movement between the two articulating surfaces would be a simple bodily movement: the disc and condyle would move in unison and in the same amount. This, however, is not the case. First, the articular eminence slopes downward, then it levels at the crest, followed by a slightly upward sloping of the anterior surface of the eminence. In order for the upper surface of the disc-condyle complex to maintain full surface contact with the temporal articular facet, *the disc must rotate anteroposteriorly on the condyle.*

It will be seen, therefore, that the disc rotates posteriorly on the condyle as the disc-condyle complex moves forward in relationship to the articular eminence. This posterior rotation continues as the crest is reached and is greatest as the forward phase of the cycle is completed (Fig 4–5). This maneuver causes the bodily forward movement of the articular disc to be considerably less than that of the condyle. This observation has been erroneously interpreted as evidence of a sliding movement between the condyle and disc—a condition rendered anatomically impossible by the discal collateral ligaments as long as they remain functional. During the return phase, the disc rotates anteriorly until the cycle is completed, thus returning the disc-condyle complex back to the resting or lightly occluded position. *It should be noted that the greater the inclination of the articular eminence, the greater the amount of posterior rotation of the articular disc on the condyle* (Fig 4–6).

An important key to the amount of rotation of the disc during the translatory cycle is the inclination and total height of the articular eminence. The greater the inclination and height of the articular eminence, the greater the demand for the rotation of the disc to accomplish smooth, silent, unobstructed translatory movements. *An extreme inclination and height of the eminence predispose to disc interference problems, and once these problems come into existence, the effects of inclination and height are augmented.* Accurate knowledge of the inclination and height of the eminence, therefore, is important in evaluating function and dysfunction of the joints.

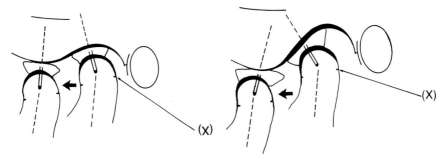

FIGURE 4–6 Effect of inclination of articular eminence on amount of rotation of the articular disc during forward translatory movement. *Left,* inclination of articular eminence about 28 degrees from horizontal supra-articular crest. *Right,* inclination of articular eminence about 52 degrees from horizontal supra-articular crest. Note that as disc-condyle complex moves forward (as in a protrusive movement), the articular disc rotates posteriorly on the condyle. By comparing the movement of the posterior edge of the articular disc toward the posterior margin of the condylar articular facet *(x),* note that the amount of such rotation in the 28-degree joint is considerably less than in the 52-degree joint. The steeper the inclination of the articular eminence, the greater the rotatory movement in the disc-condyle complex during translatory movements.

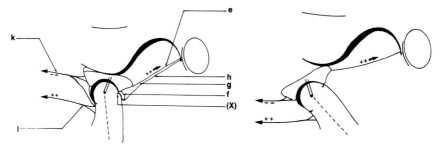

FIGURE 4–7 Comparison of maximum normal forward translatory movement and subluxation of disc-condyle complex. *Left,* maximum normal forward translatory movement (*e,* superior retrodiscal lamina; *f,* inferior retrodiscal lamina; *g,* retrodiscal loose connective tissue; *h,* posterior capsular ligament; *k,* superior lateral pterygoid muscle; *l,* inferior lateral pterygoid muscle; *x,* posterior margin of condylar articular facet). Maximum normal forward translatory movement is reached when articular disc is rotated posteriorly until its edge reaches the posterior margin of the condylar articular facet *(x),* thus arresting further rotatory movement of the disc on the condyle. In this position the dominant traction force on the articular disc is in a posterior direction due to the fully stretched superior retrodiscal lamina *(e)* against the inactive relaxed superior lateral pterygoid muscle *(k).* The dominant traction force on the condyle is in an anterior direction, owing to the actively contracted inferior lateral pterygoid muscle *(l)* against the taut posterior capsular ligament *(h). Right,* subluxated disc-condyle complex. Opening beyond the maximum normal forward translatory movement causes the disc-condyle complex to rotate on itself because of the restraining effect of the posterior capsular ligament and arrested rotatory movement in the complex. As a result, the disc-condyle complex skids bodily along the articular eminence in a rough, noisy, jerking movement.

During protrusion and lateral excursion, when separation of the jaws is minimal, the total rotation of disc on condyle is only that required to maintain surface contact between the sliding parts. Normal opening of the mouth entails, in addition, a large component of rotation sufficient to achieve full separation of the jaws. As already mentioned, rotation for both purposes is *in the same posterior direction,* relative to disc-condyle position. With a wide opening, therefore, the limit of posterior rotation of the disc may be reached, this being determined by the posterior border of the condylar articular facet. Once this limit is reached, further rotation of the disc on the condyle is impossible. An overextended opening of the mouth can move the disc-condyle complex forward beyond this point, but such a movement must take place without benefit of the articular disc rotation that is essential to surface-to-surface contact of the articular parts. Since the disc cannot rotate farther, continued movement of the complex forward causes it to skid bodily along the upper articular surface (Fig 4–7).

Pivoting of the Condyle

During a lateral excursion, the disc-condyle complex pivots on the working side, while translating on the nonworking side. The pivoting movement takes place between the upper surface of the disc and the temporal articular facet. Initially, the vertical axis of rotation passes through the center of the condyle. But, as the lateral pole rotates posteriorly, it becomes restrained by the inner horizontal fibers of the temporomandibular ligament. This shifts the vertical axis of rotation outward to the lateral pole of the pivoting condyle.[52] Normally this trochoid movement meets no resistance or interference during empty-mouth movements because of the low interarticular pressure.

Joint Stability

Although disc contour is the guiding force that positions the articular disc on the condyle as determined by passive interarticular pressure and disc-space width, joint stability is provided by the independent anteroposterior movements of the articular disc itself.[53] The anterior tractive force on the disc comes from the superior lateral pterygoid muscle, the posterior force from the elastic superior retrodiscal lamina. These linear forces are converted into rotatory sliding action by the contour of the disc as confined in the articular disc space. At rest and as translation begins, the anterior traction provided by muscle tonus of the superior lateral pterygoid muscle is dominant, because the retrodiscal lamina is relaxed and exerts no elastic traction on the disc. Soon, however, as the condyle moves forward, the elastic traction that occurs from the stretching of the lamina equals the muscle tonus effect. From that point forward, the lamina produces the dominant tractive force in a posterior direction. Therefore, at rest the disc is always in its most forward rotatory position permitted by the width of the disc space. This continues until the posterior tractive force takes over.

During forward translation and the critical turn-around phase, the disc is firmly rotated posteriorly as far as the width of the disc space permits by the fully stretched superior retrodiscal lamina. This tractive force provides increasing stability as the condyle moves forward. It is greatest in the full-forward position, and provides maximum stability to the joint when the danger of spontaneous anterior dislocation is greatest. At that point the pressure on the articulating parts to keep them in sharp contact is considerably greater than that provided by muscle tonus in the resting joint. In this way adequate joint stability is assured during the entire translatory cycle, regardless of minor variations in pressure and disc-space width. This remarkable mechanism in the TM joint should be understood and appreciated. The critical importance of disc contour in the functioning of this essential mechanism should also be appreciated.

STRESSED MOVEMENTS

When the masticatory muscles force the mandibular teeth against resistance, as happens in prehension, incising, and grinding, the biomechanics of the temporomandibular joint change. The conditions that affect articular disc function are different from those that exist during empty-mouth movements. Human activities have imposed many nonmasticatory functions upon the jaws and teeth. However, the jaws and teeth appear to behave in much the same way, although the time element may be different. Holding a pipe between the teeth simulates biting against any hard object, except that it is a prolonged activity.

Power Strokes

A complete power stroke differs from an empty-mouth translatory cycle in two ways: (1) at some point during the return phase of the cycle, resistance is met and continues to some extent for the remainder of the return phase; and (2) the cycle may terminate in maximum intercuspation of the teeth instead of in the resting position or in light occlusal contact.

The effects of biting against resistance do not involve tooth form as such, but the added sensory input from stimulated periodontal receptors may modify the guidance of muscle action in directing the chewing stroke to completion.

The particular point in the return phase at which the biomechanical factors change is determined by how far the jaws are separated when the object is engaged. This relates to the size of the object grasped and where it is located in the mouth. The continuance of such factors through the return phase of the translatory cycle depends on the intent of the effort (whether to hold, crack, bite through, incise, or grind) as well as the ability of the apparatus to accomplish such an intent. The flexion or nociceptive reflex helps protect components of the system from injury: sudden, unexpected, painful encounters of the teeth cause immediate arrest of activity in the power muscles with simultaneous contraction of antagonists.

Several factors influence the biomechanical change that occurs during a power stroke. These factors include the size and consistency of the object of resistance, the intent behind the stroke, the speed of the stroke, the distance between the object and the joint (the load moment), and the torquing effect of unilateral biting stress.

From radiographic evidence, it is known that biting hard against resistance in the third molar area causes perceptible widening of the articular disc space on the biting side. This widening continues in a diminishing way until the object is penetrated and the teeth come into full occlusion.[55] In order to prevent separation and, therefore, disarticulation of the parts, biomechanical requirements demand that continuing firm contact be maintained during this period of instability. As described by Sicher, sharp contact of the articulating surfaces results from the contraction of the superior lateral pterygoid muscle, which exerts strong holding action on the condylar neck to control the movement of the disc-condyle complex during the return phase of the power stroke and *strong anterior traction on the articular disc itself,* thus firmly rotating a thicker portion of disc into the widened articular disc space. This particular muscular activity has been confirmed electromyographically.[48, 49]

Unilateral biting on food that is forward of the third molar also causes alterations in pressure in the TM joints. Although both joints remain loaded, they are not equally so.[46] Loading changes the width of the disc space. Bilateral chewing and incising cause myriad changes in interarticular pressure with resultant variations in disc-space width. Full intercuspation loads both joints at maximum pressure with minimal width of the disc space, the articular discs being centered with the thinnest central portions between the osseous parts of the joints.

To maintain adequate stability during all the changes induced by masticatory function, the contraction of the superior lateral pterygoid muscle in conjunction with elevator muscle activity is essential. Thus, active muscle power delivers the anterior force necessary to ensure the continuous firm contact of the articulating parts during extreme variations in pressure and resultant changes in the disc-space width. A critical issue in the stabilizing mechanism of the craniomandibular articulation is the *normal contour* of the articular discs. If loss of contour permits sliding movement, stabilization cannot be maintained.

Maximum Intercuspation

When the teeth are firmly clenched in maximum intercuspation, both joints are fully loaded,[59] the disc space is of minimal width, and the articular disc is centered with its thinnest central portion interposed between the condyle and articular eminence. Following maximum intercuspation, the muscles relax, thus decreasing the interarticular pressure and proportionately increasing the width of the articular disc space. As the disc space widens slightly, the forward pull of the superior lateral pterygoid muscle (due to muscle tonus) rotates the disc anteriorly to bring a slightly thicker portion of disc firmly into the space.

When the teeth come into maximum intercuspation, the occlusion becomes a force that must be taken into account. If the condylar position dictated by the dentition is identical to that already imposed by muscle action, then only increased interarticular pressure is present, because no movement is involved. The joints ordinarily sustain such pressure very well, and no damage results. But, if the dentition-dictated position of the condyle varies from that imposed by muscle action, movement of the condyle takes place, and such movement is under increasing interarticular pressure. As the articular disc moves under pressure against the temporal articular facet, and, if weeping lubrication is exhausted, frictional abuse may predispose to damage. Once the disc becomes firmly anchored by the effect of friction, further movement forced by the dentition tends to displace the disc, thus placing considerable strain on the discal collateral ligaments. Movement under such conditions may cause injury, the severity of which depends on such factors as the force and extent of movement, the direction, the frequency and duration of such movement, and the structural form of the components involved. The damage thus sustained may cause deterioration and elongation of the discal collateral ligaments and loss of contour of the articular disc.

Bruxism

Bruxism is another situation in which stressed movement influences articular disc function. Normally, the teeth are brought into full occlusion only momentarily during chewing strokes or when the teeth are occasionally clenched.[60] Even when some occlusal disharmony is present, the joints ordinarily are able to tolerate such demands of function without sustaining appreciable damage. But, if the teeth are clenched frequently or for long periods, various muscle effects and deleterious changes may result. If gross occlusal disharmony is present, the danger increases materially. The same may be said for habitual biting and chewing with excessive force.

CLINICAL SIGNIFICANCE OF MASTICATORY PHYSIOLOGY

When viewed grossly, as, for example, radiographically, it would *appear* that, with the opening and closing of the mouth, the condyle simply rotates to separate the jaws and slides forward on the temporal bone. With protrusion, the condyle *appears* to rotate only very slightly but slides boldly forward on the temporal bone. Lateral excursion *appears* to move similarly, except unilaterally. Such visualization of temporomandibular movements would be accurate, if the condyle articulated with the temporal bone with an interposed meniscus. This, however, is not the case—the articular disc is not a meniscus.

The gross movement of the osseous parts (as viewed radiographically) *constitutes only a portion of the intricate movements that take place in the temporomandibular joint during normal functioning.* Two distinct types of rotatory movement take place, namely, rotation of the *condyle in the articular disc* and rotation of the *disc on the condyle*. Separation of the jaws calls for rotation of the condyle in the disc. As this rotation takes place, the posterior border of the condylar articular facet comes closer to the posterior edge of the articular disc. In relationship to the disc-condyle complex, the articular disc rotates *posteriorly*. In order to maintain continuous surface contact of the sliding parts during translatory movement forward, the articular disc rotates on the condyle: the steeper and higher the eminence, the greater the amount of rotation. This rotation also brings the posterior border of the condylar articular facet closer to the posterior border of the disc. In relationship to the disc-condyle complex, the disc rotates *posteriorly*. The more the condyle is moved anteriorly, the greater the rotation of the disc on the condyle. The limit of normal translation of the condyle is reached when the posterior edge of the articular disc comes in contact with the posterior border of the condylar articular facet. Protrusion and lateral excursion require only minimal rotation of the condyle in the disc but maximal rotation of the disc on the condyle. Normal opening, however, requires much of both types of rotatory movement.

A more important requirement for the rotation of the articular disc on the condyle has to do with variation in interarticular pressure in response to masticatory stresses. As pressure decreases and the articular disc space widens, the articular disc is rotated forward to fill it with a thicker portion of disc and, thus, maintain sharp contact of the articulating parts. Conversely, when the interarticular pressure increases perceptibly and the articular disc space decreases in width, the self-centering contour of the disc causes it to rotate posteriorly, leaving a thinner portion of disc in the space. The limit of this particular movement is reached when the disc is completely centered with its thinnest portion interposed between the condyle and temporal bone. The increased demands for rotation of the disc on the condyle occur during power strokes and maximum intercuspation of the teeth.

Disc-Condyle Position

In addition to disc contour, which prevents sliding movement between the articular disc and the condyle, two *active forces* relative to disc-condyle position are present, namely, the anterior traction exerted by the superior lateral pterygoid muscle and the posterior traction exerted by the elasticity of the superior retrodiscal lamina. In the resting position, the muscular pull is dominant so that at rest, the disc is rotated anteriorly as far as the width of the articular disc space permits. In forward translation the extended superior retrodiscal lamina is dominant, thus causing the articular disc to occupy the most posterior rotatory position on the condyle permitted by the width of the articular disc space. The superior lateral pterygoid muscle remains inactive during the forward phase of the translatory cycle, as well as during the critical shift from forward movement to the return phase. Thus, stability is ensured during this critical turn-around period by the maintenance of sharp contact between the articulating parts. Being firmly rotated posteriorly, the disc resists spontaneous anterior dislocation. If the superior lateral pterygoid muscle should contract prematurely at this critical time, the articular disc would be rotated anteriorly, and dislocation could result. *The primary function of the superior retrodiscal lamina is to resist spontaneous dislocation of the articular disc at the most forward point of the translatory cycle.* This condition prevails until the disc-condyle complex has begun its return phase. Then, the shift in dominance of force gradually changes back to that of the muscle, thus ensuring that the disc at rest occupies its most anterior position on the condyle permitted by the articular disc space. In this way, the stability of the joint is maintained during the complete translatory cycle by continuous sharp contact of the articulating parts.

During a power stroke, which *begins well after the extreme forward point of translation has been reached and the disc-condyle complex is safely on its return phase,* marked changes in interarticular pressure occur, which in turn alter the width of the disc space. As the elevator muscles contract to execute the power stroke, contraction of the superior lateral pterygoid muscle takes place and exerts strong holding action on the mandibular condyle. The separate attachment of this muscle to the articular disc immediately overcomes the effect of the stretched superior retrodiscal lamina and rotates the articular disc anteriorly. In this way stability of the joint is maintained by sharp contact of the articulating surfaces.

The contraction of the superior lateral pterygoid muscle continues throughout the remainder of the power stroke. It is especially active when the teeth are firmly brought into maximum intercuspation. At that time, interarticular pressure is greatest, and the articular disc space is thinnest. The articular disc is centered on the condyle, with the thinnest portion interposed between the condyle and articular eminence. With the disc thus firmly wedged between the osseous surfaces and with the superior lateral pterygoid muscle strongly contracted, *joint stability is maximal just as occlusion of the teeth takes place.* Then, as the elevator and superior lateral pterygoid muscles relax and the mandible assumes a position of rest, a state of muscular equilibrium represented by muscle tonus prevails.

With the normal relaxation of the elevator and lateral pterygoid muscles following maximum intercuspation, the resting condition of the joint is re-established. With decrease in interarticular pressure, slight widening of the articular disc space takes place. The superior lateral pterygoid muscle rotates the articular disc anteriorly as muscle tonus exceeds the traction of the relaxed superior retrodiscal lamina. As this occurs, synovial fluid penetrates the articulating surfaces, and the joint is lubricated and made ready for the next movement.

In the presence of anteroposterior traction forces exerted on the articular disc, the determinant of position between disc and condyle at any given time is the *disc contour* relative to the *width of the disc space* as determined by joint pressure. The anterior and posterior traction forces on the disc are needed to maintain continuous sharp contact of the articulating parts under all conditions of joint use.

REMODELING

Like other synovial joints, the TM joints have the propensity to adjust the shape of the osseous articular surfaces according to the demands of function—providing the requirement for change is not too great or too rapid. The TM joint normally bears the main load in its lateral part as identified by the concentration of proteoglycans in the surface layers of articular tissue.[61] Increased biomechanical loading stimulates cellular proliferation from the deeper undifferentiated mesenchymal layer that constitutes the proliferative zone.[62–64] The articular disc does not participate in the remodeling process; deterioration or loss of contour results instead.[65] The condylar and temporal surfaces, however, may undergo both progressive and regressive remodeling, providing the loading does not become excessive and the limit of weeping lubrication is not exceeded. The condylar and temporal articular surfaces of the TM joints are even capable of considerable regeneration following injury or degenerative change, if the etiologic factors are eliminated and functional conditions are favorable.

REQUIREMENTS FOR NORMAL DISC FUNCTION

In order for articular disc movements to remain free from interference, several conditions should prevail:

1. The articular surfaces should be smooth, rounded, structurally compatible in shape, and adequately lubricated.

2. Movements of the right and left joints should be reasonably symmetric.

3. Sliding movement between articulating surfaces should not take place when interarticular pressure is sufficient to cause friction.

4. Except in very flat joints, no appreciable movement between the unclenched and clenched occluded-joint positions should occur as maximum intercuspation takes place.

5. Precise coordination of muscle action should prevail at all times.

6. Joint function should be habitually restrained within its structural capability.

REFERENCES

1. Perry H.T., Harris S.C.: Role of the neuromuscular system in functional activity of the mandible. *J. Am. Dent. Assoc.* 48:665, 1954.
2. Taylor A., Cody F.W., Bosley M.A.: Histochemical and mechanical properties of the jaw muscles of the cat. *Exp. Neurol.* 38:99–109, 1973.
3. Edstrom L., Kugelberg E.: Histochemical composition, distribution of fibers and fatigability of single motor units. *J. Neurol. Neurosurg. Psychiatry* 31:424–433, 1968.
4. Gonyea W.J., Thockmorton G.S., Finn R.A., et al.: Masticatory muscles in

dentofacial deformities, in Bell W.H. (ed.): *Surgical Correction of Dentofacial Deformities*, Vol. III. Philadelphia, W.B. Saunders Co., 1985, pp. 227–258.

5. Boyd S.B., Gonyea W.J., Finn R.A., et al.: Histochemical study of the masseter muscle in patients with vertical maxillary excess. *J. Oral Maxillofac. Surg.* 42:75, 1984.
6. Throckmorton G.S., Johnston C.P., Gonyea W.J., et al.: A preliminary study of biomechanical changes produced by orthognathic surgery. *J. Prosthet. Dent.* 51:252, 1984.
7. Eriksson P.-O.: Muscle-fiber composition of the human mandibular locomotor system. *Swed. Dent. J.* (Suppl.) 12, 1982.
8. Yemm R., Berry D.C.: Passive control in mandibular rest position. *J. Prosthet. Dent.* 22:30–36, 1969.
9. Manns A., Miralles R., Palazzi C.: EMG bite force and elongation of the masseter muscle under isometric voluntary contractions and variations of vertical dimension. *J. Prosthet. Dent.* 42:674–682, 1979.
10. Hellsing G.: Functional adaptation to changes in vertical dimension. *J. Prosthet. Dent.* 52:867–870, 1984.
11. Bell W.E.: *Orofacial Pains*, ed. 3. Chicago, Year Book Medical Publishers, 1985.
12. Cailliet R.: *Neck and Arm Pain*. Philadelphia, F.A. Davis Co., 1964.
13. Coggeshall R.E., Applebaum M.L., Fazen M., et al.: Unmyelinated axons in human ventral roots, a possible explanation for the failure of dorsal rhizotomy to relieve pain. *Brain* 98:157, 1975.
14. Thilander B.: Innervation of the temporomandibular joint capsule in man. *Trans. R. School Dent.* 7:1, 1961.
15. Sicher H.: *Oral Anatomy*, ed. 3. St. Louis, C.V. Mosby Co., 1960.
16. McIntyre A.K.: Afferent limb of the myotatic reflex arc. *Nature* 168:168, 1951.
17. Hosobuchi Y.: The majority of unmyelinated afferent axons in human ventral roots probably conduct pain. *Pain* 8:167, 1980.
18. Kubota K., Masegi T.: Muscle spindle supply to human jaw muscle. *J. Dent. Res.* 56L:901, 1977.
19. Mohl N.D.: Neuromuscular mechanisms in mandibular function. *Dent. Clin. North Am.* 22:63–71, 1978.
20. Gibbs C.H., Suit S.R.: Movements of the jaw after unexpected contact with a hard object. *J. Dent. Res.* 52:810, 1973.
21. Bechtol C.O.: Muscle physiology, in The American Academy of Orthopedic Surgeons: *International Course Lectures*, Vol. 5. St. Louis, C.V. Mosby Co., 1948, Chapter 11.
22. Willis R.D., DiCosimo C.J.: The absence of proprioceptive nerve endings in the human periodontal ligament: The role of periodontal mechanoreceptors in the reflex control of mastication. *Oral Surg.* 48:108, 1979.
23. Hannam A.G., Matthews B., Yemm R.: Receptors involved in the response of the masseter muscle in tooth contact in man. *Arch. Oral Biol.* 15:17, 1970.

24. Sessle B.J., Schmitt A.: Effects of controlled tooth stimulation on jaw muscle activity in man. *Arch. Oral Biol.* 17:1587, 1972.
25. Ahlgren J.: The silent period in the EMG of the jaw muscles during mastication and its relationship to tooth contact. *Acta Odontol. Scand.* 27:219, 1969.
26. De Boever J.A.: Functional disturbances of the temporomandibular joint, in Zarb G.A., Carlsson G.E. (eds.): *Temporomandibular Joint Function and Dysfunction.* Copenhagen, Munksgaard, 1979, pp. 193–214.
27. Stohler C.S., Ash M.M. Jr.: Silent period in jaw elevator muscle activity during mastication. *J. Prosthet. Dent.* 52:729–735, 1985.
28. Lung D.T., Hwang J.C., Poon W.F.: Effect of bite force on the masseteric electromyographic silent period in man. *Arch. Oral Biol.* 27:577, 1982.
29. Bessette R., Bishop B., Mohl N.: Duration of masseteric silent period in patients with TMJ syndrome. *J. Appl. Physiol.* 30:864, 1971.
30. Bessette R.W., Mohl N.D., DiCosimo C.J. II: Comparison of results of electromyographic and radiographic examinations in patients with myofascial pain-dysfunction syndrome. *J. Am. Dent. Assoc.* 89:1358, 1974.
31. Kohno S., Freesmeyer W.B., Lindemann W.: Die veranderung der "silent period" bei wiedenholten schnellen Bewegungen in die maximale Interkuspidation. *Dtsch. Zahnarztl. Z.* Z38:560, 1983.
32. Cox P.J., Al-Khateeb T.L., Rothwell P.S., et al.: The measurement of masseteric silent periods after experimental tooth grinding. *J. Oral Rehabil.* 9:487, 1982.
33. Hellsing G., Klineberg L.: The masseter muscle: The silent period and its clinical implications. *J. Prosthet. Dent.* 49:106, 1983.
34. McNamara J.A.: Electromyography of the mandibular postural position in the rhesus monkey (Macaca mulatta). *J. Dent. Res.* 53:945, 1974.
35. Rugh J.D., Drago C.J.: Vertical dimension: A study of clinical rest position and jaw muscle activity. *J. Prosthet. Dent.* 45:670–675, 1981.
36. Bando E., Fukushima S., Kawabata H., et al.: Continuous observation of mandibular positions by telemetry. *J. Prosthet. Dent.* 28:285–290, 1972.
37. Rugh J.D., Johnson R.W.: Vertical dimension discrepancies and masticatory pain/dysfunction, in Solberg W.K., Clark G.T. (eds.): *Abnormal Jaw Mechanics.* Chicago, Quintessence Publishing Co., 1984, pp. 117–139.
38. Goldstein D.F., Kraus S.L., Williams W.B. et al.: Influence of cervical posture on mandibular movement. *J. Prosthet. Dent.* 52:421–426, 1984.
39. DuBrul E.L.: The biomechanics of the oral apparatus. Chapter IV. Postures and movement, in DuBrul E.L., Menekratis A.: *The Physiology of Reconstruction.* Chicago, Quintessence Publishing Co., 1981, pp. 39–53.
40. Nevakari K.: An analysis of the mandibular movement from rest to occlusal position. *Acta Odontol. Scand.* 14 (Suppl. 19):1, 1956.
41. Akagawa Y., Nikai H., Tsuru H.: Histologic changes in rat masticatory muscles subsequent to experimental increase of the occlusal vertical dimension. *J. Prosthet. Dent.* 50:725, 1983.
42. Carlsson G.E., Ingervall B., Kocak G.: Effect of increasing vertical dimen-

sion on the masticatory system in subjects with natural teeth. *J. Prosthet. Dent.* 41:284, 1979.

43. Ramfjord S.P., Blankenship J.R.: Increased occlusal vertical dimension in adult monkeys. *J. Prosthet. Dent.* 45:74, 1981.

44. Manns A., Miralles R., Santander H., et al.: Influence of the vertical dimension in the treatment of myofascial pain-dysfunction syndrome. *J. Prosthet. Dent.* 50:700, 1983.

45. Manns A., Miralles R., Cumsille F.: Influence of vertical dimension on masseter muscle electromyographic activity in patients with mandibular dysfunction. *J. Prosthet. Dent.* 53:243–247, 1985.

46. Hylander W.L.: Functional anatomy, in Sarnat B.G., Laskin D.M. (eds.): *The Temporomandibular Joint,* ed. 3. Springfield, Ill., Charles C Thomas, Publisher, 1979, pp. 85–113.

47. DuBrul E.L.: Origin and adaptations of the hominid jaw joint, in Sarnat B.G., Laskin D.M. (eds.): *The Temporomandibular Joint,* ed. 3. Springfield, Ill., Charles C Thomas, Publisher, 1979, pp. 5–34.

48. McNamara J.A. Jr.: The independent functions of the two heads of the lateral pterygoid muscle. *Am. J. Anat.* 138:197, 1973.

49. Lipke D.P., Gay T., Gross B.D., et al.: An electromyographic study of the human lateral pterygoid muscle. *J. Dent. Res.* 56B:230, 1977.

50. Mahan P.E., Wilkinson T.M., Gibbs C.H., et al.: Superior and inferior bellies of the lateral pterygoid muscle EMG activity of basic jaw positions. *J. Prosthet. Dent.* 50:710, 1983.

51. Gibbs C.H., Mahan P.E., Wilkinson T.M., et al.: EMG activity of the superior belly of the lateral pterygoid muscle in relation to other jaw muscles. *J. Prosthet. Dent.* 51:691, 1984.

52. DuBrul E.L.: *Sicher's Oral Anatomy,* ed. 7. St. Louis, C.V. Mosby Co., 1980.

53. Bell W.E.: Understanding temporomandibular biomechanics. *J. Craniomand. Pract.* 1(2):27, 1983.

54. Walker A.: Functional anatomy of oral tissues: Mastication and deglutition, in Shaw J.H., Sweeney E.A., Cappuccino C.C., Moller S.M. (eds.): *Textbook of Oral Biology.* St. Louis, C.V. Mosby Co., 1978, Chap. 8.

55. Scully J.J.: *Cinefluorographic Studies of the Masticatory Movements of the Human Mandible.* Thesis, University of Illinois, 1959.

56. Hylander W.L.: An experimental analysis of temporomandibular joint reaction force in Macaques. *Am. J. Phys. Anthropol.* 51:433, 1979.

57. Gibbs C.H., Mahan P.E., Lundeen H.C., et al.: Occlusal forces during chewing and swallowing as measured by sound transmission. *J. Prosthet. Dent.* 46:443, 1981.

58. Brudevold F.: A basic study of the chewing forces of a denture wearer. *J. Am. Dent. Assoc.* 43:45, 1951.

59. DuBrul E.L.: The biomechanics of the oral apparatus. Chapter III. Structural analysis, in DuBrul E.L., Menekratis A.: *The Physiology of Oral Reconstruction.* Chicago, Quintessence Publishing Co., 1981, pp. 21–38.

60. Dubner R., Sessle B.J., Storey A.T.: *The Neural Basis of Oral and Facial Function.* New York, Plenum Publishing Corp., 1978.
61. Kopp S.: Topographical distribution of sulphated glycoaminoglycans in the surface layers of the human temporomandibular joint. *J. Oral Pathol.* 7:283, 1978.
62. Blackwood H.J.J.: Pathology of the temporomandibular joint. *J. Am. Dent. Assoc.* 79:118, 1969.
63. Hansson T., Oberg T., Carlsson G.E., et al.: Thickness of the soft tissue layers and the articular disc in the temporomandibular joint. *Acta Odontol. Scand.* 35:77, 1977.
64. Carlsson G.E., Kopp S., Oberg T.: Arthritis and allied diseases of the temporomandibular joint, in Zarb G.A., Carlsson G.E. (eds.): *Temporomandibular Joint Function and Dysfunction.* Copenhagen, Munksgaard, 1979.
65. Moffett B.: Histologic aspects of temporomandibular joint derangements, in Moffett B.C. (ed.): *Diagnosis of Internal Derangements of the Temporomandibular Joint,* Vol. 1. Seattle, University of Washington, 1984, pp. 47–49.

5 | Symptoms of Masticatory Disorders

Effective management of a temporomandibular complaint rests on a knowledge of the individual patient's masticatory system. It matters little how the average craniomandibular articulation functions or what constitutes departure from normal for temporomandibular joints in general. Standards of normal should be derived and applied on an individual basis.

In order to establish a basis for judgment, it is important that we understand the functioning of the masticatory system in a way that allows for individual variations from average. Too rigid a concept of what constitutes normal should be avoided. Standards that are ideal should give way to standards that reflect considerable latitude in normal functioning of the masticatory system. Concepts of anatomical relationships without concern for their functional compatibility are neither useful nor practical.

CONCEPTS OF NORMAL

Since there is such a wide variation in morphology, in functional capability, and in musculoskeletal demands placed upon the individual masticatory apparatus, the *absence of symptoms,* rather than the presence of certain positive characteristics, should constitute the basis for judging whether the TM joints and masticatory musculature under consideration are within "normal" limits. This concept requires precision in defining masticatory symptoms.

To be considered "normal," the craniomandibular articulation (joints and muscles) should present the following features:

1. Freedom from pain or other discomfort that arises in and emanates from the TM joints or the muscles of mastication

100

2. Mandibular movements that are adequate in amplitude, that are reasonably symmetrical bilaterally, and that are not deflected during ordinary use

3. Freedom from sensations, noises, or altered movements that would indicate interference or obstruction during ordinary use

4. Freedom from acute malocclusion of the teeth that would indicate a recent symptomatic change in jaw relationship due either to a shortened muscle(s) or to change within the joint(s) proper

Joint Morphology

Early in his tomographic investigations, Ricketts[1] identified marked structural variations in nonsymptomatic TM joints. He noted variations in size and contour, in condyle-fossa relationship, in jaw movement, and in the extent of translatory movement of the disc-condyle complex. Enlow[2] pointed out that the condyle conforms to, rather than leads, growth movements of the mandibular ramus, which is a compensatory structure in face development. Care therefore should be exercised in interpreting the static radiographic appearance of the condyle without taking into consideration the growth processes that are under way or that have gone on before.

Condylar Concentricity

A judgment of abnormality of condylar position is sometimes rendered from the lack of radiographic concentricity of the condyle in the articular fossa. The variability of this relationship, however, is such that the usefulness of the method should be questioned. Dumas et al.[3] showed that in nonsymptomatic individuals with Class I occlusions the anterior joint space varied in width from 1.06 to 3.16 mm, the superior from 2.30 to 5.04 mm, and the posterior from 1.11 to 5.09 mm. Furthermore, bilateral asymmetry was the rule rather than the exception. Weinberg[4] reported that in 61 nonsymptomatic patients examined by transcranial radiography only 23% had bilateral, concentrically placed condyles, while 36% had "retruded" condyles on one or both sides. Blaschke and Blaschke[5] examined 50 nonsymptomatic patients using the tomographic method and found the range of "protruded" to "retruded" condyles to be wide, with very little correlation bilaterally. Rey and Valero[6] found no significant difference between diagnosed TM dysfunction patients and nonsymptomatic subjects. Katzberg et al.[7] reported that arthrograms of patients with clinically diagnosed protracted functional dislocation of the articular disc indicated no correlation to structural concentricity of the condyle within the fossa. Aquilino et al.[8] examined a dry skull using three different standard transcranial techniques. He found that the true anatomical position of the condyle in the glenoid fossa could not be accurately determined from the resulting radiographs. Pullinger et al.[9] did a well-controlled tomographic study of nonsymptomatic and occlusally untreated young adults and found that radiographic variability of condylar concentricity was such that it could not serve as a sole means of judging normality. They found that nonconcentricity in male patients was predominantly anterior, while that of female patients was posterior.

The proper conclusion that should be drawn from these studies is that the radiographic lack of condylar concentricity in itself is not sufficient to make a diagnosis of a TM disorder, much less a specific diagnosis of "anterior disc displacement."

Occluded Position of the Condyle

Variability of Rest Position.   A possible correlation between the resting and occlusal positions of the mandible and TM disorders has provoked considerable discussion in the past. Presently, it appears to be rather generally agreed that the rest position is too variable to be used as a means of judging normalcy. Not only does it change as muscle tonus changes, but head and body posture also cause immediate and marked alterations in the resting position of the mandible. Tilting the head forward or backward as little as 10 degrees alters rest position.[10] Rocabado et al.[11] found that 70% of patients with Class II malocclusions displayed a forward head position. Mohl[12] reported that even habitual patterns of closure and occlusal positions were altered by posture. Hairston and Blanton[13] determined that as the body reclines the EMG activity in protruder muscles increases so as to overcome the effect of gravity and, thus, prevent mandibular retrusion from becoming a threat to the airway. It is very likely that the forward head position displayed by many Class II malocclusion patients may be to avoid encroachment on the airway.

Variability of Tooth Contact.   It is now rather generally agreed that the path of mandibular closure from rest to occlusal position is not a pure hinge movement. In 1952 Alexander[14] found that this pathway could be either rotatory or translatory. In 1956 Nevakari[15] showed conclusively that the path of closure from rest to occlusal position for most people was a translatory movement of up to 1 mm. Jemt[16] reported that the mandibular position during chewing was frequently different from that assumed when swallowing solid foods, the chewing position being anterior to that of swallowing. He considered the occlusal position during chewing to be a three-dimensional zone rather than a single position. Faulkner and Atkinson[17] showed that initial tooth contact occurred in a small, well-defined area from which the mandible slid into full occlusion. They determined that "tapping" the teeth together did not make contact directly to the position of maximum occlusion. By using the Case Gnathic Replicator, Suit et al.[18] showed that all subjects displayed variable amounts of sliding in both opening and closing movements.

The conclusions that may be drawn from these reports is that the masticatory system has a compensating mechanism by which elevation of the mandible from a highly variable resting position is accomplished without incident. There is no rigid resting position, no rigid path of closure, no rigid point of initial tooth contact. Since the position of maximum intercuspation must remain fixed due to interlocking planes of implanted teeth, the flexibility of occlusal function to compensate for constantly changing postural influences on the mandibular position is mandatory—or else "normal occlusion" of the teeth would be possible in only one rigidly fixed postural attitude of the head. This, of course, is unthinkable. Variability in tooth contact that induces a slight sliding movement between the teeth as occlusal position is accomplished does much to improve masticatory efficiency, especially in grinding movements. It also reduces the chance of damage to the articular surfaces of the joints, because moving compressive force is better tolerated than static overloading. Occlusal facets that are indicative of such sliding movements should not be looked upon as evidence of abnormality or occlusal disharmony.

Balancing Contacts. Although it is generally agreed that there should be no nonworking-side tooth contacts during mastication with the natural dentition,[19] a recent EMG study of 10 nonsymptomatic subjects indicated that such contacts do occur frequently and with no apparent detrimental effects.[20]

Centric Relations Position. The use of centric relations position of the mandible for orientation purposes in occlusal therapy is well established. DuBrul[21] verified that the limit of posterior displacement of the mandible is determined by the length of the fully tensed inner horizontal portion of the temporomandibular ligament. This makes the position one that is reproducible. It is also defined as a marginal border position. Sicher[22] stated that although joints are capable of functioning from marginal border positions, they ordinarily do not do so. Even though some subjects no doubt appear to function normally at hinge axis closure,[23] it seems now to be rather generally agreed that the functional occlusal position for most people is anterior to centric relations— usually from 0.2 to 0.5 mm.[19]

Although there are advocates for the concept that the radiographic condylar position is dependable and useful in the diagnosis and treatment of TM disorders,[24, 25] the use of radiographs to establish a condylar treatment position should be discouraged because of obvious structural and functional variability.[9, 26, 27]

Too narrow and rigid a concept of what constitutes normal masticatory structure and function can lead to problems. The joints display great variability in morphology and functional behavior. Compensatory mechanisms allow for variance in functional demands as well as in continually changing head posture. As long as nutritional and lubricative capabilities of the joint are not impaired or exceeded, they do quite well. An understanding of weeping lubrication is essential to appreciating the true effect of the dentition on the craniomandibular articulation. The relationship between the dentition and the rest of the masticatory system needs to be better understood.

The conclusion that should be reached, therefore, is that occlusal function is considerably more flexible than usually defined. Concepts of TM dysfunction based on slight discrepancies in occlusal function are not justified and may be misleading. Likewise, therapeutic efforts based on the correction of such discrepancies have little rational basis. Although occlusal interference does excite muscular responses, the effect is inhibitory on elevator muscle action, not excitatory. Thus, muscle splinting may result when such effects are recent and acute, while altered patterns of muscle action may result when such effects are of long standing. Joint damage per se, however, does not occur. Occlusal function that is potentially damaging to the articular surfaces pertains to overloading, which entails the effects of maximum intercuspation. Damage sustained by the articular surfaces of the joint results from stress that exceeds the limits of weeping lubrication to maintain friction-free movements or from static overloading. Both conditions require the action of elevator muscles and relate therefore to the fully occluded position of the joint. Muscle effects may occur as a result of interference during dynamic occlusal function; structural joint damage results from static overloading or from intolerable movement induced by occlusal disharmony as maximum intercuspation is attained.

With a broader concept of "normal" structure and function, symptomatology becomes the key to judgment. An understanding of symptoms forms the foundation for diagnosis and treatment of TM disorders. For it is by symptoms that we recognize what is wrong with the masticatory system.

INCIDENCE OF SYMPTOMS

The prevalence of TM disorders in the general population is still a moot question. Many studies have been reported in recent years which supply some information, but firm conclusions cannot be drawn, largely because of lack of definition of what constitutes a true TM disorder or what symptoms are truly indicative of masticatory dysfunction. For example, one study included such symptoms as headache, face pain, ear pain, neck pain, and tinnitus—regardless of any established relationship to a TM disorder.[28] Agerberg and Carlsson[29] reported at 39% the incidence of noise with mandibular movement without qualifying the type of noise or the conditions that prevailed at the time. At least three studies[29-31] have indicated that the incidence of TM dysfunction did not significantly correlate to either the sex or the age of subjects, while the experience of clinicians is that women present with masticatory complaints at a significantly higher rate than men. Frequently, reports are based on questionnaires or other subjective evidence, or on the listing of symptoms without any objective controls to establish relevancy. For example, "restricted opening" based on some arbitrarily measured "norm" is meaningless without establishing what should be proper for that individual; the complaint of pain without establishing its true source has little relevance to masticatory problems. One report that indicated the prevalence of mandibular dysfunction at about 87% was based on the presence of one or more symptoms from a list that included such nebulous conditions as difficulty in opening, pain or soreness about the face, relative fatigue of masticatory muscles, bruxism, chronic headache, and chronic neckache.[32]

Although autopsy studies[33-38] have yielded valuable information concerning static structural changes that have occurred in the TM joints, it is well known that valid conclusions relative to musculoskeletal function cannot be drawn from cadaver material. Ascertaining whether cadaver findings truly reflect a clinical TM disorder requires considerable supporting evidence that usually is not available. It is interesting to note that autopsy studies have placed the incidence of anterior disc displacement in young adults at about 7%.[34] It is not known, of course, how many of them were symptomatic at a clinical level. In a histopathologic autopsy study of 23 elderly individuals, Castelli et al.[35] found 5 to have normal TM joints. Rohlin et al.[36] correlated TM disc sounds with joint morphology in 55 autopsy specimens. He found over half to be silent, although several anterior disc displacements were present. They did correlate discrete clicking noise with disc interference and grating noise with degenerated articular surfaces. In contrast, Hellsing and Holmlund[37] did careful autopsy studies on 115 TM joints. They found gross anterior disc displacement as well as perforation of the retrodiscal tissue to be quite rare. They concluded that minor anterior positioning of the articular disc may well be a normal variant of TM structure.

In a study of 739 college students, Solberg et al.[39] found that 26% said they had symptoms of mandibular dysfunction, but only half of the complainants considered them to be troublesome. In a group of 1,000 general dentistry patients, about 34% had joint noise or interference.[40] In another study of 324 students, 33% displayed clicking in one or both joints.[41] Farrar and McCarty[42] reported that of all their patients with TM disorders, about 70% had some form or degree of anterior disc displacement. In a study of 103 randomly selected dental clinic patients, Greene et al.[43] found that about 32% were aware of masticatory symptoms, but only about 10% displayed symptoms that were compatible with a clinical TM disorder. Westesson[44] reported that he found the evidence of adult articular disc displacement to be in the range of 56%, while Solberg et al.,[45] in a recent report of autopsy studies on young adults, found the incidence of disc displacement to be only 11.6%. Marciani et al.[46] found that in 536 elderly patients only 4.4% complained of TM pain, and only about half of those displayed joint noise.

Solberg[47] made a comprehensive review of the epidemiology, incidence, and prevalence of TM disorders which included an extensive bibliography. This should be consulted for further information.

Greene and Marbach[48] have raised several questions that affect the validity of some epidemiologic studies of mandibular dysfunction. Better definition and controls are needed before firm conclusions can be drawn from any of them. Currently, it appears that although a large segment of the population (perhaps 25% or more) may have some awareness of masticatory symptoms, probably no more than 10% actually have a condition that warrants investigation. Of these, women no doubt predominate.

STRUCTURAL HARMONY

Morphologic variation in temporomandibular joints is normal. Condyles and articular eminences vary in size and shape. This is true also of the location of the condyle within the articular fossa. Considerable variation in gross condylar position may be observed in joints that fulfill the criteria of known standards of normal. The important issue is not *morphology* so much as *compatibility* of the parts with each other. This can be summarized as follows:

1. Each temporomandibular joint should present articular surfaces that are compatible in size and shape so that they work in harmony with each other.

2. The two joints should be reasonably compatible with each other bilaterally.

3. The joints should be structurally compatible with the oral structures, particularly the dentition.

Inclination of the Articular Eminence

The most significant structural variant has to do with the inclination of the posterior slope of the articular eminence.[49] Most joints have an inclination of 30 to 60 degrees from the Frankfort horizontal. Those with inclinations of considerably less are referred to as *flat joints* (Fig 5–1). Those with considerably steeper articular eminences are referred to as *steep joints* (Fig 5–2).

The inclination of the articular eminence relates importantly to disc-condyle complex functioning during translatory movements. Since rotation of the disc on the condyle is necessary to maintain surface-to-surface contact between the disc-condyle complex and the articular eminence during translatory cycles, the flatter the joint, the less the amount of such rotation required. Conversely, the steeper the articular eminence, the greater the rotation of the disc during translation (see Fig 4–6). Very steep joints present the disc-condyle complexes with an extremely difficult task of executing smooth silent translatory cycles, especially if movements are rapid. Such joints may predispose to certain disc-interference disorders.[50] Also, very steep joints predispose to subluxation with overextended opening because of the necessary posterior rotation of the articular disc on the condyle required to execute translatory cycles.

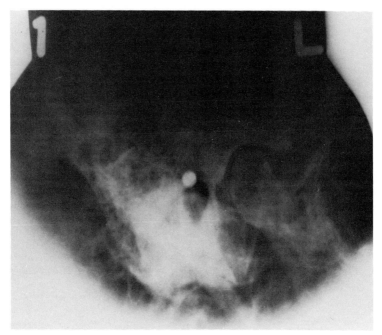

FIGURE 5–1   Radiograph illustrates a relatively flat temporomandibular joint. The inclination of the articular eminence is about 24 degrees from the horizontal supra-articular
crest.

The angle of the articular eminence is important during maximum
intercuspation if the dentition does not provide adequate stabilizing anchorage when the teeth are fully occluded. In such situations, the
steeper the inclination of the articular eminence, the more likely is the
disc-condyle complex to slide posteriorly during maximum intercuspation. This increases the burden on the lateral pterygoid muscle to hold
the condyle as well as the danger of damage to the inner horizontal
fibers of the temporomandibular ligament.

The inclination of the articular eminence also gives information on
the relationship between joint morphology, muscle action, and the dentition and oral structures.[51] Very flat joints are more expansive anteroposteriorly. The difference between the mediolateral and anteroposterior diameters of the condyle is less pronounced. The musculature
appears to function very well with a minimum of sensory guidance
from dental and oral structures, which habitually have more lateral
movement in chewing. Compatible oral structures include more expansive dental arches, flatter palate, less overbite, more shallow fossae, and

lower cusps. Such joints present considerable latitude in the occlusal relationship of the teeth in that they function well in an occlusal area, rather than in a precise occlusal position. A "tight" occlusal position actually may induce discomfort and provoke a high degree of oral consciousness.

Very steep joints are usually more compact anteroposteriorly. The difference between the mediolateral and anteroposterior diameters of the condyle is more pronounced. This causes the pivoting condyle during lateral excursions to undergo a greater shift of the vertical axis toward the lateral pole. But considerably less lateral movement is employed habitually in chewing. The musculature appears to depend more heavily on sensory and proprioceptive guidance as the occlusal position is reached. The compatible oral structures include more constricted dental arches, a higher palatal vault, and an interlocking type of dentition with considerable overbite, deeper fossae, and more prominent cusps. Such joints tolerate very little latitude in the occlusal relationship of the teeth and function best with a positive occlusal position.

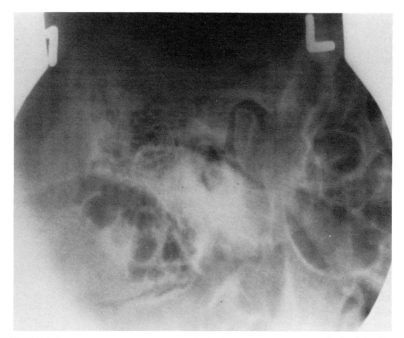

FIGURE 5–2 Radiograph illustrates a relatively steep temporomandibular joint. The inclination of the articular eminence is about 70 degrees from the horizontal supra-articular crest.

In the absence of such a position, considerable oral consciousness may develop, and the patient may complain, "I have lost my bite."

It should be noted that these morphologic relationships are evident only with extremely steep and flat joints. These relationships are not sufficiently pronounced to have clinical significance in most subjects who have an articular eminence inclination between 30 and 60 degrees from horizontal.

Bilateral Compatibility

It is important that the joints be bilaterally compatible with each other. When the difference between the inclination of the articular eminences is considerable, difficulties due to lack of structural harmony may be serious. Unilateral disc interference appears to occur chiefly in the steeper joint.[50] Other incompatible differences may result from lack of uniform development. Some problems result from the effects of trauma; some are problems of growth, such as hyperplasia of the condyle.

FUNCTIONAL HARMONY

Sliding movement that takes place between disc-condyle complex and articular eminence in any direction is functionally normal as long as it does not occur under pressure sufficient to cause frictional abuse to the moving surfaces. But sliding movement within the disc-condyle complex proper (i.e., between condyle and disc) violates its normal functional capabilities. It is resisted by disc contour and by the collateral ligaments that unite the articulating parts of the complex.

Many variations in chewing movements occur. Although some chewing strokes do end in maximum intercuspation, many do not reach even initial tooth contact, much less full occlusion. The distribution of food between the two sides alters the pattern. Incising and grinding are done differently. The degree of lateral movement utilized with chewing also varies the pattern.

Swallowing involves joint action also. Although it has been thought that swallowing is accompanied by full occlusion of the teeth, it is known that this occurs only with swallowing solid foods. Liquids and automatic swallowing of saliva do not produce this effect.[52] If there is tooth contact at all, it is very light and induces inhibitory influence on elevator muscles due to stimulation of periodontal receptors.

Bruxism, however, is quite a different matter. Whether it is clenching the teeth in firm maximum intercuspation or combined with some movement, bruxism does bring into play forces which require considerable muscle action and induce alteration of interarticular pressure. This throws a great burden of stress on the joints that may constitute overloading.

The craniomandibular articulation is unique in one respect: it must reckon with forces incidental to the occlusion of teeth. This is in addition to the forces initiated by muscle action against resistance. It has to do with forces generated by the meshing of inclined planes that comprise the occluding surfaces of teeth, i.e., the forces resulting from maximum intercuspation.

The gross position of the disc-condyle complex relative to the temporal facet at any given time throughout empty-mouth translatory cycles is determined by muscle action. The influence of the teeth is minimal, being largely inhibitory on muscle action as a result of stimulation of periodontal mechanoreceptors.

Power strokes introduce another force that alters the postural relationship between disc-condyle complex and articular eminence. This, however, is resolved by the time the teeth come into contact. Therefore, the unclenched closed position of the joint represents a relationship between the articulating parts that is the product of muscle action. By a combination of conditioned habit patterns, reflex activity, proprioceptive and sensory guidance (including that of the periodontal ligaments), and volition, the position of the disc-condyle complex relative to the articular eminence as the teeth come into contact is determined by muscle action.

As the inclined planes of the occluding teeth come under biting stress supplied by the elevator muscles, a new and irresistible force becomes the final determinant of disc-condyle complex position. This supercedes the muscular position. This force occurs suddenly as the teeth reach maximum intercuspation and disappears just as rapidly when the musculature relaxes following full occlusion of the teeth. The clenched, occluded position of the joint represents a relationship between the articulating parts that is the product of tooth form.

The act of maximum intercuspation, therefore, causes a rapid shift of postural forces from muscle action to tooth form and back to muscle action. *This takes place every time the teeth are fully occluded.* It should be obvious that any gross shifting of disc-condyle complex position by these changing forces would be conflictory and, therefore, incompatible with normal joint functioning.

Functional harmony between the masticatory muscles and the dentition, therefore, is present when the muscle-determined position of the disc-condyle complex (which represents the closed unclenched relationship of the joint) is not altered by forces generated by maximum intercuspation of the teeth (the closed clenched relationship of the joint).

Functional Incompatibility

Lack of functional harmony between the muscles and dentition may induce a variety of deleterious effects. When frictional resistance anchors the articular disc, gross movement of the condyle may induce damaging changes in the articular surfaces. Those surfaces in contact when the joint is closed are the ones that bear the burden of stress. Deleterious change causes loss of smoothness of these surfaces. This, in turn, adds to the anchoring effect of the frictional pressure, thus intensifying the possible abuse.

Because of the location of the articular eminence relative to the disc-condyle complex in the closed-joint position, gross movement of the condyle anteriorly while the disc is anchored by friction against the eminence may be damaging to the disc. Such movement of the condyle may also overload the discal collateral ligaments and, thus, permit condylar encroachment upon the thicker anterior portion of articular disc. Such damage may compromise the effectiveness of the articular disc in stabilizing the joint during the forward phase of translatory movement.

Initially, posterior displacement of the disc-condyle complex is resisted by the lateral pterygoid muscle, thus inducing muscle effects. Subsequently, it is resisted by the inner horizontal fibers of the temporomandibular ligament. As the articular disc is immobilized against the temporal articular surface by friction, overloading of the discal ligaments may cause deterioration or elongation. This may permit condylar encroachment upon the thicker posterior portion of the disc. Deleterious change in that portion of the disc reduces its effectiveness in stabilizing the joint during power strokes and maximum intercuspation. Elongation of the discal ligaments and inner horizontal fibers of the temporomandibular ligament may also permit condylar encroachment upon the retrodiscal structures.

Posterior overclosure occurs when occlusal support in the molar area is insufficient to prevent movement of the mandible during maximum intercuspation. If the remaining teeth provide sufficient anchorage to prevent movement of the mandible posteriorly, a fulcrum forward to the molar area is established. This causes the direction of force and movement of the condyle to be upward and forward, which may result in overloading against the articular eminence. If, however, the remaining teeth do not so anchor the occlusion, the disc-condyle complex is displaced posteriorly.

If displacement causes either of the discal ligaments to undergo deterioration, elongation, or detachment sufficient to impair its primary function of ensuring hinge movement in the disc-condyle complex, normal functioning may be disrupted throughout translatory cycles, especially in power strokes and maximum intercuspation. This would predispose to disc-interference disorders.

If the functional incompatibility results from recent occlusal change, structural damage to the joint is less likely to occur. Rather, the effects are predominantly muscular. Since such disharmony would constitute a recent environmental change, the altered proprioceptive and sensory input would be more likely to initiate the protective mechanism of muscle splinting. Such an effect, if protracted, may induce muscle spasm activity.

The various effects of functional disharmony between the masticatory muscles and the dentition relate to the closed relationship of the joint—unclenched to clenched occluded position. These effects do not occur when the teeth are separated or very lightly occluded. It is maximum intercuspation, whether due to power strokes and chewing movements or to bruxism, that activates the disharmony.

MASTICATORY SYMPTOMS

Lack of structural or functional harmony between components of the masticatory apparatus may lead to symptoms. Masticatory symptoms may be classified as masticatory pain and masticatory dysfunction. Different temporomandibular disorders are recognized and identified by combinations of these symptoms.

Masticatory Pain

Masticatory pain arises from the TM joints and/or the masticatory muscles. Pain of masticatory muscle origin (myalgia) is classified clinically as:

1. Protective muscle splinting
2. Muscle spasm activity
3. Local muscle soreness or inflammation

Pain of joint origin (arthralgia) emanates from a pain-sensitive structure of the TM joint. Depending on the structure(s) from which it arises, an arthralgic pain is classified as:

1. Disc attachment pain
2. Retrodiscal pain
3. Capsular pain
4. Arthritis pain

Masticatory Dysfunction

Masticatory dysfunction symptoms may be classified as restricted mandibular movement, interference during such movement, and acute malocclusion.

Restriction of Mandibular Movement. Jaw movement should be sufficient to meet the normal requirements for talking and masticating foods. Restrictions of movement are displayed as an inability to close the mouth, an inability to open the mouth adequately, or an inability to execute adequate protrusive or contralateral excursions. This may be accompanied by deflection of the opening or the protrusive path.

Interference During Mandibular Movement. Discal interference during mandibular movements may be expressed as *abnormal sensations* (sticking, binding, rubbing, slipping, hanging, catching), *abnormal noises* (clicking, popping, snapping, grating), and/or *abnormal movements* (rough, irregular, jerky, jumping movements; locking; deviation of the midline path). Westesson[53] determined that discrete clicking occurred at the moment the disc-condyle complex impacted the temporal articular surface after a mechanical obstruction had been overcome.

Acute Malocclusion. Acute malocclusion refers to some recent alteration in the occlusal relationship that is induced by an abnormal muscle action or by a change within the joint.

MASTICATORY PAIN SYMPTOMS

Pain is the most important of the various masticatory symptoms, not because it is the most serious or the most frequent, but because it is the symptom that causes the patient the greatest concern and for which he most frequently seeks treatment. Pain, therefore, is the primary issue in the management of temporomandibular disorders. It is the symptom by which most patients judge the results of treatment. It deserves first consideration in the handling of such complaints.

By definition, *masticatory pain* is discomfort about the face and mouth induced by chewing and other jaw use, but independent of local disease involving the teeth and mouth. Masticatory pain has its source in temporomandibular joints and/or masticatory muscles and, therefore, is related directly to masticatory function.[54] It does not include "chewing pains" of dental or pharyngeal origin, pains referred to the joint area, or *nonspastic* myofascial pain syndromes that cause referred pain felt elsewhere. The identification of pain as a valid masticatory symptom hinges on its source: it emanates from the joints or muscles that power the joints and relates to masticatory function.

The *site of pain* (where it is felt) is not necessarily the true *source of pain* (where it actually stems from). Pain arising in another structure may be felt in the masticatory apparatus and may seem to be related to masticatory function. For example, sternocleidomastoid muscle pain may be referred to the temporomandibular joint area. The very first judgment that should be made on pain as a masticatory symptom is whether or not it actually does have its source in temporomandibular joints or masticatory muscles.

Unfortunately, patients, and too frequently their doctors, have insufficient understanding of pain behavior. Pain tends to generate emotional response that is disproportionate to its true significance. If an aura of mystery exists as to the source of pain or its cause, considerable fear may be generated that, in turn, intensifies the pain. Thus, a vicious cycle may develop that induces symptoms bearing little relationship to the initating cause. To manage pain complaints better, it is necessary to understand some of the mechanisms of pain.

Pain Modulation

The time-honored concept of pain behavior is that noxious stimulation of peripheral structures provokes neural impulses that are conducted to the CNS, where they are perceived and reacted to. The reaction is thought to be influenced by such factors as prior conditioning, the emotional significance of the discomfort to the individual, and the general physical and emotional state of the individual at that particular time. This is the *perception-reaction concept* of pain behavior.

In recent years, this understanding of pain behavior has been replaced by the *pain modulation concept*. By pain modulation is meant that the neural impulses generated by noxious stimulation are altered (modulated) prior to being perceived and reacted to. Such modulation is accomplished by peripheral and central inhibitory and excitatory mechanisms operating prior to the noxious stimulation as well as in response to the stimulus. The effect of all modulating factors on the neural impulses is accomplished prior to being perceived. Indeed, the perception of pain is but a facet of the total reaction to those modulated impulses. Thus, when pain is perceived, all factors, including mentation and physical influences, have had their effect already. The suffering itself becomes a continuing modulating influence on the pain. This concept of pain modulation is more consistent with known neurophysiologic facts than the older perception-reaction concept, which failed to explain some features of clinical pain behavior.

The mechanisms by which pain impulses are modulated are in part theoretical. The gate-control theory proposed by Melzack and Wall in 1965 presented a model to help visualize the neural mechanisms involved.[55] Considerable difference of opinion exists as to the validity of the whole theory. In 1978, Wall reexamined the theory in light of continuing neurophysiologic investigation.[56]

Certain facts have emerged:

1. Intermittent mild stimulation of cutaneous sensory nerves exerts an inhibitory influence on pain.[57–59] This forms the basis for various treatment modalities such as massage, analgesic balms, vibration, thermal applications, vapocoolants, hydrotherapy, and counterirritation. The development of transcutaneous electrical nerve stimulation (so-called TENS units) for the symptomatic relief of pain is based on the inhibitory effect of cutaneous stimulation.

2. The stimulation of specific sites on the body surface exerts a marked inhibitory influence on pain. These acupoints have been known to the Chinese for many years. Their validity in pain control has been verified by numerous researchers.

3. Pain is increased by certain peripheral and central factors.[55] Hyperemia and inflammation of peripheral tissues reduce the inhibitory influence of the body on pain perception. It is thought that increased small afferent nociceptive fiber activity accounts for this effect. The duration of pain causes it to increase in severity, despite no added peripheral noxious input.

The discovery of endogenous opioids that act as inhibitory neuromodulators on nociceptive pathways has opened a door to pain behavior at a molecular level. Endorphin (endogenous morphine) in the cerebrospinal fluid (CSF) exerts a definite analgesic effect that is reversible by naloxone, a known morphine antagonist. Endorphins are protein molecules composed of chains of amino acids (peptides). They are secreted by brain tissue into the CSF and by the pituitary gland into the bloodstream.

Other factors on a molecular level are known to influence pain modulation. Substance P is released from primary nociceptive afferents involved in pain transmission. Substance P acts as an excitatory neuromodulator that facilitates pain impulses. Its release is suppressed by β-endorphin as well as by morphine. The suppressive effect is reversed by naloxone.[60]

Certain information concerning pain modulation has evolved:

1. Placebo has a therapeutic inhibitory influence on pathologic pain, reducing the pain level by 30% or more.[61] Distraction of the subject's attention also has a therapeutic inhibitory effect as is witnessed by hypnotic suggestion and such techniques as "white sound."

2. Endorphin level decreases with the duration of pain and, therefore relates importantly to chronic pain syndromes.[62, 63]

3. Endorphin level is increased by acupuncture and electroanalgesia. These pain inhibitory effects are reversible by naloxone.[64, 65] Cerebrospinal fluid endorphin does not appear to be increased by transcutaneous electrical nerve stimulation, however, unless it is applied at acupoints.[66] Nevertheless, such stimulation does inhibit pain conduction by another mechanism.

Secondary Effects of Deep Pain

Another pain mechanism that has clinical importance, both diagnostically and therapeutically, has to do with secondary effects of deep pain input.[54] Unfortunately, the neurophysiologic mechanisms are obscure and poorly understood. The clinical behavior of these effects, however, is well known. Secondary effects induced by deep pain include (1) referred pain with, and without, secondary hyperalgesia, and (2) skeletal muscle effects.

In general, these effects occur as a CNS phenomenon. They probably result from the convergence of impulses conducted by primary afferent neurons onto other interneurons that ordinarily would not be stimulated. Continued deep-pain input appears to cause hyperexcitability of such neurons. These phenomena are referred to as *central excitatory effects*.

Several clinical features of these secondary effects are known:

1. They appear to require continuity of deep-pain input. Some effects, such as referred pain, remain wholly dependent on the primary pain input and disappear when the primary pain is arrested, even temporarily, as with local analgesic blocking. Some effects, such as secondary hyperalgesia, are dependent on the primary pain but may persist for a while after the primary initiating pain ceases. If secondary muscle contraction develops into a cycling muscle spasm, it becomes independent of the initiating pain and behaves instead as a new deep-pain source with the same potentiality of inducing other secondary effects as deep pain elsewhere. Intermittent input does not seem to induce secondary central excitatory effects. The greater the severity and duration, the greater the likelihood that secondary effects will occur.

2. Secondary effects of deep-pain input occur in otherwise *normal* structures. The sites where such effects are seen should be quite innocent and therapy directed toward them is not effective, except for cycling myospasms.

3. The primary pain input may or may not be felt on a conscious level. If the primary pain is silent, the secondary pain may be mistaken for the true source of pain.

4. Secondary effects are most likely to occur in peripheral structures innervated by other fibers of the same major nerve. If trigeminal secondary effects are expressed in adjacent divisions of the nerve that mediates the input, the effects follow a vertical pattern. If structures innervated by a different neural segment become involved, the secondary effects occur predominately in a cephalad direction.[67] Ordinarily, trigeminal pain input does not induce secondary effects outside the vast trigeminal region.

Referred Pain.   Heterotopic pain is that which is felt in an area other than the true site of origin. Heterotopic pain may be expressed as *projected pain* which is felt in the peripheral distribution of the same nerve that mediates the primary pain input. It may be expressed as *referred pain* which is felt in an area that is not innervated by the nerve that mediates the primary pain input.[54]

Referred pain frequently complicates masticatory pain symptoms and therefore should be understood and differentiated clinically from other heterotopic pains. *It requires CNS synapse.* The primary pain responsible for the condition is of deep origin and is mediated in the usual way to the trigeminal nucleus. There the transfer is made (presumably as the result of convergence) in such a way that it is felt as coming from a different site. The *primary pain* is the true source of the complaint; the *secondary pain* is felt in the referred pain site. Provocation of the primary pain site initiates or aggravates both primary and secondary pains; provocation of the secondary pain site does nothing. Analgesic blocking of the pathway that mediates the primary pain arrests both primary and secondary pains; blocking the pathway that subserves the secondary pain site arrests neither pain.

Secondary Hyperalgesia. Referred pains may or may not be accompanied by areas of secondary hyperalgesia located superficially or deeply in the body structures. Hyperalgesia is defined as excessive sensitivity or sensibility to stimulation (provocation). It may be primary or secondary. *Primary hyperalgesia* results from a local cause that has lowered the pain threshold of the structures that hurt. In *secondary hyperalgesia,* no local cause exists for the condition. The pain threshold in the area is essentially normal. It occurs in conjunction with the phenomenon of referred pain and is a true central excitatory effect.

Secondary hyperalgesia follows the same general rules that apply to other central excitatory effects, except that it may persist for a while after the primary pain ceases. The area of hypersensitivity may be situated on the surface, or it may occur more deeply in the tissues. Superficial secondary hyperalgesia is felt as *excessive sensitivity to touch.* As such, it usually presents no diagnostic problem. But, if located deeply, it is felt as *tenderness to palpation* and may be confused with other primary pain sources, such as spasm or inflammation of muscle tissue. It is important to be able to differentiate deep secondary hyperalgesia from a true primary-pain source. This may be done by analgesic blocking which completely arrests primary pain but only partially reduces the discomfort of secondary hyperalgesia.

Muscle Effects. Deep pain input may cause certain effects in skeletal muscles due to central hyperexcitability. Such effects are predominantly contractile and tend to induce myospasm. If myospasm persists long enough to become painful, a cycling myospasm may develop and remain as a separate clinical entity indefinitely—as a self-perpetuating, pain-dysfunction syndrome.

Muscle effects occur especially in muscles innervated by the same neural segment that mediates the initiating primary pain. Therefore, the muscles innervated by the trigeminal nerve (i.e., the masticatory muscles plus the mylohyoid, anterior digastric, tensor palati, and tensor tympani muscles) are the ones affected by pain from the vast trigeminal region. Since effects of central hyperexcitability occur almost exclusively in a cephalad direction (when extrasegmental reference occurs), other deep-pain sources of facial and cervical origin also may cause muscle effects in trigeminal innervated muscles.

Although muscle effects due to central excitation are usually contractile, it appears from clinical evidence that myofascial trigger-point pain may be initiated in like manner. Such syndromes may also persist quite independently of the initiating deep-pain input. When this occurs, the referred pain that characterizes nonspastic myofascial pain syndromes often is felt at or near the site of the initiating primary-pain source. Pain of myofascial origin arises from trigger points located within the muscle or its tendinous attachments. Such trigger points, when stimulated by normal functional activities, cause referred pain that is felt elsewhere outside the muscle proper. These trigger sites, however, are locally tender to manual palpation, with or without simultaneous reference of pain. The patient may be wholly unaware of the muscular source of the pain and may think the site of pain represents the cause of his complaint. The involved muscle(s) may otherwise be quite normal. The zones of reference for such trigger points have been well charted by Travell and Simons.[68] That such triggers do exist and cause referred pain is unmistakable, even though the mechanism involved is not clear. Analgesic blocking of such trigger points arrests the reference of pain.

It should be understood that myofascial trigger-point pain does not display increased EMG activity and therefore does not constitute muscle spasm activity. The significance of trigger-point pain involving masticatory muscles lies in its *potentiality* to induce myospastic activity. Painfully stretching a myofascial trigger site may induce muscle spasm.[68] No doubt, many muscle spasm disorders of the masticatory system arise in this way, and quite correctly are termed *myofascial* pain-dysfunction syndromes. But, muscle spasm activity from other causes (such as from conditions that begin as protective muscle splinting or as a central excitatory effect from deep pain input) are not examples of myofascial pain. Since myofascial trigger-point pain is usually felt as referred pain or secondary hyperalgesia in areas outside the muscle, and, since dysfunction is minimal, nonspastic myofascial trigger-point pain involving a masticatory muscle should not be taken as a clinical symptom of a TM disorder. Such pain conditions relate to TM disorders only etiologically.

CRITERIA FOR IDENTIFYING MASTICATORY MYALGIA

Myogenous pain that is symptomatic of a masticatory muscle disorder can be identified as deep somatic pain of musculoskeletal type (Fig 5–3). Effective management of a masticatory muscle disorder requires that the particular clinical type of myogenous pain be identified as accurately as possible. This can usually be done by observing certain criteria.

Protective Muscle Splinting

Etiology. Muscle splinting is thought to occur in response to afferent input that signals the presence of injury or threat of injury (i.e., a marked change from the usual sensory or proprioceptive input). The history, therefore, should indicate prior injury, change in the oral environment, dental treatment (especially with local anesthesia), increased oral consciousness (e.g., evoked volitional chewing that conflicts with established habitual patterns), or stress-induced bruxism.

Symptoms. Onset of pain is sudden. It occurs when muscles are contracted. Moderate muscle stiffness and a feeling of a muscular weakness usually are present.

Muscular Dysfunction. Muscle splinting causes slightly increased resistance to passive stretch. Except for the inhibitory influence of pain and the sensation of muscular weakness, little or no structural dysfunction is present.

Clinical Course. Muscle splinting disappears when the injury or threat resolves. Abusive use or injudicious therapy may protract the splinting effect. *Protracted splinting may induce muscle spasm.*

Myospastic Activity

Etiology. Myospasm may occur spontaneously, especially in tense individuals. By way of protracted muscle splinting, many local conditions may induce muscle spasm. These include minor strains, abusive use, bruxism, and muscle fatigue. Myospastic activity may occur with or without a prior stage of nonspastic myofascial pain due to systemic

OROFACIAL PAIN SYNDROMES

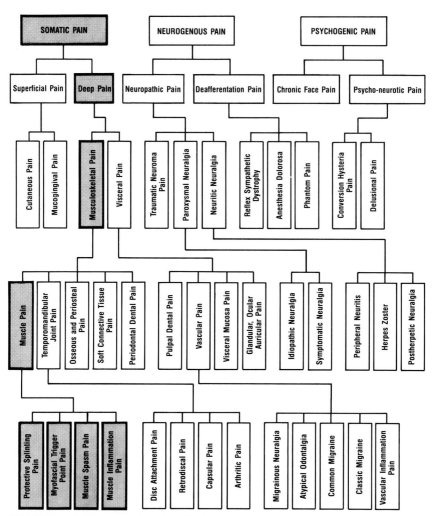

FIGURE 5–3   Chart showing classification relationship of muscle pains to other orofacial pain syndromes. (From Bell W.E.: *Orofacial Pains: Classification, Diagnosis, Management,* ed. 3. Chicago, Year Book Medical Publishers, 1985. Reproduced with permission.)

causes such as illness, infection, or emotional stress. It may occur as a side effect of certain medications (e.g., phenothiazines). A frequent cause of masticatory myospasm is a continuous input of deep pain located elsewhere (as a central excitatory effect). This may occur not only as the result of deep trigeminal pain, but also in response to facial, glossopharyngeal, and particularly cervical pain sources. It should be noted that in all cases of cycling muscle spasm, the mere presence of myospastic activity does not indicate its proximate cause or even if a cause persists, since such conditions become self-perpetuating and wholly independent of the initiating cause.

Symptoms.   Sudden onset, with or without prior occurrence, is characteristic. Pain is felt with stretching or contraction of the spastic muscle.

Muscular Dysfunction.   Muscle spasm causes structural dysfunction, the type depending on the muscle(s) involved and the kind of spasm (isotonic or isometric). Isotonic spasm shortens the muscle. Isometric spasm induces resistance to stretch and some muscular rigidity.

Clinical Course.   Cycling myospasm becomes self-perpetuating and therefore tends to persist. If abused or injudiciously treated (especially by excessive exercising), protracted myospasm may become inflammatory and present as masticatory myositis.

Muscle Inflammation

Etiology.   Masticatory myositis may result from any local cause, such as unaccustomed use, abuse, injury, infection, or adjacent disease. It may be secondary to another inflammatory condition due to surgery, trauma, or infection. By way of muscle splinting and protracted myospasm, myositis may result from any and all causes of muscle pain.

Symptoms.   Pain occurs with the muscle at rest and with all use. It parallels the clinical course of the inflammatory process.

Muscular Dysfunction.   The stiffness and swelling due to the inflammatory process cause trismus if elevator muscles are involved.

Clinical Course.   The incidence, development, leveling off, and resolution of the condition are timed to the determinants of severity and phase of the inflammatory process.

CRITERIA FOR IDENTIFYING ARTHRALGIA

Effective management of TM arthralgia depends on precise knowledge of the type of pain and from what structure(s) it emanates (Fig 5–4). This information usually can be determined by observing certain identifying criteria.

Disc-Attachment Pain

Etiology.   Pain that emanates from the collateral ligaments that attach the articular disc to the medial and lateral poles of the mandibular condyle occurs as a result of strain on those ligaments as they resist displacement between disc and condyle.

Symptoms.   Pain occurs in conjunction with the discal interference present. Momentary pain with or immediately prior to symptoms of discal interference usually is indicative of functional strain on the ligaments. More constant pain that is aggravated by such interference suggests the presence of inflammatory change. If the disc-attachment pain relates intimately to maximum intercuspation, it may be reduced by biting against a separator that prevents such intercuspation.

Dysfunction.   Joint dysfunction consists of disc interference during mandibular movements.

Clinical Course.   The ligaments are innervated with receptors that may induce a variety of muscle effects (muscle splinting, etc.) Inflamed collateral ligaments may induce capsulitis secondarily.

Retrodiscal Pain

Etiology.   Pain emanating from the retrodiscal tissue is chiefly inflammatory and due to injury inflicted by encroachment of the mandibular condyle. Extrinsic trauma is a frequent cause. But, if the dentition is such that it does not satisfactorily anchor the mandible in maximum intercuspation, abusive strain on the inner horizontal fibers of the temporomandibular ligament may result. This may lead to elongation or

OROFACIAL PAIN SYNDROMES

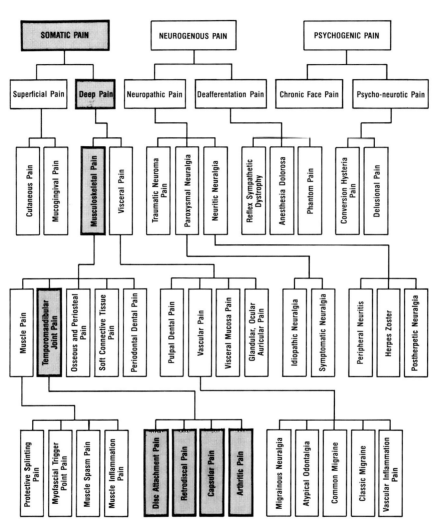

FIGURE 5–4 Chart showing classification relationship of temporomandibular joint pains to other orofacial pain syndromes. (From Bell W.E.: *Orofacial Pains: Classification, Diagnosis, Management*, ed. 3, Chicago, Year Book Medical Publishers, 1985. Reproduced with permission.)

degenerative change that permits condylar encroachment on the retrodiscal tissue.

Symptoms. Retrodiscal pain occurs during maximum intercuspation. It may be reduced by biting against a separator that prevents full intercuspation.

Dysfunction. Retrodiscal swelling and/or excessive intracapsular fluid may displace the condyle in the resting closed position of the joint, thus causing acute malocclusion.

Clinical Course. The pain follows an inflammatory pattern if the condition is due to acute extrinsic trauma. Hemarthrosis may predispose to fibrous adhesions. Degeneration or elongation of the temporomandibular ligament predisposes to chronic disc interference symptoms.

Capsular Pain

Etiology. Capsular pain is due to synovitis or inflammation of the capsule as the result of (1) trauma, (2) direct extension of inflammation from injured discal collateral ligaments or temporomandibular ligament, (3) arthritis or periarticular inflammation, or (4) abuse to preexistent capsular fibrosis.

Symptoms. Capsulitis is characterized by palpable tenderness directly over the joint proper. Pain is increased with movements that stretch the capsule. If the capsulitis is due to discal or temporomandibular ligament injury, pain also increases in maximum intercuspation and is decreased by biting against a separator.

Dysfunction. Including the inhibitory influence of pain, dysfunction due to capsulitis may range from minor restriction of function, noticeable only in extended movements, to immobilization of the joint. Excessive intracapsular fluid may cause acute malocclusion. If the condition is secondary to articular disc interference, inflammatory arthritis, inflamed capsular fibrosis, or periarticular conditions, other dysfunction consistent with such conditions may be observed and no doubt will persist after the capsular inflammation resolves.

Clinical Course. Persistence of capsular inflammation predisposes to capsular fibrosis.

Arthritis Pain

Etiology. The pain is due to (1) inflammatory arthritis or (2) inflammation of adhesions of ankylosis that are injured by abusive chewing movements or other jaw use.

Symptoms. The pain relates to the kind, degree, duration, and phase of the inflammatory condition present. There is usually some secondary capsulitis present also.

Dysfunction. Restriction and interference relate to the type of arthropathy present. Intracapsular inflammatory effusion may cause acute malocclusion.

Clinical Course. Chronicity is characteristic. If pain is due to inflamed ankylosis, restricted movement will remain after the pain disappears.

MASTICATORY DYSFUNCTION SYMPTOMS

Most TM complaints have a component of dysfunction that is expressed as (1) inability to move the jaw normally, (2) various noises and sensations of interference that occur during jaw movements, or (3) some recent alteration in the way the teeth come together. Effective management of temporomandibular disorders depends on precise identification of the kind of dysfunction present in the complaint, where it is located, and what chiefly is responsible for it.

Restriction of Movement

The normal range of movement of the mandible is that which is adequate for the purpose intended—mastication and talking. Abnormality in this regard is an individual matter. For a particular individual, restriction of mandibular movement is symptomatic of masticatory dysfunction when it interferes in some way with his usual masticatory activities.

Pseudoankylosis. If mandibular movement is restricted for reasons independent of the TM joint and/or the masticatory muscles, the condition is usually termed *pseudoankylosis*. It may occur from a variety of causes.

Cicatricial tissue involving the lips can cause microstomia that restricts mouth opening. This may occur as the result of burns especially. Extensive ulceration of the oral mucosa may cause contractures to form between the maxillary and mandibular arches; this can impose severe limitation on mouth opening (Fig 5–5). Depressed fractures of the zygomatic arch and traumatic displacement of the coronoid process may cause interference with normal mandibular movements. Hypertrophy of the coronoid process may interfere with jaw functioning.[69–71] Tumor formation, especially malignant invasion (Figs 5–6 and 5–7), and inflammatory conditions of the face and jaws (Fig 5–8) may seriously interfere with movements of the mandible.

All such complaints due to pseudoankylosis should be recognized and differentiated from the true temporomandibular disorders.

Restriction of mandibular movement more frequently results from causes related directly to the joint and particularly to the masticatory muscles. Depending on where the cause is located, such limitation of movement is classified as extracapsular, capsular, or intracapsular. It is of considerable diagnostic and therapeutic importance that the location of restraint be identified properly. This can be done by observing certain clinical criteria. Confirmation, if needed, can be done radiographically.

Extracapsular Restraint.   Although an occasional nonmasticatory extracapsular cause for restricted jaw movement does occur, the usual

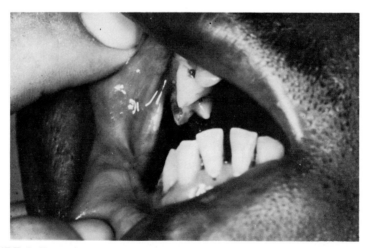

FIGURE 5–5 Mouth opening is restricted to 20-mm interincisal distance because of cicatricial contracture in the right buccal mucosa that developed as a result of extensive ulceration from mercurial poisoning.

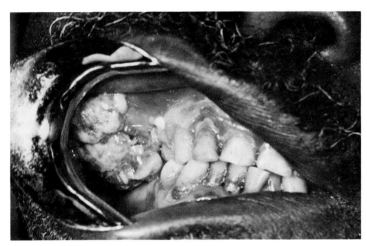

FIGURE 5–6 Mouth opening is restricted to a few millimeters due to invasive adeno-carcinoma involving the posterior maxillary and mandibular area.

cause is a shortened or immobilized elevator muscle due to spasm, inflammation, or contracture.

A shortened elevator muscle restricts mouth opening without appreciably affecting protrusion or lateral excursion. Therefore, the clinical symptoms of myogenous restriction of mandibular movement are:

1. Restricted opening, but fairly normal protrusion and lateral excursion to the opposite side.

2. Deflection of the midline incisal path with opening, but not with protrusion.

3. Pain, if any, increasing with opening widely (due to stretching the painful muscle) and with biting (due to contracting the painful muscle).

Deflection of the incisal path is to be distinguished from deviation. *Deflection* refers to a continuing eccentric displacement of the midline incisal path and is symptomatic of restriction of movement. *Deviation* refers to discursive movement that ends in the centered position and is indicative of interference during movement.

When opening is restricted, deflection of the midline incisal path may occur. Shortening of an elevator muscle arrests opening without affecting the capability of the disc-condyle complex to execute translatory movements. Unless inhibited by the effect of pain, protrusive and lateral movements remain normal. But, if an attempt is made to open the mouth widely, the mandible deflects, thus permitting the teeth to be separated farther. This deflection is due to lateral excursive movement. *The direction that it takes depends on the location of the shortened muscle(s).* The masseter and temporalis muscles are located lateral to the condyle. A shortened masseter or temporalis muscle does not inhibit freedom of lateral excursion in the opposite joint. Because of such translatory movement in the opposite joint, a shortened masseter or temporalis muscle permits deflection of the midline incisal path ipsilaterally (to the same side). This is not true, however, of the medial pterygoid muscle. Being located medial to the condyle, a shortened medial pterygoid muscle causes translatory movement in the ipsilateral rather than the opposite joint, a movement similar to that of the nonworking condyle in a normal lateral excursive movement. The opposite condyle remains seated. Thus, the midline incisal path is deflected contralaterally (to the opposite side). It should be noted, however, that contralateral deflection induced by a shortened medial pterygoid muscle may be observed only *if that is the sole muscle involved.*

Deflection of the incisal path begins immediately as the restraining effect of a shortened elevator muscle arrests the opening effort. Thus,

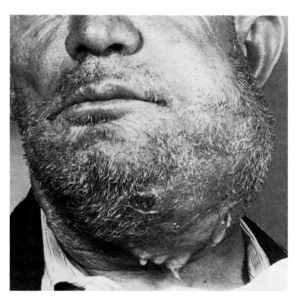

FIGURE 5–7   Left temporomandibular joint is immobilized by invasive squamous cell carcinoma.

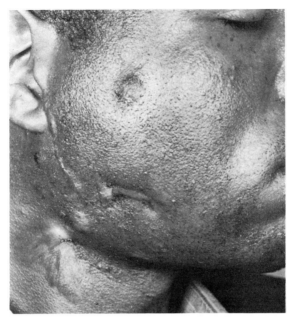

FIGURE 5–8 Mouth opening is restricted by actinomycosis involving the right facial, cervical, and masseter muscle area.

the point at which obvious deflection commences indicates the degree of shortening of the muscle. Since the deflection itself is due to lateral excursion of the mandible, the amount of deflection is indicative of the degree of lateral excursion that takes place.

Deflection with opening may not occur, or does so very slightly, (1) if the medial pterygoid muscle is involved in conjunction with the masseter or temporalis muscles, (2) if bilateral extracapsular restraint involves both joints, or (3) if the opposite joint is incapable of significant lateral movement.

Deflection with opening can occur, *but it may not do so* if the musculature (usually the opposite temporalis muscle) holds the opposite condyle in sympathetic posture with the affected side. This usually is due to the inhibitory influence of pain. When deflection does not take place, the separation of the teeth is less, and the resultant trismus is relatively greater.

Radiographic confirmation of extracapsular restriction of mandibular movement is done by comparing the condylar position in maximum opening with that of lateral excursion to the opposite side. The condyle position in lateral excursion will appear normal, whereas in the open position it will be considerably less (Fig 5–9).

Capsular Restraint. Reduction in the size and flexibility of the capsular ligament imposes limitation on the extent of translatory movement of the disc-condyle complex. Such limitation occurs whether the translatory movement is for opening, protrusion, or lateral excursion, and condylar restriction exists to the same degree for all such movements. When capsular restraint is minor, condylar restriction may be evident in the outer ranges of movement only. The degree of restraint depends on the amount of change in capsular size and flexibility. Capsular restraint of mandibular movement may result from inflammatory swelling of the capsule (capsulitis due to various causes) or to fibrotic contracture of the capsule (capsular fibrosis due to prior capsulitis or scarring from injury or surgery).

The most reliable clinical indication of capsular restraint is that its effect on condylar movement remains exactly the same, whether it is for opening, protrusion, or contralateral excursion. Rotatory opening is not affected, unless inhibited by pain or intracapsular effusion. Therefore, an opening capability of 25 mm (more or less) is present, even though the patient may be reluctant to move the jaw to that extent.

Radiographic confirmation is accurate due to the sameness of the

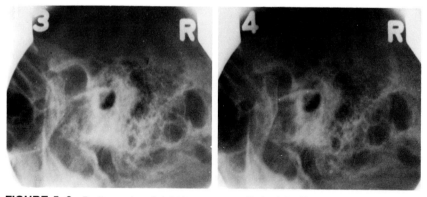

FIGURE 5–9 Radiographs of right temporomandibular joint illustrate extracapsular restriction of mandibular movement. *Left,* lateral excursion to the opposite side. *Right,* maximum opening. Note that condylar movement in lateral excursion is within normal limits, while in maximum opening it is less than that of lateral excursion. (From Bell W.E.: Management of temporomandibular joint problems, in Goldman H.M., Gilmore H.W., Royer R.Q., et al. (eds.): *Current Therapy in Dentistry.* St. Louis, C.V. Mosby Co., 1970, vol. 4. Reproduced with permission.)

restraining effect on condylar movement in the different positions. It is usually sufficient to compare the open and lateral excursion joint positions. The condyle shadows will exactly superimpose in the two views. In capsular restraint of moderate degree, the condylar position may be just short of the crest of the articular eminence (Fig 5–10).

Capsular restraint due to capsulitis, as a progressive effect of inflammation of the discal collateral ligaments (discitis) or the inner portion of the temporomandibular ligament, may complicate some disc-interference disorders. The pain of such capsulitis is increased with maximum intercuspation and reduced by biting against a separator. Capsular restraint due to capsulitis may also accompany inflammatory arthritis. It is important therapeutically that such restraint be clearly differentiated from extracapsular restrictions due to secondary muscle spasm or other causes.

Intracapsular Restraint. The most frequent cause of intracapsular restriction of mandibular movement is obstruction of the articular disc, which tends to prevent further movement of the condyle. This can occur for different reasons, including (1) excessive passive interarticular pressure, (2) structural incompatibility of the articulating parts, (3) impairment of disc-condyle complex function, especially a damaged articular disc in conjunction with dysfunctional discal collateral ligaments, and (4) gross change in the joint due to arthritis. A significantly

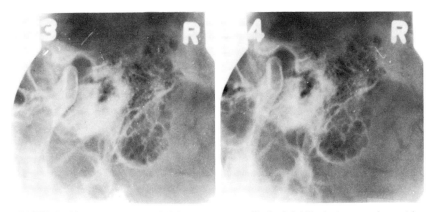

FIGURE 5–10 Radiographs of right temporomandibular joint illustrate capsular restriction of mandibular movement. *Left,* lateral excursion to the opposite side. *Right,* maximum opening. Note that condylar movement in lateral excursion is short of the crest of the articular eminence. The restriction in maximum opening is exactly the same. (From Bell W.E.: Management of temporomandibular joint problems, in Goldman H.M., Gilmore H.W., Royer R.Q., et al. (eds.): *Current Therapy in Dentistry.* St. Louis, C.V. Mosby Co., 1970, vol. 4. Reproduced with permission.)

important cause of intracapsular restriction of mandibular movement has to do with blockage of forward translation of the condyle by a dislocated articular disc due to functional displacement[72] or trauma.[73] Fibrous or osseous ankylosis also induces restriction of movement.

Any condition that positively arrests translatory movement within the joint affects all movements—opening, protrusion, and lateral excursions. This accounts for the clinical symptoms, namely:

1. Restriction of opening to the amount permitted by rotatory movement, plus whatever translatory movement occurs before arrest takes place.

2. Arrested protrusive movement.

3. Arrested contralateral excursive movement.

4. Deflection of the midline incisal path ipsilaterally (toward the symptomatic side) with opening and with protrusion.

Deflection of the midline incisal path relates precisely to the point of arrested forward movement of the disc-condyle complex. Some variation in symptoms may occur, especially with disc obstruction and protracted anterior functional dislocation as different mandibular movements are examined. These different movements are not identical, and the conditions that cause discal obstruction may vary. This applies especially to the significant difference that exists between empty-mouth movements and power strokes.

Radiographic confirmation of intracapsular restriction of movement is accurate. Such confirmation is done by comparing the restricted condylar positions in open and lateral views with the closed-joint position. The location of the condyle in open and lateral positions nearly superimpose, and both remain fairly close to the closed position (Fig 5–11).

Interference During Movement

Normally, movements of the disc-condyle complex along the articular eminence take place without any interference that would cause abnormal sensations, noises, movements, deviations of the midline incisal path, or pain. Interference between the disc-condyle complex and the temporal articular surface presents clearly identifiable clinical evidence, namely:

1. Abnormal sensations that can be felt, such as sticking, rubbing, slipping, binding, or catching sensations.

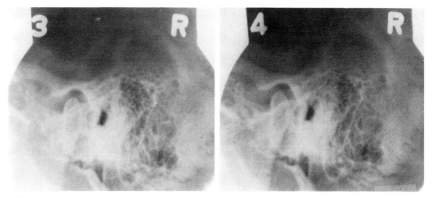

FIGURE 5–11 Radiographs of right temporomandibular joint illustrate intracapsular restriction of mandibular movement. *Left,* lateral excursion to the opposite side. *Right,* maximum opening. Note that condylar movement in lateral excursion remains close to the closed position of the joint. The restriction in maximum opening is exactly the same. (From Bell W.E.: *Orofacial Pains: Differential Diagnosis,* ed. 2. Chicago, Year Book Medical Publishers, 1979. Reproduced with permission.)

2. Abnormal sounds that can be heard, such as clicking, popping, snapping, and grating noises.

3. Abnormal movements that can be seen, such as jerky or irregular movement or deviation of the midline incisal path.

4. Pain, if any, related temporally to the interference—either just prior to, with, or immediately following such interference.

Interference during mandibular movement is identified by various combinations of these symptoms as they relate to each other. *They should be considered together, not as isolated symptoms.* Good clinical evaluation of joint function requires that the interference responsible for such abnormal sensations, sounds, and movements be identified correctly. It is not enough just to recognize them; it is necessary to relate them to the functional abnormality that provokes them.

Although translatory cyclic movements of the disc-condyle complex are quite similar, whether they are for opening, protrusion, or lateral excursion, they are not necessarily identical. Likewise, symptoms of interference are not necessarily identical in the different jaw movements. Consideration should be given to interference behavior relative to lateral excursion to the opposite side. In lateral excursion the nonworking condyle follows a path of movement that is not straight forward, but moves medially. This movement is influenced by (1) the opposite joint (due to the effect of pivoting, restraint by the temporomandibular ligament, and sideways shift) and (2) the shape of the medial aspect of the articular eminence surface over which the translating disc-condyle complex moves. The difference between opening and lateral excursive movement, even in empty-mouth efforts, causes a difference in interference behavior also. These considerations should be kept in mind when comparing evidence of interference during the various movements of the mandible.

It should be noted that deviation of the midline incisal path during opening and closing is different from deflection, as described above. Deviation is thought to occur as a neuromuscular pattern that develops in response to interference during mandibular movement. It may be considered a kind of compensatory mechanism for abnormality in the functioning of the disc-condyle complex. Deviation is discursive movement from the normal straight-line opening that returns again to the normal centered position.

Interference during mandibular movement should be considered according to how it relates to the translatory cycle.

Interference During Maximum Intercuspation.   Normally, intercuspation of the teeth and resumption of a resting closed-joint position is wholly free of symptoms because the act of clenching the teeth should embody no strain on, or gross movement of, the articulating parts. It should consist only of a momentary increase in interarticular pressure as power is delivered by contraction of elevator muscles to bring the teeth into their fully occluded relationship.

But, if functional harmony is lacking between the muscle position of the joint (unclenched closed relationship) and the tooth form position (maximum intercuspation), the act of clenching the teeth causes movement between the disc-condyle complex and the articular eminence. As interarticular pressure increases due to elevator muscle action, such movement may exhaust weeping lubrication and induce friction, which tends to immobilize the articular disc against the eminence. Complications that develop depend on such factors as the inclination of the articular eminence, the force of the clenching effort, and the direction of movement so induced. As a result, frictional abuse may lead to deleterious change in the articular disc and the osseous-supported articular surface.

The clinical symptoms of interference of this type consist of:

1. A momentary sensation of stress or movement as the teeth are firmly clenched.

2. Discal noise, which may be heard as the teeth are brought into maximum intercuspation or immediately as biting force is released.

3. Pain, if any, is a momentary disc-attachment arthralgic pain that occurs with maximum intercuspation. All the symptoms are prevented by biting against a tongue blade ipsilaterally.

Radiographic confirmation is available if the occlusal disharmony is sufficiently great to cause radiographically visible displacement of the condyle from unclenched to clenched occluded position and if such displacement takes place in the sagittal plane (Figs 5–12, 5–13).

Interference Following Maximum Intercuspation. After the teeth are brought into maximum intercuspation, the elevators and superior lateral pterygoid muscles normally relax back to a state of muscle tonus, thus permitting the joint to resume its resting closed position. When this takes place, the interarticular pressure returns to empty-mouth level, the articular disc space widens slightly, the superior lateral pterygoid muscle (by muscle tonus) rotates the articular disc anteriorly

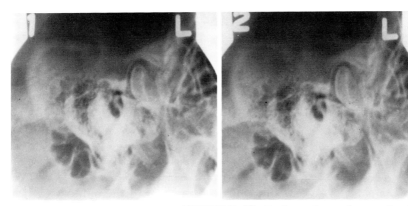

Left T-M Joint

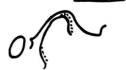

FIGURE 5–12 Radiography confirms occlusal disharmony sufficient to displace condyle anteriorly when the teeth are clenched. *Top,* radiographs of left temporomandibular joint in unclenched closed position *(left)* and clenched occluded position *(right).* *Bottom,* tracings made from these films show condylar position in unclenched closed position as a *solid line,* in clenched occluded position as a *broken line.* Note that clenched occluded position is slightly anterior to the unclenched closed position. (From Bell W.E.: *Orofacial Pains: Differential Diagnosis,* ed. 2. Chicago, Year Book Medical Publishers, 1979. Reproduced by permission.)

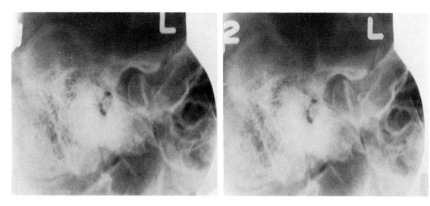

Left T-M Joint

FIGURE 5–13 Radiography confirms occlusal disharmony sufficient to displace condyle posteriorly when the teeth are clenched. *Top,* radiographs of left temporomandibular joint in unclenched closed position *(left)* and clenched occluded position *(right.) Bottom,* tracings made from these films show condylar position in unclenched closed position as a *solid line,* in clenched occluded position as a *broken line.* Note that the clenched occluded position is slightly posterior to the unclenched closed position. (From Bell W.E.: *Orofacial Pains: Differential Diagnosis,* ed. 2. Chicago, Year Book Medical Publishers, 1979. Reproduced with permission.

to properly fill the widened disc space, and synovial fluid lubricates the joint surfaces. Thus, the joint is prepared for the next translatory cycle.

If, however, there is sufficient deterioration of the articular surfaces, this normal sequence may be interfered with. Maximum intercuspation may cause the articular disc to stick to the temporal surface. In that case, the following translatory cycle cannot begin from the lubricated resting closed position. Instead, as the condyle moves forward, the discal collateral ligaments pull the disc free, thus emitting noise as it is suddenly replaced in position. Once this occurs, the disc-condyle complex completes a normal translatory cycle.

The chief cause of this type of interference is alteration in the articular surfaces at the closed-joint position. Several etiologic factors can cause such damage, namely

1. Trauma to the joint sustained when the teeth are in occlusion
2. Habitual hard biting force
3. Bruxism
4. Chronic occlusal disharmony, especially lack of firm molar occlusal contact

Such interference occurs after maximum intercuspation. Ordinarily, the symptoms take place as a new translatory movement is initiated following a biting stroke. They may also follow voluntary clenching of the teeth or bruxing. Or, they may consist of a single incidence of discal noise following a period of inactivity (e.g., first thing in the morning). The symptoms do not occur if the translatory movement begins from the resting closed position. Such interference does not relate so much to protrusive or lateral excursions as to opening the mouth. Although the disc symptoms occur as the translatory cycle begins, the mouth may be opened several millimeters before the noise is heard.

The severity of the deterioration in the articular surfaces in the closed position has considerable bearing on the symptoms produced. If such change is minor, it may require vigorous maximum intercuspation to induce interference. If the damage is greater, less vigorous intercuspation of the teeth is required to initiate the symptoms.

The clinical symptoms of interference that occur just as the translatory cycle begins (following maximum intercuspation, voluntary clenching, or after a long period of inactivity) are a sensation of sticking, which is felt as condylar movement begins, followed by a click. It may be associated with momentary pain. Following the initial symptoms, joint functioning appears to be normal.

The symptoms are prevented by an occlusal stop that increases vertical dimension or slightly protrudes the mandible, which prevents the condyle from returning to the closed position.

Interference During Normal Translatory Cycle. If there is structural compatibility between the moving parts and if there is normal interarticular pressure, empty-mouth translatory cycles and power strokes are smooth and relatively silent. The inclination of the articular eminence bears importantly on joint function. Any discrepancy assumes greater significance in steeply inclined joints.

Interference that occurs during normal translatory cycles and power strokes stems from a variety of causes, some of minor significance, some constituting calamitous conditions of the joint. The causes may be grouped under three main headings, namely,

1. Excessive passive interarticular pressure
2. Structural incompatibility between the sliding parts
3. Impairment of disc-condyle complex function

Excessive passive interarticular pressure predisposes to interference during sliding and, therefore, may activate an otherwise nonsymptomatic condition into a clinical complaint.

If all conditions of the temporomandibular joint are normal, increased interarticular pressure alone does not induce interference with movement. The joints are constructed to function well under varying degrees of pressure. But, if some abnormality that predisposes to interference is present, increased interarticular pressure may become the *activating factor* that initiates symptoms.

The level of *passive* interarticular pressure, at the resting closed position of the joint and during empty-mouth translatory cycles, depends on *muscle tonus* of elevator masticatory muscles. Such tonus is not constant. It varies especially with emotional tension. During periods of increased emotional stress, the tonicity of elevator muscles increases, thus increasing the passive interarticular pressure within the joints. During such periods, interference may occur as symptoms of discal noise, sensations of interference, or even discomfort. Persons with conditions of this sort have a history of intermittent, recurring episodes of interference that relate to recurring periods of elevated emotional stress. A single emotional crisis can be sufficient to precipitate a symptomatic condition in the absence of a history of any prior occurrence.

Conditions that induce muscle splinting and myospasm activity also increase the passive interarticular pressure within the joints. Changes in the oral environment, sensed as injury or threat of injury, and increased oral consciousness may be answered by muscle splinting. Increased emotional tension may accentuate the problem. Thus, interarticular pressure may be increased sufficiently to activate symptoms of interference. Protracted muscle splinting may develop myospastic activity. Myospasm of elevator masticatory muscles, regardless of cause, predisposes to such interference.

The clinical indications that interference may be due to excessive passive interarticular pressure are:

1. Occurrence of symptoms with or following increased emotional stress or crisis.

2. Sudden onset of symptoms that accompany an acute muscle disorder of the masticatory apparatus.

3. Variability, recurrence, or periodicity in symptom behavior.

Structural incompatibility between the sliding surfaces may cause interference that occurs each time a similar movement is made. Such interference persists and usually becomes gradually worse.

The chronic nature of interference of this kind appears to favor the development of habit patterns of opening and closing that compensate for the interference in the form of deviation of the incisal path. It should be noted, however, that if movements are speeded up, the interference may become more evident. Interference due to structural incompatibility relates not only to the force and speed of movements, but also to the interarticular pressure within the joint.

Some structural incompatibility relates to the inclination of the articular eminence. As has been discussed previously, the steeper the articular eminence, the greater the functional burden placed on the disc-condyle complex to execute translatory cycles smoothly and silently. Extremely steep joints may show evidence of minor interference, especially when movements are rapid or forceful.

Some structural interference may occur as the result of a developmental anomaly, such as a gross malformation, lack of harmony in the size or shape of the sliding parts as they relate to each other and to the opposite joint, and aberrations of growth from any cause. Some structural interference is acquired as the result of trauma. A fairly frequent cause of interference has to do with minor trauma sustained when the jaws are separated, thus causing the damage to occur along the incline of the articular eminence. Interference is noticed when the disc-condyle complex slides over the site of damage during translatory cycles. More severe trauma may lead to hypertrophic growth and other deformation at the site of injury. Some sequelae of trauma are sufficiently great to be visible radiographically.

Structural interference may occur as the result of deleterious change in response to such things as habitual abusive use, mannerisms, and unusual functional conditions imposed on the masticatory apparatus. Most such etiologic factors are obvious, e.g., habitually biting on a pipestem, cigar, pencil, or other object held between the teeth; chewing on fingernails, tooth picks, rubber bands, or bubble gum; and mannerisms involving protrusive or lateral movements due to nervousness, oral consciousness, or dental appliances. Chronic occlusal interference during lateral excursions that cause abnormal movements in the nonworking joint may cause some deterioration. Another cause is restricted translatory movement in the opposite joint. When normal movement is restrained, the act of opening and closing causes the unrestrained condyle to move medially. Such unnatural movement tends to induce deleterious changes in the translating joint, thus leading to functional interference. Another cause of structural disharmony between the sliding articular surfaces is change in the subarticular osseous structure due to degenerative or rheumatoid arthritis.

It should be noted that when the interference is due to structural incompatibility of the sliding surfaces, any decrease in the interarticular pressure decreases the symptoms. This may take place on the biting side during power strokes. *Therefore, patients with this complaint may find themselves doing their hard chewing on the symptomatic side.*

The clinical indications that interference is due to structural incompatibility between the sliding surfaces are:

1. Discrete, precise, and unchanging symptoms that occur with little or no variation as similar movements are executed.

2. Deviations of the incisal path that minimize the interference. (More rapid movements may make the symptoms more evident. Patient is usually unaware of such deviation.)

3. Chronicity, persistence, or resistance to therapy.

4. Decrease in interference by chewing on the symptomatic side.

5. Reciprocal interference symptoms during opening and closing occurring at the same point relative to the translatory cycle; the closing symptoms cannot be varied by altering the timing of biting efforts.

Impaired disc-condyle complex may be expressed as (1) adhesions between the disc and condyle, (2) damage to the articular disc, (3) functional displacement/dislocation of the disc, or (4) dysfunctional superior retrodiscal lamina.

Adhesions between the disc and condyle prevent normal rotatory movements that are essential to the functioning of the temporomandibular joint. This can occur as the result of trauma, surgery, infection, or rheumatoid arthritis. When rotatory movement does not occur, translation of the condyle cannot incorporate smooth gliding action that results from surface-to-surface contact of articular disc with the articular eminence. Rather, the immobilized disc remains in a fixed relationship with the condyle, thus skidding forward with only a portion of the disc in contact with the temporal articular surface. The whole translatory cycle consists of an irregular, noisy, skidding movement forward and backward which predisposes to degenerative arthritis.

The clinical indication of this condition is the presence of symptoms similar to those of joint hypermobility, except that they occur throughout the translatory cycle rather than with extended opening only.

Damage to the articular disc may consist of roughening, thinning, perforation, or fracture. Roughening of the upper surface of the disc causes a grating interference *throughout the translatory cycle;* deterioration of the inferior surface of the disc causes grating noise during *rotatory opening*. Thinning does very little to increase symptoms unless it involves the anterior or posterior areas disproportionately. If a loss of contour occurs in conjunction with elongation of discal ligaments, then thinning anteriorly predisposes to functional displacement of the disc posteriorly during full forward translatory cycles, whereas thinning posteriorly predisposes to anterior functional displacement during power strokes. Perforations of the disc may alter joint function through disruption of normal hydrodynamics of synovial fluid. Fracture of the disc adds little to the symptoms unless the fractured parts are separated or override each other. Both conditions cause acute malocclusion of the ipsilateral posterior teeth, sensed during maximum intercuspation. Separated fragments cause a sensation of overstressed posterior teeth; overriding fragments cause disclusion of the posterior teeth.

Deleterious change in the articular disc occurs as the result of microtraumas from abusive use, structural interference during jaw movements, frictional displacement during maximum intercuspation, and overloading. The most important predisposing factor is chronic occlusal disharmony, and paramount among exciting causes are bruxism and habitual hard chewing. Acute trauma occasionally is a factor. It should be noted that damaged articular discs and dysfunctional discal ligaments are facets of a common problem of functional abuse.

The clinical indications suggestive of a damaged articular disc are:

1. Grating noise throughout the translatory cycle or during restrained rotatory opening movements.

2. Functional displacements of the disc during power strokes and/or full forward translatory movements.

3. Acute malocclusion sensed as overstressed or disoccluded ipsilateral posterior teeth during maximum intercuspation.

All stresses that tend to displace the disc from the condyle are brought to bear on the discal ligaments. This includes the conditions that cause deleterious changes in the disc proper, namely, abusive use, structural interference during jaw movements, frictional displacement during maximum intercuspation, and overloading. Occlusal disharmony, accentuated especially by habitual hard chewing and bruxism, is the chief condition responsible for deleterious changes in the ligaments. Acute trauma may be a factor.

Resultant damage to the discal ligaments may consist of elongation, structural change that renders them less effective as ligamentous structures, or actual detachment from the condyle. Although such change almost invariably affects both ligaments to some degree, the extent may be disproportionate between the two, usually affecting the lateral ligament more. All such damage seriously disrupts functioning and is irreversible.

It should be noted that these ligaments, like all true ligaments, are composed of nonelastic collagenous tissue. Under stress, they do not stretch. When stress is excessive over a period of time, they may lengthen *permanently*. Such elongation permits sliding movement between the disc and condyle, depending on the extent of elongation and the loss of disc contour. The disc may be displaced posteriorly by traction of the superior retrodiscal lamina during forward phases of the translatory cycle. It may be displaced anteriorly by contraction of the superior lateral pterygoid muscle during power strokes and maximum intercuspation.

It should be noted that, in most functional displacements of the articular disc, dislocation of the disc in front of the condyle does not take place. Although displacement consists of linear sliding movement between the disc and condyle, the disc continues to remain in contact between the condylar and temporal articular surfaces, thus preventing collapse of the articular disc space and entrapment. The interference symptoms therefore consist of obstruction of movement during the translatory cycle, and are frequently reciprocal. This differs from the reciprocal symptoms induced by incompatibility of the sliding surfaces, however, in that with functional displacement the closing symptoms usually occur at a different point relative to the translatory cycle from that of the opening symptoms. Also, the timing of the closing symptoms can be altered by manipulating the functional demands. This is due to the fact that the displacement of the disc during closing that causes the reciprocal obstruction is induced by contraction of the superior lateral pterygoid muscle, which can be altered by different biting efforts. It should be noted that the symptoms of disc displacement are discrete—definite clicking noise, catching sensations, momentary locking, or hard locking. These symptoms are usually accentuated by chewing on the symptomatic side.

Functional anterior dislocation is different. It may occur (1) when the loss of contour is sufficient to permit the disc to be pulled through the articular disc space, (2) when the discal collateral ligaments are sufficiently elongated to permit such gross displacement, *and* (3) when the inferior retrodiscal lamina is no longer functional. The actual dislocation usually occurs during a power stroke or clenching as a result of strong contraction of the superior lateral pterygoid muscle. This is especially so if the biting is on the symptomatic side. With dislocation the disc space collapses, and the disc is trapped in front of the condyle. Reduction is accomplished only by action of the superior retrodiscal lamina during a full forward translatory movement of the condyle. It should be noted that if the entrapped disc blocks normal condylar movement, reduction is impossible. The symptoms of anterior functional dislocation of the articular disc are quite different from those of displacement, namely:

1. No discrete symptoms of any kind. If locking occurs, it is "soft" and near full opening.

2. Irregular translatory movements.

3. Variable degree of retrodiscitis.

4. Sensation of overstressed ipsilateral posterior teeth when clenched.

A dysfunctional superior retrodiscal lamina may cause noisy, irregular movements during the forward phase of the translatory cycle. The danger of spontaneous anterior dislocation is increased. Traumatic severance from the articular disc renders any anterior displacement or dislocation of the disc permanent, because it is the only joint structure capable of effecting a reduction.

Interference Due to Hypermobility.   Smooth, relatively silent sliding movement in the TM joint depends on normal rotation of the articular disc on the condyle to maintain surface-to-surface contact between the sliding parts. Wide opening entails posterior rotation of the disc. When the combined posterior rotatory movement from opening and translation reaches the limit imposed by the posterior border of the condylar articular facet, further rotatory movement is arrested. Then, extended opening of the mouth exceeds normal translatory movement. When mouth-opening exceeds this limit, it takes place without benefit of continuous surface contact of the sliding parts. The disc-condyle complex skids along the anterior slope of the articular eminence with only its posterior border in contact (see Fig 4–7). This partial dislocation (subluxation) induces clinical symptoms, consisting of an initial pause, then a sudden jumping forward of the condyle, accompanied by noise and sometimes discomfort. This condition is referred to as joint hypermobility.

The etiology of such interference is habitual overextension of opening beyond normal limits. It does not usually occur with protrusive or lateral movements. It is more likely to occur with very steep joints. Hypermobility predisposes to spontaneous anterior dislocation.

The clinical symptoms of interference of this kind include the following:

1. As the mouth is opened fully, a momentary pause is followed by the condyle skidding forward to its full anterior limit.

2. This jerky movement of the condyle is accompanied by noise and sometimes minor discomfort.

3. These symptoms do not take place with protrusive or lateral excursive movements unless the mouth is opened also.

Interference Due to Spontaneous Dislocation.   When the mouth is opened widely, the disc-condyle complex is situated at the full forward position of the translatory cycle with the disc rotated posteriorly by the stretched superior retrodiscal lamina. At this critical moment when forward condylar movement is arrested by the taut posterior capsular ligament, further effort to open the mouth or any *premature* contraction of the superior lateral pterygoid muscle may result in spontaneous anterior dislocation of the disc (see Fig 7–1).

The clinical symptoms of spontaneous anterior dislocation are:

1. Inability to close the mouth after an overextended opening. As the posterior teeth (or edentulous ridges) come into contact, the anteriors remain widely apart.

2. Discomfort, if any, due to an attempt to force a closure of the mouth.

Acute Malocclusion

Another symptom of masticatory dysfunction is acute malocclusion—that which occurs suddenly in conjunction with other evidence of dysfunction and about which the subject is fully aware. Such malocclusion is sensed subjectively as a change in the way the teeth occlude. It usually is accompanied by some discomfort when the teeth are brought forcefully into maximum intercuspation. Such discomfort usually is reduced by biting against a tongue blade that prevents bringing the teeth into their fully occluded relationship.

Acute malocclusion may be induced (1) by muscle action or (2) by a change in the relationship of the disc-condyle complex to the articular eminence.

Muscle-Induced Malocclusion.   Most muscle-induced acute malocclusion results from spasm of the lateral pterygoid muscle. The condyle is drawn forward on the affected side, thus causing disclusion of the posterior teeth and premature contact of the anteriors contralaterally. This condition can be confirmed radiographically by comparing the unclenched closed position with the clenched position. The condyle is displaced anteriorly in the resting closed position (Fig 5–14).

Myospasm involving elevator muscles may induce acute malocclusion of a less dramatic type. Such may be evident only subjectively. Spasm of the masseter muscle tends to displace the mandible laterally; spasm of the medial pterygoid displaces it medially.

Joint-Induced Malocclusion.   A change in the relationship of the disc-condyle complex with the articular eminence causes acute malocclusion. This may occur as the result of gross trauma to, or rapid deterioration of, the osseous surfaces (Figs 5–15 and 5–16), overriding or separation of the parts of a fractured articular disc, dislocation of the disc from the condyle, swelling of the retrodiscal tissue, or accumulation of excessive fluid within the joint cavity from inflammatory effusion or hemarthrosis (Fig 5–17). It may occur iatrogenically as a result of local anesthesia of the joint or the injection of a solution into the joint cavity.

The clinical indications suggestive of acute (symptomatic) malocclusion that may be a symptom of masticatory dysfunction are:

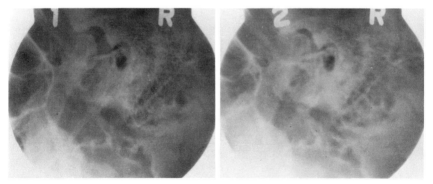

FIGURE 5–14   Radiographs of right temporomandibular joint illustrate muscle-induced acute malocclusion caused by myospastic activity in the right lateral pterygoid muscle. *Left,* unclenched closed position; *right,* clenched occluded position. Note that the unclenched closed position is anteriorly displaced by contraction of the right lateral pterygoid muscle. Maximum intercuspation forces condyle posteriorly into its usual occluded relationship.

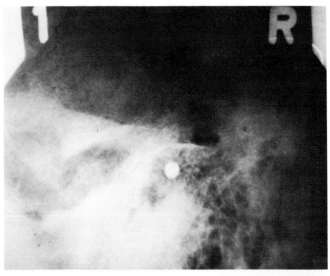

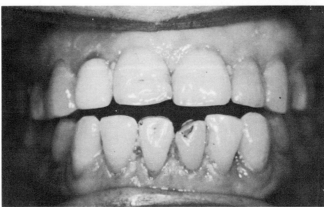

FIGURE 5–15   Illustration of joint-induced acute malocclusion caused by rapid resorption of condylar osseous structure from rheumatoid arthritis. *Top,* radiograph of temporomandibular joint showing bizarre osseous resorption that reduces vertical height of mandibular ramus. (From Bell W.E.: *Orofacial Pains: Differential Diagnosis,* ed. 3. Chicago, Year Book Medical Publishers, 1985. Reproduced by permission.) *Bottom,* photograph of resulting progressive anterior open-bite. (From Bell W.E.: Management of temporomandibular problems, in Goldman H.M., Gilmore H.W., Royer R.Q., et al. (eds.): *Current Therapy in Dentistry.* St. Louis, C.V. Mosby Co., 1970, vol. 4. Reproduced with permission.)

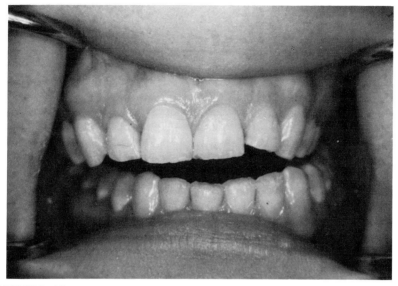

FIGURE 5–16 Acute malocclusion due to rheumatoid arthritis in a 24-year-old woman. Anterior open-bite was rapidly progressive.

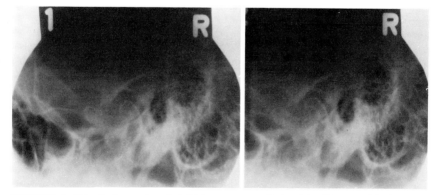

FIGURE 5–17 Radiographs of right temporomandibular joint illustrate joint-induced acute malocclusion caused by inflammatory effusion of fluid within the joint cavity. *Left,* unclenched closed position; *Right,* clenched occluded position. Note that unclenched closed position is inferiorly displaced by the presence of excessive intracapsular fluid. Maximum intercuspation forces the condyle superiorly into the usual occluded relationship.

1. Recent obvious change in the occlusion, of which the patient is aware and about which he complains.

2. Such altered occlusion occurring in conjunction with other evidence of masticatory dysfunction or pain.

3. Accompanying pain increasing with maximum intercuspation and decreasing by biting against a separator ipsilaterally.

REFERENCES

1. Ricketts R.M.: Laminography in the diagnosis of temporomandibular disorders. *J. Am. Dent. Assoc.* 46:620, 1953.
2. Enlow D.H.: Role of the TMJ in facial growth and development, in *The President's Conference on the Examination, Diagnosis and Management of Temporomandibular Disorders.* Chicago, American Dental Association, 1983, pp. 13–16.
3. Dumas A.L., Neff P., Moaddab M.B., et al.: A combined tomographic-cephalometric analysis of the TMJ. *J. Craniomand. Pract.* 1(3):23, 1983.
4. Weinberg L.A.: Role of condylar position in TMJ dysfunction-pain syndrome. *J. Prosthet. Dent.* 41:636, 1979.
5. Blaschke D.D., Blaschke T.J.: Normal TMJ bony relationships in centric occlusion. *J. Dent. Res.* 60:98, 1981.
6. Rey R., Valero J.: TMJ radiograph of subjects with/without dysfunction in Mexican population. *J. Dent. Res.* 61 (Special issue) Abst. No. 232, 1982.
7. Katzberg R.W., Keith D.A., Ten Eick W.R., et al.: Internal derangements of the temporomandibular joint: An assessment of condylar position in centric occlusion. *J. Prosthet. Dent.* 49:250, 1983.
8. Aquilino S.A., Matteson S.R., Holland G.A., et al.: Evaluation of condylar position from temporomandibular joint radiographs. *J. Prosthet. Dent.* 53:88–97, 1985.
9. Pullinger A.G., Hollender T., Solberg W.K., et al.: A tomographic study of mandibular condyle position in an asymptomatic population. *J. Prosthet. Dent.* 53:706–713, 1985.
10. Troendle R., Troendle K., Rugh J.D.: Electromyographic and phonetic rest position changes with head posture. *J. Dent. Res.* 59:494 (Special issue A), 1980.
11. Rocabado M., Johnston B.E. Jr., Blakney M.G.: Physical therapy and dentistry: An overview. *J. Craniomand. Pract.* 1(1):47, 1982.
12. Mohl N.D.: The role of head posture in mandibular function, in Solberg W.K., Clark G.T. (eds.): *Abnormal Jaw Mechanics.* Chicago, Quintessence Publishing Co., 1984, pp. 97–116.
13. Hairston L.E., Blanton P.L.: An electromyographic study of mandibular position in response to changes in body position. *J. Prosthet. Dent.* 49:271, 1983.

14. Alexander P.C.: Movements of the condyle from rest position to initial contact and full occlusion. *J. Am. Dent. Assoc.* 45:284, 1952.
15. Nevakari K.: An analysis of the mandibular movement from rest to occlusal position. *Acta Odontol. Scand.* 14 [suppl. 19]:1, 1956.
16. Jemt T.: Positions of the mandible during chewing and swallowing recorded by light-emitting diodes. *J. Prosthet. Dent.* 48:206, 1982.
17. Faulkner K.D.B., Atkinson H.F.: An analysis of tooth position on initial tooth contact. *J. Oral Rehabil.* 10:257, 1983.
18. Suit S.R., Gibbs C.H., Benz S.T.: Study of gliding tooth contacts during mastication. *J. Periodontol.* 47:331, 1975.
19. Ramfjord S.P.: Goals for an ideal occlusion and mandibular position, in Solberg W.K., Clark G.T. (eds.): *Abnormal Jaw Mechanics.* Chicago, Quintessence Publishing Co., 1984, pp. 77–95.
20. Mohamed S.E., Christensen L.V., Harrison J.D.: Tooth contact patterns and contractile activity of the elevator jaw muscles during mastication of two different types of food. *J. Oral Rehabil.* 10:87, 1983.
21. DuBrul E.L.: The biomechanics of the oral apparatus. Chapter IV. Postures and movement, in DuBrul E.L., Menekratis A.: *The Physiology of Oral Reconstruction.* Chicago, Quintessence Publishing Co., 1981, pp. 39–53.
22. Sicher H.: Positions and movements of the mandible. *J. Am. Dent. Assoc.* 48:620, 1954.
23. Graham M.M., Buxbaum J., Staling L.M.: A study of occlusal relationships and the incidence of myofascial pain. *J. Prosthet. Dent.* 47:549, 1982.
24. Farrar W.B., McCarty W.L.: *A Clinical Outline of Temporomandibular Joint Diagnosis and Treatment.* Montgomery, Ala., Normandie Publications, 1982.
25. Mongini F.: Abnormalities in condylar and occlusal positions, in Solberg W.K., Clark G.T. (eds.): *Abnormal Jaw Mechanics.* Chicago, Quintessence Publishing Co., 1984, pp. 23–50.
26. Gilboe D.B.: Centric relation as the treatment position. *J. Prosthet. Dent.* 50:685, 1983.
27. Sheppard S.M.: Asymptomatic morphologic variations in the mandibular condyle-ramus region. *J. Prosthet. Dent.* 47:539, 1982.
28. Gelb H., Bernstein I.: Clinical evaluation of two hundred patients with temporomandibular joint syndrome. *J. Prosthet. Dent.* 49:234, 1983.
29. Agerberg G., Carlsson G.E.: Functional disorders of the masticatory system. 1. Distribution of symptoms according to age and sex as judged from investigation by questionnaire. *Acta Odontol. Scand.* 30:597, 1972.
30. Helkimo M.: Studies on function and dysfunction of the masticatory system. IV. Age and sex distribution of symptoms of dysfunction of the masticatory system in Lapps in the north of Finland. *Acta Odontol. Scand.* 32:255, 1974.
31. Rieder C.E., Martinoff J.T., Wilcox S.H.: The prevalence of mandibular dysfunction. Part I: Sex and age distribution of related signs and symptoms. *J. Prosthet. Dent.* 50:81, 1983.
32. Rieder C.E., Martinoff J.T.: The prevalence of mandibular dysfunction. Part II: A multiphasic dysfunction profile. *J. Prosthet. Dent.* 50:237, 1983.

33. Hansson T., Solberg W.K., Penn M.K., et al.: Anatomic study of the TMJs of young adults: A pilot investigation. *J. Prosthet. Dent.* 41:556, 1979.

34. Hansson T.L., Solberg W.K., Penn M.K.: Temporomandibular joint changes in young adults. *J. Dent. Res.* 58 (Special issue A):267, 1979.

35. Castelli W.A., Nasjleti C.E., Diaz-Perez R., et al.: Histopathologic findings in temporomandibular joints of aged individuals. *J. Prosthet. Dent.* 53:415–419, 1985.

36. Rohlin M., Westesson P., Eriksson L.: The correlation of temporomandibular joint sounds with joint morphology in fifty-five autopsy specimens. *J. Oral Maxillofac. Surg.* 43:194–200, 1985.

37. Hellsing G., Holmlund A.: Development of anterior disk displacement in the temporomandibular joint: An autopsy study. *J. Prosthet. Dent.* 53:397–401, 1985.

38. Isberg-Holm A.M., Westesson P.L.: Movement of disc and condyle in temporomandibular joints with clicking. An arthrographic and cineradiographic study on autopsy specimens. *Acta Odontol. Scand.* 40:151, 1982.

39. Solberg W.K., Woo M., Houston J.: Prevalence of signs and symptoms of mandibular dysfunction. *J. Dent. Res.* 54 (Special issue A): abstract No. 432, Feb. 1975.

40. Gross A., Gale E.N.: A prevalence study of the clinical signs associated with mandibular dysfunction. *J. Am. Dent. Assoc.* 107:932, 1983.

41. Bush F.M., Butler J.H., Abbott D.M.: The relationship of TMJ clicking to palpable facial pain. *J. Craniomand. Pract.* 1(4):43, 1983.

42. Farrar W.B., McCarty W.L.: The TMJ dilemma. *J. Ala. Dent. Assoc.* 63:19, 1979.

43. Greene C.S., Turner C., Laskin D.M.: Mandibular dysfunction symptoms in a random population. *J. Dent. Res.* 62 (special issue) Abst. No. 1218, 1983.

44. Westesson P.: Double contrast arthrography and internal derangement of the temporomandibular joint. *Swed. Dent. J.* Supplement 13, 1982.

45. Solberg W., Hansson T., Nordstrom B.: Morphologic evaluation of young adult TMJs at autopsy. *J. Dent. Res.* 63:228, Abst. No 518, 1984.

46. Marciani R.D., Haley J.V., Roth G.I.: Facial pain complaints in the elderly. *J. Oral Maxillofac. Surg.* 43:173–176, 1985.

47. Solberg W.K.: Epidemiology, incidence and prevalence of temporomandibular disorders: A review, in *The President's Conference on the Examination, Diagnosis and Management of Temporomandibular Disorders.* Chicago, American Dental Association, 1983, pp. 30–39.

48. Greene C.S., Marbach J.J.: Epidemiologic studies of mandibular dysfunction: A critical review. *J. Prosthet. Dent.* 48:184, 1982.

49. Bell W.E.: *Temporomandibular Joint Disease.* Dallas, Egan Press, 1960.

50. Hall M.B., Gibbs C.H., Sclar A.G.: Association between the prominence of the articular eminence and displaced TMJ disks. *J. Craniomand. Pract.* 3:238–239, 1985.

51. Ingervall B.: Relationship between height of the articular eminence of the

temporomandibular joint and facial morphology. *Angle Orthod.* 44:15, 1974.

52. Dubner R., Sessle B.J., Storey A.T.: *The Neural Basis of Oral and Facial Function.* New York, Plenum Publishing Corp., 1979.
53. Westesson P.: Cineradiographic, arthrographic and high-speed cinematographic analysis of the mechanics of clicking temporomandibular joints, in Moffett B.C. (ed.): *Diagnosis of Internal Derangements of the Temporomandibular Joint,* Vol. 1. Seattle, University of Washington, 1984, pp. 35–41.
54. Bell W.E.: *Orofacial Pains,* ed. 3. Chicago, Year Book Medical Publishers, 1985.
55. Melzack R., Wall P.D.: Pain mechanisms: A new theory. *Science* 150:971, 1965.
56. Wall P.D.: The gate control theory of pain mechanisms: A reexamination and restatement. *Brain* 101:1, 1978.
57. Kane K., Taub A.: A history of local electrical analgesia. *Pain* 1:125, 1975.
58. Long D.M., Hagfors N.: Electrical stimulation in the nervous system: The current status of electrical stimulation of the nervous system for relief of pain. *Pain* 1:109, 1975.
59. Sternbach R.H., Ignelzi R.J., Deems L.M., et al.: Transcutaneous electrical analgesia: A follow-up analysis. *Pain* 2:34, 1976.
60. Jessell T.M., Iverson L.L.: Opiate analgesics inhibit substance P release from rat trigeminal nucleus. *Nature* 268:549, 1977.
61. Beecher H.K.: The use of chemical agents in the control of pain, in Knighton R.S., Dumke P.R. (eds.): *Pain.* Boston, Little, Brown & Co., 1966, pp. 221–239.
62. Almay B.G.L., Johansson F., Von Knorring L., et al.: Endorphins in chronic pain: I. Differences in CSF endorphin levels between organic and psychogenic pain syndromes. *Pain* 5:153, 1978.
63. Terenius L.: Endorphins in chronic pain, in Bonica J.J., Liebeskind J.C., Albe-Fessard D.G. (eds.): *Advances in Pain Research and Therapy,* Vol. 3. New York, Raven Press, 1979, pp. 459–471.
64. Sjolund B.H., Ericksson M.B.E.: Electroacupuncture and endogenous morphine. *Lancet* 2:1085, 1976.
65. Pomerantz B., Cheng R.: Suppression of noxious impulses in single neurons of cat spinal cord by electroacupuncture and its reversal by opiate antagonist naloxone. *Exp. Neurol.* 64:327, 1979.
66. Sjolund B.H., Ericksson M.B.E.: Endorphins and analgesia produced by peripheral conditioning stimulation, in Bonica J.J., Liebeskind J.C., Albe-Fessard D.G. (eds.): *Advances in Pain Research and Therapy,* Vol. 3. New York, Raven Press, 1979, pp. 587–592.
67. Dalessio D.J.: *Wolff's Headache and Other Head Pain,* ed. 3. New York, Oxford University Press, 1972.
68. Travell J.G., Simons D.G.: *Myofascial Pain and Dysfunction.* Baltimore, Williams & Wilkins Co., 1983.
69. Westesson P.: Clinical and arthrographic findings in patients with TMJ

disorders, in Moffett B.C. (ed.): *Diagnosis of Internal Derangements of the Temporomandibular Joint,* Vol. 1. Seattle, University of Washington, 1984, pp. 59–71.

70. Rusconi L., Brusati R.: Restricted opening of the mouth from symmetrical bilateral hyperplasia of the coronoid process. *J. Oral Surg.* 32:452–456, 1974.

71. Praal F.R.: Limitation of mandibular movement due to bilateral mandibular coronoid process enlargement. *J. Oral Maxillofac. Surg.* 42:534, 1984.

72. Farrar W.B.: Diagnosis and treatment of anterior dislocation of the articular disc. *N.Y. J. Dent.* 41:348, 1971.

73. Shira R.B., Alling C.C.: Traumatic injuries involving the temporomandibular joint articulation, in Schwartz L.L., Chayes C.M. (eds.): *Facial Pain and Mandibular Dysfunction.* Philadelphia, W.B. Saunders Co., 1968, pp. 129–139.

6 | Etiology

The musculature, ligaments, and articular structures of synovial joints, like many other body tissues, may react either physiologically or pathologically to altered functional conditions. Many times, it is difficult to identify such conditions clinically. For example, joints being driven by muscle action are normally under muscular control that is constantly monitored by a proprioceptive and sensory feedback mechanism. Thus, altered functional demands are answered by appropriate muscle action in α motor neurons initiated by the CNS. Some alterations in afferent input initiate a protective response that is clinically discernible as so-called muscle splinting. Yet, the step from splinting to myospastic activity may be a subtle one in which there may be little or no change in afferent input. And, again, the step from myospasm to an inflammatory condition of the muscle may occur without appreciable change in cause.

Likewise, the tissues of the joint proper normally react to functional demands by both atrophic and hypertrophic changes. Increased loading normally is answered by remodeling processes whereby joint morphology is harmonized to function physiologically with the biomechanical forces that act on the articular surfaces. This constitutes adaptation of form to function. Yet, the step from remodeling to degenerative change may be very subtle, in which no appreciable change in loading is discernible.

Consideration of etiologic agents therefore becomes a complex matter of judgment between numerous factors, many of which fall within the category of normal joint function. Conditions which shift normal physiologic response to the abnormal pathologic type may rest upon such factors as the inherent constitutional make-up of the indi-

155

vidual person and his structural components. It may relate to the duration and timing of the functional demands. It may be in response to psychologic influences, emotional stress, or tension—determinants that we are just beginning to understand, if, indeed, we understand them at all. For example, it has been determined that EMG activity in the resting temporalis muscle is reduced appreciably simply by closing the eyes.[1] Sex may be an important determinant in TM disorders. Gerschman et al.[2] found that, in 40,000 orofacial pain patients, 76% were women. It is well known that clinicians everywhere report that patients who seek treatment for TM disorders are predominantly female. Even the effect of direct external trauma may be modulated by systemic and constitutional factors. Seldom, if ever, should one look for a single isolated etiologic agent. In a general way one should think in terms of predisposing conditions, activating factors, and perpetuating influences.

GENERAL PRINCIPLES OF ETIOLOGY

Although it is impossible to separate the joint proper functionally from its power supply, the musculature, for purposes of analysis and description it is helpful to consider them as separate entities. Etiologically, we can think in terms of muscle effects and joint effects.

Muscle Effects

Conditions that alter muscle action predominate as etiologic agents in the extra-articular TM disorders. These conditions have to do with afferent neural input that supplies information needed to properly coordinate joint movements. Altered proprioceptive and sensory input may be recent and acute, or it may be more persistent and chronic. The resultant effects are not the same.

Altered Patterns of Movement. It is now well established that long-term altered input which informs the CNS concerning the conditions that prevail induces marked change in muscle action. When function is arrested, atrophic change in the muscle begins almost immediately. If such restriction of movement prevents normal stretching of the muscle, the elimination of the inverse stretch reflex may induce myostatic contracture of the muscle and thus reduce its resting length. Conversely, increased muscle function, especially isometric exercise, tends to build up muscle tissue.

Unless volition is imposed, chewing movements normally follow deeply engrained patterns of behavior which are CNS generated. It is thought that the basic cyclic design of chewing muscle action is derived reflexly from a central neural pattern generator located in the brain stem.[3] Although this central generator can function independently of sensory feedback, Sessle[4] has shown that marked variability in chewing movements occurs in response to sensory input from peripheral receptors and in response to influences from the higher centers involved in volitional behavior. Chewing patterns also are altered by the consistency of the foodstuff being masticated.[5] It is confirmed that occlusal alterations can modify chewing patterns, and avoidance reflexes are known to protect sensitive teeth.[3] Increased vertical dimension of occlusion that alters the resting length of elevator muscles is rapidly adjusted to.[6]

Long-term altered afferent input tends to induce changes in the chewing pattern that satisfactorily compensate for such input. If the muscles are able to adapt, clinical symptoms as such usually do not occur; altered patterns of movement may develop instead. Thus, we may see deviations of the midline incisal path induced by proprioceptive input from the joints and muscles. We may see unusual patterns of closure and occlusal positions develop in response to occlusal interferences. When any such alteration in habitual movement is recognized, it should be evident that the condition that produced it has been there a long time, and that, if change is occurring at all, it is doing so very slowly. Recent, variable, and rapidly changing conditions do not produce such effects; muscle splinting occurs instead.

Muscle Splinting Effects. Recent, sudden alteration of afferent input is nearly always answered in the same way—by so-called muscle splinting. This is characterized by pain that is elicited when the muscle is contracted. It is usually accompanied by a sensation of muscular weakness. Pain alone reduces biting force from 30% to 50%.[7] Thus, normal function is inhibited, presumably as a protective mechanism. Although muscle hypertonicity is present and some resistance to stretch may be displayed, there is no significant increase in EMG activity. Splinting, however, may develop into myospastic activity which does show a marked increase in EMG activity.[8]

Several different conditions tend to produce this effect, namely:

1. Altered proprioceptive and/or sensory input from the joint ligaments, muscles, periodontal mechanoreceptors, and other oral structures from functional activities.

2. Oral consciousness (awareness of masticatory functioning) which provokes voluntary chewing movements that may override normal habitual jaw movements.

3. Emotional tension, illness, and other systemic conditions.

4. Fatigue, strain, trauma, and nearby inflammatory conditions.

5. Dental treatment, local anesthesia, and iatrogenic alterations in occlusal function.

Delayed Local Muscle Soreness.   Unaccustomed use of a muscle may cause localized soreness that is felt the next day and may persist for a while. This effect is different from muscle splinting, which displays no discomfort in the resting state of the muscle. Such delayed soreness has been poorly understood. It has been attributed to the accumulation of metabolites, even though nociceptive impulses are not generated in the absence of algogenic substances such as bradykinin.[9, 10] Nor is the pain explained on the basis of ischemia.[11] No histologically identifiable inflammatory change is evident. Recent histochemical and electron microscopy research into this enigmatic problem, however, has revealed that, even though there is no evidence of ischemic necrosis or actual fiber rupture, there is some unmistakable mechanical disruption in the ultrastructure of the muscle fibers.[12] Whether this change is a primary one or secondary to some other unidentified factor has not been decided, but it does represent a new concept in muscle behavior. Its true significance is not yet understood.

Effect of Deep Pain Input.   Deep pain input may induce, as a central excitatory effect, either a myofascial trigger-point mechanism or myospastic activity. Such a myofascial trigger does not display appreciable muscular dysfunction or show increased EMG activity in the involved muscle.[13] Symptoms from such a trigger point are expressed primarily as referred pains. A pain-induced myospasm, however, displays clinically evident muscular dysfunction and elicits pain when the muscle is stretched or contracted. It is characterized by a marked increase in EMG activity.[8] Such a cycling painful myospasm may initiate other central excitatory effects.

Effect of Phenothiazine Medication.   The extrapyramidal action of the phenothiazines may induce muscle symptoms such as dyskinesia and myospastic activity, especially in the facial and masticatory muscles.[14] Prolonged medication has caused irreversible rhythmic involuntary movements of the facial and masticatory musculature—a condition known as tardive dyskinesia.[15]

Effect of Trauma. External trauma, including surgical trauma, may induce an inflammatory reaction in muscle tissue that terminates as myofibrotic contracture. Such contracture involving an elevator muscle causes a permanent decrease in the resting length of the muscle and imposes a measure of painless hypomobility on the TM joint.

Joint Effects

Conditions that induce deleterious effects in the joint proper relate to direct trauma, infection, growth aberrations, functional overloading, frictional movements, and systemic disorders.

Trauma. The application of traumatic force can injure any or all components of the joint. Traumatic dislocation or fracture may occur. Injured subarticular bone may react by resorption or by overgrowth, either of which may reduce the functional compatibility of the articular surfaces. If the blow is sustained when the teeth are in occlusion, the effect will occur at the closed position of the joint; as such it may predispose to a Class II disc-interference disorder. If it is sustained when the teeth are separated, the effect will occur along the articular eminence; as such it may predispose to a Class III disc-interference disorder of the type that results from incompatibility of the sliding surfaces.

Bruising and laceration of articular surfaces, ligaments, and/or retrodiscal tissue, with or without hemarthrosis, may result in damage to the joint. Such sequelae could include capsular fibrosis, fracture or detachment of the articular disc, deformed articular surfaces, detachment of the discal collateral ligaments, rupture of the temporomandibular ligament, detachment of the superior retrodiscal lamina, or adhesions. Cicatrization following lacerating injuries including surgery may be complicated by traumatic neuroma formation, thus causing sharp lancinating neurogenous pain each time the capsule is stretched during functional movements. Katzberg et al.[16] reported that of 89 patients with arthrographically positive internal derangements, 25% had a history of jaw trauma immediately prior to the onset of the TM disorder. Trauma is a significant etiologic factor in ankylosis of the mandible.[17] It should be noted that experimental hemarthrosis failed to produce fibrous ankylosis.[18] In view of this, Laskin[19] proposed that bony contact due to dislocation of the articular disc may predispose to fibrotic union of the articular surfaces. Immobilization of the moving parts during the healing process is thought to contribute to the danger of adhesions. Several cases of synovial chondromatosis of the TM joint have been reported.[20, 21]

Infection.   Inflammatory involvement of the joint by both local and systemic conditions may be important etiologically. Infectious arthritis is occasionally seen. Psoriatic arthritis of the TM joint has been reported.[22] Infection is a frequent cause of ankylosis.[17] The TM joint may become involved by direct extension from a nearby inflammatory condition.

Structural Aberrations.   A variety of developmental and acquired alterations of joint morphology may occur which can cause loss of structural symmetry or incompatibility of the articular surfaces. Developmental anomalies include hypoplasia, hyperplasia, dysplasia, and dysmorphia, while postnatal growth abnormalities include inadequate growth due to hypothyroidism, hypopituitarism, and nutritional deficiency as well as overgrowth due to gigantism or acromegaly.[23] A number of benign neoplasms involve the TM joint. Trismus from a benign parotid tumor has been reported.[24] Occasionally, malignancy invades the TM joint. Trotter's syndrome is such an example.[25] Pseudoankylosis that restricts normal joint movement due to an abnormality in extra-articular structures may be encountered and must be distinguished from true articular disorders. Bilateral union between the coronoid processes and the maxilla has been reported.[26]

Functional Overloading.   If loading of an articular surface is protracted, deformation of the tissue will continue to increase as the synovial fluid is expressed by compressive force.[27, 28] Determinant factors include the amount of force as well as the rate of application and duration. Movement reduces the deforming effect as the force is shifted from one part of the articular surface to another. The osseous-supported articular surfaces have the propensity to remodel and therefore adjust to compressive force, provided it does not exceed the adaptability of the articular tissue; otherwise, degenerative change takes place. The articular disc, however, does not have this capability. It does not undergo cellular remodeling.[29] Excessive pressure causes deformation or deterioration instead.

As far as ordinary masticatory function is concerned, damage from overloading or frictional abuse occurs in the occluded position, which requires contraction of elevator muscles to bring the teeth into maximum intercuspation. Nonmasticatory abuse, such as habitual biting on an object such as a pipe stem, may cause the compressive force to be directed at some point along the opposite articular eminence. Hypomobility in one joint forces a lateral excursion in the opposite joint each time the mouth is opened. Such unnatural movement may result in damage to the moving joint. Overloading does not result so much from occlusal discrepancies that cause interference during chewing movements. Abnormal stress under those conditions tends to affect the muscles or the dentition more than the joints proper. Synovial joints are structured to tolerate moving compressive force without sustaining injury by their unique system of weeping lubrication.[30] Abusive compressive force occurs in TM joints especially when the teeth are clenched and when biting hard against resistant objects. Damage may occur as a result of either static overloading, impact loading, or frictional movement.

Static overloading has its main deleterious effect on the articular disc; the condylar and eminence articular surfaces may adapt by remodeling. Static overloading is the stationary application of excessive pressure. The usual cause is a slight deficiency in molar occlusal support which permits upward condylar pressure on the articular disc rather than having it dissipated to the maxillary bones through the teeth. Bruxism is no doubt the primary activating factor, while emotional stress and habitual hard chewing may contribute.

Static overloading causes deformation of the articular disc which deepens the central bearing area and may roughen the articular surface. There is no loss of disc contour that would predispose to disc displacement. Static overloading predisposes to a grating noise with purely rotatory movement, to Class II disc-interference disorders, and to a perforation or fracture of the disc that would lead to degenerative joint disease. It does not predispose to reciprocal clicking or locking of the disc during mandibular movements.

Impact loading occurs especially during maximum intercuspation when the condyle is displaced medially or anteriorly, thus bringing undue compressive force against the anchored articular disc. This is the result of occlusal disharmony and occurs only when the teeth are clenched. Bruxism is no doubt the primary activating factor. Occlusal disharmony that displaces the condyle anteriorly or medially in maximum intercuspation is not rare. Weinberg[31] reported that 18% of his TM dysfunction patients displayed anterior condylar displacement. Weinberg and Lager[32] reported that anterior condylar displacement occurred about half as often as posterior displacement.

Another cause of impact loading is anchored posterior overclosure. When molar teeth are missing, the condyle is not arrested by the occluded dentition but continues upward when the teeth are clenched. This is known as posterior overclosure. If the remaining bicuspids sufficiently anchor the occlusion, the condyle cannot be displaced posteriorly. Rather, a fulcrum is formed at the bicuspid tooth around which the condyle moves upward and forward, impacting the articular disc.[33]

Impact loading causes the loss of disc contour, flattening it medially or anteriorly, as the case may be. Thus, it causes the disc to lose some of its self-centering capability. Impacting medially predisposes to perforation of the disc. Impacting anteriorly predisposes to posterior displacement of the articular disc during the forward phase of the translatory cycle (Class III disc-interference disorder). Westesson[34] reported that he had arthrographically identified posterior displacement of the disc in less than 2% of his cases. Impact loading may also predispose to Class I and II disc-interference disorders as well as to grating noise during sliding movements, a symptom of degenerative joint disease.

Frictional movement is due to overloaded movement that exceeds the ability of weeping lubrication to prevent damage to the articular surfaces from friction. It is impact loading under gross movement. This can occur only in maximum intercuspation. It is due to gross occlusal disharmony that displaces the condyle when the teeth are firmly clenched. The displacement may be in any direction. The movement of the condyle is gross enough to be sensed subjectively by the patient, to be seen at the midline (if the displacement is laterally), or felt with the fingers, and to be recorded radiographically (if the displacement is in the sagittal plane). Bruxism no doubt is the primary activating agent. The most common causes of gross posterior condylar displacement are nonanchored posterior overclosure and Class II Division 2 malocclusion. The damage that is sustained includes abrasive injury to the disc and to the articular surface of the eminence, loss of disc contour, elongation of the discal collateral ligaments, and, ultimately, if in a posterior direction, elongation of the inner horizontal portion of the temporomandibular ligament with traumatic encroachment of the condyle onto the retrodiscal tissue. Damage to the eminence articular surface may be minimized by remodeling, but damage to the disc is permanent. It predisposes to functional displacement of the disc and degenerative joint disease. Loss of disc contour and elongation of the discal ligaments permit sliding movement to take place between the disc and condyle, thus predisposing to Class III disc-interference disorders. Anterior condylar displacement predisposes to posterior disc displacement during forward ranges of the translatory cycle. Posterior condylar displacement predisposes to anterior disc displacement in the closed resting position of the joint.

At a clinical level, various combinations of static overloading, impact loading, and frictional movement may be identified.

Constitutional Factors.   Various systemic factors may have etiologic significance in TM disorders. There appears to be some inherited predisposition to certain types of disorders. Illness, such as diabetes, affects tissue reactivity. Rheumatoid arthritis and hyperuricemia involve the TM joints. All such factors may affect not only the diagnostic identification of TM disorders but the effectiveness of therapy as well.

ROLE OF EMOTIONAL TENSION

Sustained emotional tension plays an important etiologic role in many TM disorders.[35, 36] Such tension has to do with stressful life situations and results from the burden of being human. The masseter is among the first of the skeletal muscles to undergo protracted contraction as a result of stressful life situations.[37]

The presence of emotional tension should not imply that a serious psychologic problem exists. All persons are subject to emotional stress. The signs of elevated emotional tension may develop quickly. Usually, however, a less obvious, slow, smoldering build-up of tension accumulates from a variety of stressful situations, with no one incident being particularly decisive. Consequently, the emotional level rises and falls in a somewhat rhythmic pattern. Then some situation may arise that adds just enough to an already high level of emotional tension so that a crisis ensues. It may appear that such an incident was solely responsible for the crisis, when actually it was but the "last straw."

Emotional stress increases muscle tonus, which alters the resting position of the mandible. It also increases the passive interarticular pressure within the joint. As such, it may activate an otherwise nonsymptomatic condition and therefore appear to be a direct cause of a disc-interference disorder.

There is considerable support for the psychophysiologic theory of masticatory dysfunction. Psychologic stress does increase muscle activity, which can in turn lead to myogenous pain and dysfunction, thus accounting for some symptoms that are displayed.[38] It is thought that bruxing may represent an involuntary tension-relieving mechanism that leads to muscular fatigue and myospastic activity.[36] Psychologic testing using Holmes and Rahe's *Social Readjustment Rating Scale* indicates that patients with TM complaints rate higher than control groups.[39, 40] This would indicate a higher level of emotional stress and suggests that such stress may play a significant role in muscular disorders. Greene et al.[41] concluded that evidence is abundant that psychologic factors have an important role in the etiology, progression, and treatment of myofascial pain-dysfunction symptoms.

Emotional stress may be a primary etiologic factor in muscle splinting and myospastic TM disorders. It can very well be a decisive activating factor in otherwise dormant and nonsymptomatic conditions. It can also be important as a perpetuating influence in many TM disorders.

ROLE OF OCCLUSAL DISHARMONY

Since dentists are conditioned to think in terms of the dentition, they naturally turn to what they know best when it comes to managing masticatory problems. And, in truth, the TM joints and musculature do relate primarily to masticatory function in which the teeth play the most visible part. Yet, there appears to have developed no real concensus as to just what part occlusal discrepancies play etiologically in TM disorders.

Okeson stated:[42] "When a patient presents an occlusal position that is neither optimal nor normal, the tendency is to assume that it is the major contributing factor. Although logical, this assumption cannot be substantiated by research studies." The wide disparity in thought on this subject is reflected by contrasting Schwartz's[43] research (1959) with current concepts of management: He considered occlusal conditions to be of insufficient importance to warrant inclusion in his studies while currently many advocate occlusal manipulation as the chief therapeutic tool. In commenting on the role of malocclusion, Loiselle[44] reported that of 2,000 Veterans Administration patients 48% exhibited malocclusion, but none had TM dysfunction.

Many years ago, the standard for judging normal occlusion was quite rigid, with some leaders in the field insisting on an occlusal position that precisely coincided with centric relations.[45] In 1957 Posselt[46] reported that a slide from centric relations to centric occlusion was present in approximately 90% of the population. Okeson[42] reported that the relations position was from 1 to 2 mm posterior to intercuspal position. Ramfjord[47] placed the functional occlusal position some 0.2 to 0.5 mm anterior to centric relations. Although Ingervall and Carlsson[48] found that EMG activity in the masticatory muscles did not change following the occlusal adjustment of interferences on the nonworking side, Williamson and Lundquist[49] found that such interference increased the EMG activity in elevator muscles. In a review of the literature on this subject, Carlsson and Droukas[50] concluded that occlusal factors may be masked by other etiologic components, being of minor importance in some and perhaps a major etiologic factor in others.

Since clinical experience testifies to the importance of occlusal disharmony in TM disorders, it would be well to determine, if possible, why no concensus has developed. Perhaps one reason is the failure to properly recognize the significant difference between the effect of dynamic occlusal interference that occurs during mandibular movements and that of static positional disharmony that asserts itself only when the teeth are firmly clenched.

As previously discussed, occlusal interferences that occur prior to maximum intercuspation do not particularly damage the articular surfaces or joint ligaments. Such interference has its effect primarily on the muscles and the teeth. Since chronic conditions provoke muscular changes that affect habit patterns (changes that may be entirely nonsymptomatic as far as masticatory complaints are concerned), only recent changes in the occlusion should be expected to induce such conditions as muscle pain and dysfunction. As such, occlusal interference that results from trauma or dental treatment may be important etiologically in muscle complaints. In the absence of recent change or recent activation, evidence of occlusal disharmony in acute muscle disorders may be disregarded etiologically. Such occlusal disharmony at least in part may likely be the result, rather than the cause, of the disorder and therefore should be regarded as symptomatic rather than etiologic.

Occlusal disharmony that is potentially damaging to the joint proper asserts itself as the teeth are clenched into full maximum intercuspation. The disharmony must be such as to induce overloading. Such disharmony may cause no damage at all unless activated by voluntary clenching, by habitual hard biting, by elevated emotional tension including oral consciousness, or by bruxism.

It is important to distinguish between the effects of occlusal disharmony and other manipulations of the jaws and/or dentition that may be of etiologic significance. For example, the damaging effects of habits such as biting against hard objects should not be confused with that of occlusal disharmony per se. Nor should the damaging effects of nonsymmetrical chewing be confused with an occlusal discrepancy simply because chewing is involved. For example, if one joint is hypomobile for any reason, the opening-closing movements in the opposite joint are not straight forward, but are lateral excursions. Thus, the opposite joint may eventually sustain enough damage to become symptomatic. Correction of the occlusion would yield no benefit; only correcting the hypomobility would be effective.

In reality, the etiologic role of occlusal disharmony is a very important one; some discrepancies are important in muscle complaints; some are important in disorders of the joint proper. But, they are not the same. Occlusal interference serves primarily as a predisposing factor that requires activating before it becomes etiologically important. Emotional tension and bruxism are the important activating factors.

ROLE OF BRUXISM

Bruxism is defined[51] as rhythmic or spasmodic grinding of the teeth in other than chewing movements of the mandible, especially such movements performed during sleep. The word is used broadly to include all forms of involuntary parafunctional mandibular activity—both clenching and grinding, and both nocturnal and diurnal. It is accomplished by active contractions of the elevator muscles, and no doubt entails coincidental activity in the superior lateral pterygoid muscles. It is thought to occur chiefly during the REM (rapid eye movement) phase of sleep.[42] It is likely due at least in part to partial arousal from some stimulating influence such as emotional tension.[52] Since serotonin acts as a neurotransmitter in the descending inhibitory system of the brain stem to suppress afferent stimuli of different types, bruxism likely represents a relative serotonin deficiency.[53]

Nocturnal bruxism cannot be elicited by the experimental introduction of deflective occlusal contacts.[54] There is no experimental evidence to support the hypothesis that occlusal disharmony causes bruxism.[55] Since tooth contact stimulates periodontal mechanoreceptors which exert inhibitory influence on elevator muscle action,[56] bruxism can hardly be the product of occlusal function or dysfunction.

It has been established that increasing the vertical dimension of occlusion actually induces a reduction in elevator muscle activity.[57] Occlusal splinting effectively arrests the nocturnal EMG activity of bruxism, but only as long as the appliance is worn.[58] A splint of 6-mm thickness is more effective than one 2 mm thick.[59] Biofeedback techniques of muscle relaxation also reduce the muscle activity of bruxism.[55]

It appears at this time that bruxism is a CNS generated state of increased activity in elevator masticatory muscles that may reflect such conditions as elevated emotional tension and other psychologic states that provoke arousal. The increased EMG activity can be controlled by occlusal splinting, by relaxation techniques, and by massed practice therapy.[60]

The role of bruxism as an activator of predisposing etiologic factors in TM disorders is of prime importance. The effect of occlusal disharmony on the muscles, on the teeth, and on the joints depends largely on bruxism. Emotional tension, in turn, appears to be a dominant factor in bruxism. Thus, the prime targets that require attention in the management of most TM disorders are identified—bruxism and emotional tension.

It has been speculated that bruxism may act as a direct cause of anterior displacement of the articular disc through action of the superior lateral pterygoid muscle.[61, 62] Although such muscle action, no doubt, is decisive in displacing the disc anteriorly in the closed position of the joint, this effect would be impossible as long as normal disc contour is present. Before the muscle can displace the disc, a loss of disc contour and an elongation of the discal collateral ligaments must have occurred. These conditions are the product of an abusive compressive force acting on the structures involved as previously described. It is extremely unlikely that the action of the superior lateral pterygoid alone, even in a state of spasticity, causes the sort of destruction within the joint that is required for gross displacement of the articular disc. Bruxism is certainly a more decisive factor in disc-interference disorders. It is related more to the action of elevator muscles that generate the compressive forces that damage the joint.

ROLE OF POSTURE

Head posture influences the resting position of the mandible, the path of closure, and the site of initial occlusal contact of the teeth.[63–66] Body posture also has its effect: As the body reclines, the inferior lateral pterygoid muscles draw the mandible forward to safeguard the airway.[67] Rocabado et al.[68] have reported that there is correlation between Class II malocclusion and forward head position about 70% of the time. Although this is given as evidence of a relationship between head posture and malocclusion, there is no indication that this represents more than a compensating mechanism to protect the airway.

Currently, there appears to be little documented evidence that relates TM disorders etiologically to head or body posture other than the occurrence of related myospastic activity that may involve the neck and head region. The masticatory mechanism is structured to function normally with a changing head position. Immobilization, however, may be a different matter. Not only does immobilization predispose to muscle atrophy, it is also a major factor in the progression of painful muscle spasm to painless muscle contracture.[69] Postural vertigo may arise from a trigger-point mechanism situated in the posterior clavicular division of the sternocleidomastoid muscle.[70]

REFERENCES

1. Widmalm S.E., Ericsson S.G.: The influence of eye closure on muscle activity in the anterior temporal region. *J. Oral Rehabil.* 10:25, 1983.
2. Gerschman J., Burrows G., Reade P.: Chronic orofacial pain, in Bonica J.J., Liebeskind J.C., Albe-Fessard D.G. (eds.): *Advances in Pain Research and Therapy,* Vol. 3. New York, Raven Press, 1979, pp. 317–323.
3. Dubner R., Sessle B.J., Storey A.T.: *The Neural Basis of Oral and Facial Function.* New York, Plenum Publishing Corp., 1978.
4. Sessle B.J.: How are mastication and swallowing programmed and regulated?, in Sessle B.J., Hannam A.G. (eds.): *Mastication and Swallowing: Biological and Clinical Correlates.* Toronto, University of Toronto Press, 1976, pp. 161–171.
5. Ahlgren J.: Mechanisms of mastication. *Acta Odontol. Scand.* 24:1–109 (Suppl. 44), 1966.
6. Carlsson G.E., Ingervall B., Kocak G.: Effect of increasing vertical dimension on the masticatory system in subjects with natural teeth. *J. Prosthet. Dent.* 41:284, 1979.
7. Molin C.: Vertical isometric muscle forces of the mandible: A comprehensive study of subjects with and without manifest mandibular pain dysfunction syndrome. *Acta Odontol. Scand.* 30:485, 1972.
8. Travell J.G., Simons D.G.: *Myofascial Pain and Dysfunction.* Baltimore, Williams & Wilkins Co., 1983.
9. Mense S., Meyer N.: Bradykinin-induced sensitization of high-threshold muscle receptors with slowly conducting afferent fibers. *Pain* Supplement 1:S204, 1981.
10. Higgs G.A., Moncada S.: Interactions of arachidonate products with other pain mediators, in Bonica J.J., Lindblom U., Iggo A. (eds.): *Advances in Pain Research and Therapy,* Vol. 5. New York, Raven Press, 1983, pp. 617–626.
11. Christensen L.V., Mohamed S.E., Harrison J.D.: Delayed onset of masseter muscle pain in experimental tooth clenching. *J. Prosthet. Dent.* 48:579, 1982.
12. Friden J., Sjostrom M., Ekblom B.: A morphological study of delayed muscle soreness. *Experientia* 37:506, 1981.
13. Simons D.G., Travell J.: Letter to the editor. *Pain* 10:106, 1981.
14. Kraak J.G.: A drug-initiated dislocation of the temporomandibular joint: Report of case. *J. Am. Dent. Assoc.* 74:1247, 1967.
15. U.S. Department of Health, Education and Welfare, Food and Drug Administration: *FDA Drug Bulletin,* May 1973.
16. Katzberg R.W., Dolwick M.F., Helms C.A., et al.: Arthrotomography of the temporomandibular joint. *Am. J. Roentgenol.* 134:944, 1980.

17. Adekeye E.O.: Ankylosis of the mandible: Analysis of 76 cases. *J. Oral Maxillofac. Surg.* 41:442, 1983.
18. Hoaglund F.T.: Experimental hemarthrosis. *J. Bone Joint Surg. (Am.)* 49-A:285, 1967.
19. Laskin D.M.: Role of the meniscus in the etiology of posttraumatic temporomandibular joint ankylosis. *Int. J. Oral Surg.* 7:340, 1978.
20. Morrish R.B. Jr., Hansen L.S., Ware W.H.: Synovial chondromatosis of the temporomandibular joint. *J. Craniomand. Pract.* 2(1):64, 1983.
21. Eriksson L., Westesson P., Henrikson H.: A 66-year-old man with limited jaw opening and temporomandibular joint pain, clicking, and crepitation. *J. Craniomand. Pract.* 3:184–188, 1985.
22. Stimson C.W., Leban S.G.: Recurrent ankylosis of the temporomandibular joint in a patient with chronic psoriasis. *J. Oral Maxillofac. Surg.* 40:678, 1982.
23. Keith D.A.: Etiology and diagnosis of temporomandibular pain and dysfunction: Organic pathology (other than arthritis), in *The President's Conference on the Examination, Diagnosis and Management of Temporomandibular Disorders.* Chicago, American Dental Association, 1983, pp. 118–122.
24. Tovi F., Zirkin H., Sidi J.: Trismus resulting from a parotid hemangioma. *J. Oral Maxillofac. Surg.* 41:468, 1983.
25. Gorlin R.J., Pindborg J.J.: *Syndromes of the Head and Neck.* New York, McGraw-Hill Book Co., 1964.
26. Super S., Cotten J.S. Jr.: Bilateral pseudoankylosis of the temporomandibular joint due to synostoses between the mandible and maxilla. *J. Oral Maxillofac. Surg.* 40:590, 1982.
27. Frankel V.H., Nordin M.: *Basic Biomechanics of the Skeletal System.* Philadelphia, Lea & Febiger, 1980.
28. Moffett B.: Questions and answers, Session 4, in Moffett B.C. (ed.): *Diagnosis of Internal Derangements of the Temporomandibular Joint,* Vol. 1. Seattle, University of Washington, 1984, pp. 103–108.
29. Moffett B.: Histologic aspects of temporomandibular joint derangements, in Moffett B.C. (ed.): *Diagnosis of Internal Derangements of the Temporomandibular Joint,* Vol. 1. Seattle, University of Washington, 1984, pp. 47–49.
30. DuBrul E.L.: The biomechanics of the oral apparatus. Chapter III. Structural analysis, in DuBrul E.L., Menekratis A.: *The Physiology of Oral Reconstruction.* Chicago, Quintessence Publishing Company, 1981, pp. 21–38.
31. Weinberg L.A.: Role of condylar position in TMJ dysfunction pain syndrome. *J. Prosthet. Dent.* 41:636–643, 1979.
32. Weinberg L.A., Lager L.A.: Clinical report on the etiology and diagnosis of TMJ dysfunction pain syndrome. *J. Prosthet. Dent.* 44:642, 1980.
33. Mahan P.E.: The temporomandibular joint in function and pathofunction, in Solberg W.K., Clark G.T. (eds.): *Temporomandibular Joint Problems.* Chicago, Quintessence Publishing Company, 1980, pp. 33–42.
34. Westesson P.: Questions and answers, Session 3, in Moffett B.C. (ed.): *Diagnosis of Internal Derangements of the Temporomandibular Joint,* Vol. 1. Seattle, University of Washington, 1984, pp. 91–94.
35. Greene C.S.: Myofascial pain-dysfunction syndrome: The evolution of

concepts, in Sarnat B.G., Laskin D.M. (eds.): *The Temporomandibular Joint,* ed. 3. Springfield, Ill., Charles C Thomas, Publisher, 1979, pp. 277–288.

36. Laskin D.M.: Etiology of the pain-dysfunction syndrome. *J. Am. Dent. Assoc.* 79:147, 1969.
37. Wolff H.G.: *Headache and Other Head Pain,* ed. 2. New York, Oxford University Press, 1963.
38. Rugh J.D.: Psychological factors in the etiology of masticatory pain and dysfunction, in *The President's Conference on the Examination, Diagnosis and Management of Temporomandibular Disorders.* Chicago, American Dental Association, 1983, pp. 85–94.
39. Stein S.S., Loft G., Davis H., et al.: Symptoms of TMJ dysfunction as related to stress measured by the Social Readjustment Rating Scale. *J. Prosthet. Dent.* 47:545, 1982.
40. Fearon C.G., Serwatka W.J.: Stress: A common denominator for nonorganic TMJ pain-dysfunction. *J. Prosthet. Dent.* 49:805, 1983.
41. Greene C.S., Olson R.E., Laskin D.M.: Psychological factors in the etiology, progression and treatment of MPD syndrome. *J. Am. Dent. Assoc.* 105:443, 1982.
42. Okeson J.P.: *Fundamentals of Occlusion and Temporomandibular Disorders.* St. Louis, C.V. Mosby Co., 1985.
43. Schwartz L. (ed.): *Disorders of the Temporomandibular Joint.* Philadelphia, W.B. Saunders Co., 1959.
44. Loiselle R.J.: Relation of occlusion to temporomandibular joint dysfunction: The prosthodontic viewpoint. *J. Am. Dent. Assoc.* 79:145, 1969.
45. McCollum B.B., Stuart C.E.: *A Research Report.* South Pasadena, Calif., Scientific Press, 1955.
46. Posselt U.: Movement areas of the mandible. *J. Prosthet. Dent.* 7:375, 1957.
47. Ramfjord S.P.: Goals for an ideal occlusion and mandibular position, in Solberg W.K., Clark G.T. (eds.): *Abnormal Jaw Mechanics.* Chicago, Quintessence Publishing Company, 1984, pp. 77–95.
48. Ingervall B., Carlsson G.E.: Masticatory muscle activity before and after elimination of balancing-side occlusal interference. *J. Oral Rehabil.* 9:183, 1982.
49. Williamson E.H., Lundquist D.O.: Anterior guidance: Its effect on electromyographic activity of the temporal and masseter muscles. *J. Prosthet. Dent.* 49:816, 1983.
50. Carlsson G.E., Droukas B.C.: Dental occlusion and the health of the masticatory system. *J. Craniomand. Pract.* 2(2):141, 1984.
51. *Dorland's Illustrated Medical Dictionary,* ed. 26. Philadelphia, W.B. Saunders Co., 1981.
52. Kreisberg M.K.: Alternative view of the bruxism phenomenon. *Gen. Dentistry* Mar.–Apr. 1982, p. 121.
53. Basbaum A.I.: Brainstem control of nociception: The contribution of the monoamines. *Pain* Supplement 1:S231, 1981.
54. Rugh J.D., Barghi N., Drago C.J.: Experimental occlusal discrepancies and nocturnal bruxism. *J. Prosthet. Dent.* 51:548, 1984.

55. Clarke N.G.: Occlusion and myofascial pain dysfunction: Is there a relationship? *J. Am. Dent. Assoc.* 104:443, 1982.

56. Hannam A.G., Matthews B.. Yemm R.: Receptors involved in the response of the masseter muscle in tooth contact in man. *Arch. Oral Biol.* 15:17, 1970.

57. Kovaleski W.C., DeBoever J.: Influence of occlusal splints on jaw position and musculature in patients with temporomandibular joint dysfunction. *J. Prosthet. Dent.* 35:321–327, 1975.

58. Solberg W.K., Clark G.T., Rugh J.D.: Nocturnal electromyographic evaluation of bruxing patients undergoing short-term splint therapy. *J. Oral Rehabil.* 2(3):215, 1975.

59. Drago C.J., Rugh J.D., Barghi N.: Night-guard vertical thickness effects on nocturnal bruxism. *J. Dent. Res.* 58:316 (Special issue A), 1979.

60. Ayer W.A., Gale E.N.: Extinction of bruxism by massed practice therapy. *J. Can. Dent. Assoc.* 35:492, 1969.

61. Dolwick M.F.: Diagnosis and etiology, in Helms C.M., Katzberg R.W., Dolwick M.F. (eds.): *Internal Derangements of the Temporomandibular Joint.* San Francisco, Radiology Research and Education Foundation, 1983, pp. 31–41.

62. Jankelson B.: Modern diagnosis and management of musculoskeletal dysfunctions of the head and neck, in Morgan D.H., House L.R., Hall W.P., et al. (eds.): *Diseases of the Temporomandibular Apparatus,* ed. 2. St. Louis, C.V. Mosby Co., 1982, pp. 591–599.

63. Mohl N.D.: The role of head posture in mandibular function, in Solberg W.K., Clark G.T. (eds.): *Abnormal Jaw Mechanics.* Chicago, Quintessence Publishing Company, 1984, pp. 97–116.

64. Troendle R., Troendle K., Rugh J.D.: Electromyographic and phonetic rest position changes with head posture. *J. Dent. Res.* 59:494 (Special issue A), 1980.

65. Goldstein D.F., Kraus S.L., Williams W.B., et al.: Influence of cervical posture on mandibular movement. *J. Prosthet. Dent.* 52:421, 1984.

66. Rocabado M.: Diagnosis and treatment of abnormal craniocervical and craniomandibular mechanics, in Solberg W.K., Clark G.T. (eds.): *Abnormal Jaw Mechanics.* Chicago, Quintessence Publishing Company, 1984, pp. 141–159.

67. Hairston L.E., Blanton P.L: An electromyographic study of mandibular position in response to changes in body position. *J. Prosthet. Dent.* 49:271, 1983.

68. Rocabado M., Johnston B.E. Jr., Blakney M.G.: Physical therapy and dentistry: An overview. *J. Craniomand. Pract.* 1(1):47, 1982–83.

69. Travell J.: Temporomandibular joint pain referred from muscles of the head and neck. *J. Prosthet. Dent.* 10:745, 1960.

70. Weeks V.D., Travell J.: Postural vertigo due to trigger areas in the sternocleidomastoid muscle. *J. Pediatrics* 47:315, 1955.

7 | Classification of Temporomandibular Disorders

Currently, there is no generally accepted classification of TM disorders. Indeed, there is little agreement as to just what constitutes masticatory dysfunction. That an acceptable definition and classification of masticatory disorders is eminently needed, there can be little doubt.

The craniomandibular articulation, which is composed of two TM joints and the masticatory musculature, like other components of the musculoskeletal system, is subject to a variety of disorders, many of which relate to function—masticatory function. Such disorders may induce muscle symptoms, joint symptoms, or both. Muscle disorders result especially when functional activity involves such factors as proprioceptive and sensory feedback mechanisms, while joint disorders relate primarily to biomechanical factors such as loading and movement. An interplay between joint and muscle symptoms is normal and expected. This articulation is subject to the ills common to other synovial joints, plus a few that are unique because of the TMJ's highly specialized function.

SYNDROME CONCEPT

A notion has persisted for half a century that dysfunctions of the masticatory apparatus comprise a "syndrome"—initially referred to as Costen's syndrome[1] or the temporomandibular syndrome.[2] In 1956 Schwartz introduced the TM pain-dysfunction syndrome.[3] Then came the myofascial pain-dysfuntion (MPD) syndrome in 1969.[4] The term *craniomandibular syndrome* is now used quite frequently.

172

It should be interesting to note that in the medical dictionary[5] the only joint disorder listed as a *syndrome* is Costen's. This syndrome concept has no doubt contributed to the one-disease-one-treatment myth. It also, perhaps, has given some credence to the notion that the TM joint is not a true synovial joint and therefore follows a different set of rules from other synovial joints of the body.

The clinical signs and symptoms displayed by masticatory disorders are much too varied to be classified as a "syndrome." According to medical definition, a *syndrome* is a set of symptoms which occur together; a symptom complex.[5] The term applies to symptoms as such. A *disorder* is a derangement or abnormality of function; a morbid physical or mental state.[5] This term applies not to symptoms but to conditions. The general term *temporomandibular disorders* should be adopted to designate the conditions that comprise complaints of the masticatory system involving the craniomandibular articulation and its musculature. A definite trend in this direction is evident from recent dental literature, which stresses the multifactorial nature of such conditions.[6–10]

DEVELOPING A CLASSIFICATION

The first serious attempt to classify TM disorders was in 1970.[11] This divided the disorders into six groups, as follows:

1. Spontaneous dislocation
2. Traumatic joint
3. Masticatory pain-dysfunction syndrome
4. Temporomandibular arthritis
5. Chronic mandibular hypomobilities
6. Developmental anomalies and neoplasms

This classification entailed implications of etiology which, of course, required diagnostic differentiation. *Being dependent on diagnosis*, it could not become a very useful diagnostic tool.

In 1980 the American Academy of Craniomandibular Disorders proposed an elaborate classification of masticatory disorders that has been well received.[12] It, however, is complex and is not based on symptomatology.

At the 1982 President's Conference on the Examination, Diagnosis and Management of Temporomandibular Disorders sponsored by the American Dental Association, this author[13] presented a classification of

TM disorders that was published earlier that year.[14] Although embracing this classification in some respects, the one that the Association adopted still continued to reflect etiologic considerations.[15] It is a constructive step forward, but the American Dental Association's classification of TM disorders lacks precise definition and falls short of being a useful diagnostic tool.

Classification Based on Clinical Symptoms

A truly useful classification of TM disorders should be based on clinical symptoms, so that it can serve as a sort of diagnostic "road map" to help guide the examiner toward accurate identification of the patient's complaint.

If a classification is to be based on clinical symptoms, however, first those symptoms must be clearly defined. As previously discussed, the symptoms (using the term broadly, to include both subjective and objective evidence) that designate a masticatory disorder are:

1. *Masticatory pain,* identified as primary pain that emanates from the TM joints and/or the masticatory muscles

2. *Restriction* (limitation) of mandibular movement

3. *Interference* during mandibular movement (sensations that are felt, noises that are heard, altered movements that are felt and seen)

4. *Acute malocclusion* identified as a symptomatic change in the occlusion due to abnormal muscle action or changes within the joint

By utilizing these four cardinal symptoms, TM disorders can be classified into one or more of five general categories, as follows:

1. Masticatory muscle disorders
2. Disc-interference disorders
3. Inflammatory disorders of the joint
4. Chronic mandibular hypomobilities
5. Growth disorders of the joint

Each of these five categories displays symptoms that are characteristic, even though there may be considerable variation in both the incidence and the intensity of the symptoms. The characteristic identifying clinical symptoms for each group of disorders should be understood and appreciated.

Masticatory Muscle Disorders

Masticatory pain: (A predominant symptom) The pain is myogenous. (When continuous, secondary central excitatory effects may add symptoms that must be recognized and evaluated.)

Restricted movement: (A predominant symptom) The limitation of mandibular movement is extracapsular.

Interference: Discal interference (if any) is muscle-induced, due to excessive passive interarticular pressure.

Acute malocclusion: Symptomatic alteration of the occlusion is muscle-induced, due to a shortened muscle(s). (Preexistent malocclusion is irrelevant unless recently induced.)

Disc-Interference Disorders

Masticatory pain: The pain (if any) is disc-attachment arthralgia that is coincident with other interference symptoms. (Being intermittent, no central excitatory effects are displayed.)

Restricted movement: Arrested movement (if any) is intracapsular and due to obstruction of the disc.

Interference: (The predominant symptom) Disc-interference symptoms reflect the severity, the location, and the duration of discal obstruction. (If the interference is of recent origin, protective muscle splinting may occur.)

Acute malocclusion: Symptomatic malocclusion (if any) may result from a fractured or dislocated articular disc. (Considerable relevant preexistent malocclusion may be present.)

Inflammatory Disorders of the Joint

Masticatory pain: (The predominant symptom) The pain is retrodiscal, capsular, or arthritic arthralgia of inflammatory type. (If the pain is continuous, secondary central excitatory effects may add symptoms that must be recognized and evaluated.)

Restricted movement: Restriction of movement (if any) is capsular.

Interference: There is none, except that due to trauma or preexistent noninflammatory degenerative joint disease.

Acute malocclusion: Symptomatic malocclusion (if any) is joint-induced, due to excessive intracapsular fluid, swelling of the retrodiscal tissue, or rapid osteolysis. (Considerable relevant preexistent malocclusion may be present.)

Chronic Mandibular Hypomobilities

Masticatory pain: The condition is painless unless it becomes inflamed from excessive or abusive movement.

Restricted movement: (The predominant symptom) The location of restriction identifies the particular disorder: Extracapsular restriction signifies elevator muscle contracture; capsular restriction signifies capsular fibrosis; intracapsular restriction signifies ankylosis.

Interference: There is none, unless it is preexistent.

Acute malocclusion: There is none. (Irrelevant preexistent malocclusion may be present.)

Growth Disorders of the Joint

Masticatory pain: None would exist, unless it would be due to marked structural change or malignancy.

Restricted movement: The limitation of movement correlates to the extent of the structural abnormality.

Interference: Discal interference correlates to the altered functional relationship of the disc-condyle complex.

Acute malocclusion: None would be found, unless the structural change is rapid, as with malignancy. (Considerable relevant chronic malocclusion may be displayed.)

Each of the major categories comprises a number of disorders that are identifiable clinically by such features as location, extent of dysfunction, and etiology. There may be considerable variation in severity, duration, and incidence of the symptoms, however.

CLASSIFICATION OF TM DISORDERS

    I. MASTICATORY MUSCLE DISORDERS
      1. Protective muscle splinting
      2. Muscle spasm activity
        a) Elevator muscle spasm
        b) Inferior lateral pterygoid muscle spasm
        c) Superior lateral pterygoid muscle spasm
      3. Muscle inflammation
    II. DISC-INTERFERENCE DISORDERS
      1. Class I interference (during maximum intercuspation)
      2. Class II interference (following maximum intercuspation)

    3. Class III interference (during *normal* translatory cycle)
       a) Due to excessive passive interarticular pressure
       b) Due to structural incompatibility between the sliding surfaces
       c) Due to impaired disc-condyle complex
          (1) Adhesions between disc and condyle
          (2) Damaged articular disc
          (3) *Functional* displacement/dislocation of the disc
          (4) Dysfunctional superior retrodiscal lamina
    4. Class IV interference (joint hypermobility)
    5. Class V interference (*spontaneous* dislocation)
III. INFLAMMATORY DISORDERS OF THE JOINT
    1. Synovitis and capsulitis
    2. Retrodiscitis
    3. Inflammatory arthritis
       a) Traumatic arthritis
       b) Degenerative arthritis
       c) Infectious arthritis
       d) Rheumatoid arthritis
       e) Hyperuricemia
IV. CHRONIC MANDIBULAR HYPOMOBILITIES
    1. Contracture of elevator muscle(s)
       a) Myostatic contracture
       b) Myofibrotic contracture
    2. Capsular fibrosis
    3. Ankylosis
       a) Fibrous
       b) Osseous
V. GROWTH DISORDERS OF THE JOINT
    1. Aberration of development
    2. Acquired change in joint structure
    3. Neoplasia
       a) Benign
       b) Malignant

CATEGORIES OF TM DISORDERS

Identification of a particular condition requires the examiner to be conversant with the possible disorders he may encounter. It is necessary to obtain a good understanding of the various categories of disorders that afflict the masticatory apparatus. It is not enough to merely establish that a problem of the temporomandibular joint exists.

Disorders of the masticatory apparatus have similarities and differences. It is by their similarities that they can be grouped into various classes of conditions. It is by their differences that individual disorders within each group can be identified. Establishing an accurate clinical diagnosis demands knowledge of the similarities and differences of various masticatory disorders. One cannot hope to recognize a condition that he does not know exists; nor can he identify it accurately if he does not know how it compares with other disorders of the system.

Although disc-interference disorders, chronic mandibular hypomobilities, and growth disorders have clinical features that clearly identify them individually, acute muscle disorders and inflammatory conditions of the joint may have clinical symptoms that are much alike and therefore may be confused diagnostically. Accurate identification, however, is necessary, because the treatment is not the same.

MASTICATORY MUSCLE DISORDERS

The masticatory muscle disorders are characterized by sudden onset, changeableness, and recurrence. The myogenous pain and extracapsular restriction of movement dominate the symptom complex. The acute disorders are classified as (1) protective muscle splinting, (2) muscle spasm activity, and (3) muscle inflammation. These terms are not intended to signify the histopathologic changes that may take place in the muscle tissue—conditions that cannot be discerned clinically. Rather, they designate conditions that are expressed clinically and that require different forms of therapy. Since these conditions may form a sort of continuum, transitional phases may occur that make differentiation difficult.

Protective Muscle Splinting

Muscle splinting is regarded *clinically* as a CNS-induced hypertonicity of a muscle(s) that occurs in response to altered proprioceptive and sensory input as a protective mechanism to restrain the use of the threatened muscle or part. It may occur as the result of (1) altered sensory or proprioceptive input from any cause, e.g., altered dentition, dental treatment, local anesthesia, or unusual jaw position or movement; (2) volitional jaw movements that conflict with preexisting habit patterns or that arise from oral consciousness; (3) injury or threat of injury, strain, abusive use, or muscle fatigue; and (4) increased bruxism associated with emotional tension or illness.

Muscle splinting occurs insidiously but becomes symptomatic rapidly. Normally it is of short duration, lasting only a few days, and tends to disappear quickly when the etiologic factors resolve. Abusive use or injudicious therapy, however, may protract the splinting effect, which can terminate in myospasm. The clinical effects of muscle splinting are observed chiefly in the elevator muscles. On some occasions, the lateral pterygoid muscles may be involved, and myospasm can develop if such splinting is protracted.

The clinical symptoms by which protective muscle splinting may be recognized are:

Masticatory pain: Pain occurs with contraction of the muscle and is usually accompanied by a sensation of weakness. (When an elevator muscle is involved, pain occurs with biting; with the inferior lateral pterygoid muscle, there is pain with protrusion against resistance.)

Restricted movement: There is no limit on movement, except that due to the inhibitory influence of pain and sensation of weakness.

Interference: None.

Acute malocclusion: None.

Muscle Spasm Activity

Muscle spasm is regarded *clinically* as a CNS-induced involuntary tonic contraction of a muscle(s). It may occur as the result of several conditions, such as (1) protracted muscle splinting from any of the causes mentioned above, (2) preexisting nonspastic myofascial pain syndrome (involving that muscle) from any cause, (3) myospasm activity secondarily induced as a central excitatory effect from deep pain input elsewhere in the trigeminal area or secondary to deep facial, glossopharyngeal, or cervical pain syndromes, and (4) systemic illness, emotional tension, physical fatigue, or as an extrapyramidal effect of certain medications.

When myospastic activity develops a component of pain, it becomes an independent self-perpetuating cycling myospasm, no longer dependent on any cause. *As such it can cycle indefinitely.*

A simple cycling spasm of a masticatory muscle should present no problem, diagnostic or therapeutic. Unfortunately, spastic activity of elevator muscles increases the passive interarticular pressure, thus altering or interfering with normal biomechanics of the joint. As such, it predisposes to discal interference during mandibular movements. Also, spastic activity in the lateral pterygoid muscle induces acute malocclusion, thus initiating a chain of masticatory problems that involve the joint proper and the musculature. Therefore, it is the *secondary effects* of what initially may be a simple muscle problem that complicate the biomechanical functioning of the masticatory apparatus and cause management problems. This is sufficient reason to manage acute myospasms of masticatory muscles with dispatch.

It should be understood that what initially may be nothing more than a simple muscle disorder may *activate* an otherwise dormant non-symptomatic temporomandibular disorder and, therefore, become the dominant etiologic factor in a considerably more serious masticatory problem.

To treat such conditions effectively, it is necessary to distinguish between muscle disorders and the more serious structural disorders of the joint proper.[16] The secondary effects of cycling muscle spasm activity may present the real challenge to the therapist. *Myospastic activity in masticatory muscles may cycle indefinitely, especially if subjected to continued painful use or to injudicious therapy.* Protracted or abused myospasm may develop into an inflammatory condition, myositis.

The symptoms displayed depend on which muscle(s) is involved, the type of contraction (isotonic or isometric), and to what extent.

Elevator Muscle Spasm.   The clinical symptoms by which spastic activity in an elevator muscle may be recognized are:

Masticatory pain: Pain occurs with contracting (biting) and stretching (opening). The biting pain is not decreased by biting against a tongue blade. No pain occurs with protruding against resistance.

Restricted movement: Being extracapsular, opening is restricted, but not protrusion or contralateral excursion (unless inhibited by pain). The opening midline path deflects, but the protrusive midline path does not. (Note: Acting singly, a shortened medial pterygoid muscle deflects contralaterally. When several muscles are involved, there may be little or no deflection of the midline path.)

Interference: There is none, unless spasm causes excessive passive interarticular pressure.

Acute malocclusion: Slight muscle-induced malocclusion may be sensed subjectively.

Inferior Lateral Pterygoid Spasm   The clinical symptoms by which spastic activity in the inferior lateral pterygoid muscle may be recognized are:

Masticatory pain: Occurs when the muscle is contracted (protruding against resistance) and when stretched (firm maximum intercuspation).

The biting pain is reduced by biting against a tongue blade (which prevents intercuspation of the teeth).

Restricted movement: None.

Interference: None.

Acute malocclusion: Muscle-induced malocclusion is sensed as disclusion of the ipsilateral posteriors and premature occlusion of the contralateral anteriors.

Superior Lateral Pterygoid Spasm. The clinical symptoms by which spastic activity in the superior lateral pterygoid muscle may be recognized are:

Masticatory pain: Pain occurs when the muscle is contracted (biting) and when stretched (maximum intercuspation). The biting pain is not reduced by biting against a tongue blade. Protruding against resistance causes no pain.

Restricted movement: None.

Interference: Spontaneous anterior dislocation is likely to occur. Anterior functional displacements/dislocations, if any, will not be reduced automatically by a forward translatory movement.

Acute malocclusion: Muscle-induced malocclusion (if any) is sensed as ipsilateral disclusion of the posterior teeth and contralateral premature occlusion of the anterior teeth.

When several masticatory muscles are involved in myospastic activity, a bizarre symptom picture may be displayed. Diagnosis may require skillful functional manipulation and careful identification of pain source by analgesic blocking.

Muscle Inflammation

Inflammation of a masticatory muscle is regarded *clinically* as a localized reaction in the muscle in response to (1) local injury from such causes as unaccustomed or abusive use, strain, infection, and adjacent disease, (2) direct extension of inflammation from another inflammatory condition in a nearby structure, or (3) protracted or abused myospastic activity from any of many possible causes.

The symptoms are those of an inflammatory condition and reflect the type, degree, and phase of inflammatory reaction present. The symptoms tend to follow an inflammatory curve in incidence, development, plateauing, and resolution. Generally, alteration in function outlasts pain as resolution takes place. Protracted myositis predisposes to muscular contracture. Clinically, myositis involves the elevator muscles chiefly. It tends to induce some associated secondary muscle splinting effects also.

The clinical symptoms by which an inflamed muscle may be recognized are:

Masticatory pain: The pain is inflammatory in type and is expressed as persistent soreness in the resting muscle. It is increased by all use. The chewing pain is not decreased by biting against a tongue blade. Secondary central excitatory effects and protective muscle splinting may complicate the symptom picture. The pain follows an inflammatory time frame.

Restricted movement: Extracapsular restriction limits opening without altering protrusion and contralateral excursion, unless inhibited by pain or unless the inflammatory condition immobilizes the joint.

Interference: None.

Acute malocclusion: None.

DISC-INTERFERENCE DISORDERS

Disorders due to interference with normal functioning of the articular disc occupy a position among temporomandibular complaints second in incidence only to muscle disorders. In fact, if nonsymptomatic conditions of the masticatory apparatus are included, interference disorders of the joint no doubt rank first. This group includes particularly the noisy, clicking, popping joints, with or without a component of pain.

The term sometimes used to designate such complaints is "degenerative joint disease." It is satisfactory only if it is clearly understood that these conditions represent the noninflammatory phase of degenerative joint disease, not true inflammatory degenerative arthritis. In recent years such conditions have been referred to as *internal derangements of the joint.* They are morphofunctional disorders of the disc-condyle complex.

Disorders of this sort are grouped together because they have clinical features that are similar, and they appear to be related in that they frequently represent a progressive series of deleterious changes of the joint. Pain may or may not accompany the masticatory dysfunction symptoms that dominate the clinical symptom picture.

Extrinsic trauma may damage the joint proper. Violent injury, including fracture and fracture-dislocation, may result in structural disorders such as deformation, chronic mandibular hypomobility, or traumatic arthritis. Less severe trauma may cause capsulitis or retrodiscitis. Minor external trauma may initiate deleterious changes in the joint surfaces.

More frequently the initiating factor that leads to interference disorders of the joint has to do with *microtraumas* sustained by the articulating parts of the joint as a result of structural or functional incompatibilities. Insidious damage may result from the habitual use of excessive biting force. It may relate to abusive habits, mannerisms, or use of the mouth and jaws for special purposes other than talking and mastication. But the most important parafunctional abuse no doubt relates to bruxism, both static and moving. In either case, the decisive factor that most significantly predisposes to deleterious change is occlusal disharmony—lack of functional compatibility between the unclenched and clenched positions during maximum intercuspation. An important clinical feature common to interference disorders of the joint is intermittency.

The similarities by which interference disorders of the joint are grouped together are as follows:

1. Noninflammatory dysfunction symptoms dominate the complaints. These are interferences during movements expressed as sensations, noises, and alterations of movement. If any restriction of mandibular movement occurs, it is due to associated obstruction or blockage by the articular disc.

2. Pain, if any, relates to strained discal ligaments. It is disc-attachment arthralgia that results from injury involving the collateral ligaments as they offer resistance to the interference. Being intermittent, it does not tend to induce secondary central excitatory effects.

Chronic interference disorders of the joint do not induce muscle splinting or myospasm activity in the masticatory muscles. However, a recently instituted occlusal disharmony (e.g., from recent change in the dentition due to trauma, extraction of teeth, or dental treatment) or recent activation of a preexisting but nonsymptomatic interference disorder (as a result of abuse or excessive passive interarticular pressure, as from an emotional crisis or an episode of oral consciousness) may institute muscle splinting. If protracted, it may develop myospastic activity. When an acute muscle disorder initially complicates a disc-interference disorder, it is a good assumption that the interference disorder preexisted and was activated into a symptomatic complaint. If, however, the symptoms of interference follow in the wake of protracted myospasm, one may assume that deleterious change is taking place in the joint as a direct result of the myospastic activity. When acute muscle symptoms subsequently occur during a prolonged period of disc-interference symptoms, it may be assumed that the condition has progressed to the inflammatory stage, and that the muscle symptoms represent the effect of continuous deep pain input.

Disc-interference disorders may become inflammatory. When this occurs, the condition should be reclassified as an *inflammatory disorder of the joint.*

In recent years two terms have become popular to describe certain disc-interference disorders: "reciprocal clicking" has been termed *disc displacement with reduction,* and so-called "closed lock" has been termed *disc displacement without reduction.* Although these terms may have some value arthrographically, they are not precise enough to have diagnostic value, because reciprocal clicking may or may not be due to anterior displacement of the disc and arrested opening may or may not be due to protracted dislocation of the disc. Since they refer to symptoms rather than to conditions, they are unsuitable terms for designating specific TM disorders.

The clinical symptoms by which disc-interference disorders of the joint may be recognized are:

Masticatory pain: The pain is intermittent, disc-attachment pain that is coincident with other disc-interference symptoms. Secondary central excitatory effects usually do not occur. If discal collateral ligaments or the inner horizontal portion of the TM ligament become inflamed, capsular-type pain symptoms are displayed.

Restricted movement: Severe obstruction of an articular disc can induce discrete, "hard" locking of the joint. Functional dislocation that blocks condylar movement induces "soft" locking near full opening.

Interference: Sensations of binding or catching, clicking or grating noises, and/or irregular movement, momentary locking, or deviations of the incisal path occur, depending on the degree of obstruction to movement. If opening symptoms are followed by symptoms during closing movement, they are said to be reciprocal.

Acute malocclusion: If the disc is fractured or functionally dislocated, malocclusion may be sensed as altered occlusal stress on ipsilateral posterior teeth. Spontaneous anterior dislocation causes gross malocclusion with only the posterior teeth touching while the anteriors remain apart.

Internal derangements are classified as they relate to the translatory cycle. Precise identification is needed because the treatment is not the same for the different types of interference. Since some disc-interference disorders, expecially those that stem from occlusal disharmony, form a sort of continuum, transitional phases may occur during which precise differentiation may be difficult.

Class I Interference

The symptoms of Class I interference occur in the closed position of the joint as the result of maximum intercuspation of the teeth. The basic cause of this disorder is chronic occlusal disharmony of a kind and magnitude that displaces the disc-condyle complex from the unclenched closed position when the teeth are brought into maximum intercuspation. The condition that results depends on the degree, direction, duration, and frequency of such abnormal movement. Any movement of the disc-condyle complex that exhausts weeping lubrication is potentially damaging to the articular surfaces.

If such disharmony has been created recently, as with changes in the dentition from trauma, extraction of posterior teeth, or dental treatment, an acute muscle disorder is more likely to result. Likewise, if a preexistent, dormant, nonsymptomatic, chronic occlusal disharmony is activated by bruxism due to an emotional crisis or by a period of oral consciousness, an acute muscle disorder may result. All such recently activated occlusal disharmony relates more closely to masticatory muscle spasm activity than to the subtle, less dramatic complaints that comprise disc-interference disorders.

The typical symptoms of Class I interference are a sensation of tightness or movement when the teeth are firmly clenched, frequently accompanied by momentary sharp pain, and then a discrete clicking sound just as the biting pressure is released. These symptoms can be prevented by biting ipsilaterally on a separator.

This type of discal interference predisposes to and may develop into a clinically identifiable Class II disc-interference disorder. Class I interference also predisposes to deleterious changes in the disc-condyle complex and as such may develop progressively into a Class III disc-interference disorder. Transitional phases between different classes of interference disorders may be difficult to define clinically. If such differentiation can be made, clinical management of the complaint is facilitated. It should be understood, however, that although etiologic factors responsible for Class I interference disorders may be reversible, the damage thus sustained by the joint structures may not be. *This is sufficient reason to understand and identify disc-interference disorders at their earliest stage of development, so that more recalcitrant conditions are avoided.*

Class II Interference

The symptoms of Class II interference occur as the mouth is opened immediately following maximum intercuspation. The typical symptoms consist of an initial sensation of the joint "sticking," followed by a discrete click, which may be accompanied by momentary discomfort. The rest of the translatory cycle is quite normal, and the symptoms do not recur unless the teeth are again brought firmly into maximum intercuspation. Similarly, this may occur as the first jaw movement that takes place following an extended period of inactivity, especially if bruxing has occurred. The entire symptom complex can be prevented by inserting an occlusal stop between the teeth that prevents the condyle from returning to the fully occluded position or by biting in a slightly protruded position.

Although Class II interference may develop from Class I as the result of occlusal disharmony that displaces the condyle during clenching, another frequent cause is the lack of firm occlusal contact between the molar teeth. This occurs usually as a result of dental restorations, replacements, or partial dentures with a posterior extension saddle. Other causes are trauma sustained with the teeth occluded, habitual use of excessive biting force, and bruxism.

Class II interference places considerable strain on the articular disc and its collateral ligaments. Therefore, it predisposes to Class III interference disorders if disc contour is lost and the ligaments undergo deterioration and elongation. Class II interference may be difficult to distinguish from early Class III functional displacement of the disc. Class II interference occurs, however, during the first few millimeters of opening and follows maximum intercuspation only while Class III disc displacement symptoms permit rotatory opening and may occur from the resting position.

Class III Interference

Symptoms of Class III disc-interference disorders occur during the course of normal translatory cycles—*after it begins, but not including strained movements or overextended opening*. Symptoms that occur as a result of forced, strained, or otherwise unnatural joint function are irrelevant to diagnosis.

Interference during translatory cycles may result from catching of the articular disc between the condyle and eminence. The result of such interference may be momentary locking. The inclination of the articular eminence should be considered, since the steeper the joint, the greater the likelihood of discal interference, and therefore the greater the importance of other factors that predispose to such interference.

Class III interference disorders occur for three basic reasons, namely, (1) excessive passive interarticular pressure, (2) lack of compatibility in the shape of the articulating surfaces, so that they hang as they glide over each other, and (3) some derangement or impairment of function involving the disc-condyle complex.

Excessive Passive Interarticular Pressure. The passive interarticular pressure in the joint reflects muscle action. Minimal passive interarticular pressure is that exerted by muscle tonus. It is increased by emotional tension and by the spasm of elevator muscles. Excessive passive pressure is an activating factor in all other causes of discal interference, sometimes making symptomatic a condition that otherwise might remain quite dormant. Discal interference due to this cause may show sudden onset, variability and, sometimes, a pattern of recurrence that parallels the rise and fall of emotional tension.

Structural Incompatibility of the Sliding Surfaces. Structural incompatibility between the articulating surfaces (articular eminence and upper surface of the disc-condyle complex) sufficient to cause catching of the articular disc during translatory cycles may result from several causes. These include developmental anomalies, growth aberrations, trauma, remodeling, and change due to such things as abusive use, mannerisms, chronic occlusal disharmony, and unusual functional demands. Trauma to the mandible sustained when the teeth are separated is a frequent cause. Immobilization of the opposite joint for any reason causes movements that may induce deterioration within the joint. All such interference due to structural incompatibility relates intimately to the degree of passive interarticular pressure as well as to the speed and force of movement.

Interference due to this cause has a pattern of sameness and chronicity, unless varying interarticular pressure gives it an episodic quality. Due to the sameness of behavior, interference of this type may be compensated for by deviation of the midline incisal path, which is considered to be an attempt on the part of muscles to find a way around the interference. When rapid movements are made, however, the initiating interference usually will become evident. Interference from structural incompatibility is less pronounced on the biting side.

Many times, interference symptoms are reciprocal—occurring with both opening and closing movements. When this takes place, it will be observed that the closing symptoms occur at about the same point in the translatory cycle as the opening symptoms, and the timing of the closing symptoms is precisely the same regardless of the speed of closure. These diagnostic points are the chief means of distinguishing between interference caused by structural incompatibility and that due to functional displacement of the articular disc. This differentiation is essential, because the treatment for the two conditions that display quite similar clinical symptoms is not the same. It should be noted that so-called "reciprocal clicking" from structural incompatibility occurs frequently.

Concerning the loud, audible, cracking noises that occur with chewing strokes, it should be noted that when such discrete symptoms are due to interference from structural incompatibility, it usually occurs as the result of biting on the opposite side. When due to disc displacement, however, the interference usually is accentuated by biting on the same side. This is due to active interarticular pressure and its effect on the width of the articular disc space.

Another point of differentiation is that symptoms due to structural incompatibility may include a definite deviation of the midline opening path that the patient is entirely unaware of. Deviations due to disc displacement are usually volitional. Unconscious midline deviations do not ordinarily develop from disc displacement disorders because of the variability of the interference as it relates to functional demands.

Impaired Disc-Condyle Complex. The more refractory Class III interferences occur as a result of functional impairment of the disc-condyle complex. Malfunctioning of the complex may be due to different structural abnormalities that result from chronic occlusal disharmony, trauma, or abusive use. These changes include (1) adhesions between the articular disc and mandibular condyle, (2) deterioration or fracture of the articular disc, (3) loss of disc contour and elongation of the discal ligaments, and (4) dysfunction of the superior retrodiscal lamina. Interference from such causes is usually progressive, thus predisposing to degenerative arthritis. The particular structural problem represented by a given complaint may not be clearly discernible diagnostically because of transitional phases and the various possible combinations that can occur. It is important, however, that Class III interference from structural failure of disc-condyle complex functioning be identified, because such judgment is the basis for choosing a treatment modality for managing the complaint.

Adhesions between articular disc and condyle. Hemarthrosis induced by trauma or surgery may cause fibrous adhesions that unite the condylar articular facet with the lower surface of the articular disc.[17, 18] The elimination of hinge movement in the disc-condyle complex disrupts normal joint functioning during translatory movements. Smooth, silent, surface-to-surface gliding of the articular disc along the articular eminence is impossible, and such movement becomes a bodily skidding of the immobilized disc. The result is rough, irregular, noisy movement throughout all translatory cycles. This condition predisposes to degenerative arthritis.

Damaged articular disc. Roughening of the superior surface of the articular disc due to trauma or deleterious change provokes interference throughout the translatory cycle. This is manifested as a more or less continuous grating noise punctuated at points of greater resistance by discrete noise and sensations of catching. Similar deterioration in the lower compartment of the joint elicits a grating sound when the mouth is opened and closed in pure rotation. Grating sounds during jaw movements result from some breakdown of articular tissue and are clinically indicative of degenerative joint disease.[19] Thinning of the disc due to continuing destructive change may result in perforation. This may alter internal hydrodynamic action of the synovial fluid, about which little is presently known. Thinning also predisposes to disc fracture. Separated fragments of a fractured disc lead to acute malocclusion, sensed as overstressed ipsilateral posterior teeth during maximum intercuspation. Overriding fragments cause acute malocclusion, manifested as disclusion of the posterior teeth.

Functional displacement/dislocation of the disc. Along with disc contour, the ligaments that firmly attach the articular disc to the medial and lateral poles of the condyle are the structures that make the disc and condyle into a hinge-joint unit. When disc contour is lost and the functional capability of the ligaments is compromised by deterioration, elongation, or detachment, normal hinge movement in the complex disappears, and linear sliding movement between the condyle and articular disc takes place. When the disc fails to follow the condyle closely, its essential function of maintaining sharp surface contact between the moving parts is impaired. It tends to catch and hang, thus causing irregular, rough, noisy movements. Discrete noises, catching sensations, and disc locking may take place. Noise and other symptoms of discal interference are likely to occur at the beginning of a power stroke when the superior lateral pterygoid muscle suddenly overcomes

the posterior traction of the superior retrodiscal lamina. All such interference is particularly sensitive to other contributing factors, such as
the steepness of the articular eminence, excessive interarticular pressure, structural incompatibility, and the speed and force of the jaw
movement. Interference symptoms tend to become reciprocal.

Two kinds of Class III disorders that involve dysfunctional discal
ligaments in conjunction with the loss of contour of the articular disc
are (1) functional displacements and (2) functional dislocations of the
articular disc.

1. Functional displacement of the disc: The sequence of clicking,
popping, or snapping noises emitted by the disc-condyle complex during opening and closing depends on the *location of destructive change* in
the articular disc, the *extent of elongation* of discal ligaments, and the
kind of movements made. Thinning of the posterior portion of the disc
permits functional displacement in an anterior direction; thinning of
the anterior portion permits displacement posteriorly. The extent of
elongation of the discal ligaments determines the amount of displacement possible. The kind of mandibular movement as it relates to the
action of the superior lateral pterygoid muscle and the superior retrodiscal lamina determines the incidence of displacement.

a) *Posteriorly thinned articular disc:* When loss of disc contour is located posteriorly, the articular disc is displaced anteriorly in the resting,
closed position by the muscle tonus action of the superior lateral pterygoid muscle. Since the lateral discal ligament is usually elongated
more than the medial one, the articular disc in the closed resting position of the joint may not be displaced straight forward, but may be
twisted around the medial attachment to the condyle.[20] Then, as the
translatory cycle begins, the condyle is obstructed by the twisted articular disc. Condylar movement is thus decelerated and momentarily arrested as the obstruction is met.[21, 22] The disc space widens as the condyle engages the thicker twisted disc.[22] Additional force is applied to
overcome the resistance of obstruction. The symptoms of interference
(clicking, catching, locking, pain) occur as the obstruction is overcome
and are coincident with a renewed burst of speed.[21, 22] The width of
the articular disc space returns to normal.[22]

Toller[21] has shown that disc interference symptoms result from the
mechanical obstruction of disc movement rather than from the condyle
merely slipping over different bands of the disc, as has been believed
by many in the past. From extensive cadaver studies, Hellsing and
Holmlund[23] have shown that gross anterior displacement of the articular disc actually occurs rarely, and that the usual hypothesis of the

condyle slipping behind the disc and then pushing it forward is improbable indeed. In fact, their studies suggested that some anterior positioning of the disc should be looked upon as a normal variant.

The timing of the opening symptoms relates to the degree of impairment in the disc-condyle complex. Minimal elongation of the ligaments and minimal loss of disc contour cause the symptoms to occur immediately after rotatory opening or just as protrusion begins. Greater elongation and loss of contour permit more opening or protrusion before symptoms occur. Marked elongation and severe loss of contour permit still more opening or protrusion before symptoms occur.

The character of the symptoms also relates to the degree of deterioration in the disc-condyle complex. When damage is slight and symptoms occur promptly, the noise and locking sensation are more discrete, pain is greater, and muscle effects (splinting, etc.) are more likely to occur. But, the prognosis for therapeutic correction is proportionately better. As elongation and loss of contour take place, and the symptoms occur later in the translatory cycle, the clicking and locking become less discrete, the discomfort is considerably less, and fewer muscle effects are displayed. This is because deterioration in the discal ligaments makes them less restrictive, and there is an appreciable decrease in innervation, both nociceptive and proprioceptive. As further damage is sustained by the disc-condyle complex, disc noise becomes more diffuse, locking is "softer," and the condition may become quite painless and free of secondary muscle effects. It should be noted, however, that, in turn, the prognosis for therapeutic correction without surgical intervention becomes all the more unfavorable.

After the initial symptoms, translation proceeds normally, unless there is some other disorder such as structural incompatibility. This is because, once the obstruction due to the twisted, anteriorly displaced disc is overcome, the disc-condyle relationship is normal and remains so by the tractive force of the elastic superior retrodiscal lamina as it stretches during forward translatory movement. If no power stroke or rapid closure ensues, no reciprocal symptoms will occur until just prior to reaching the closed joint position, when muscle tonus in the superior lateral pterygoid muscle again displaces the disc anteriorly. This has been observed arthrographically.[24] But, reciprocal symptoms can be produced at will by inducing a power stroke during which the active contraction of the superior lateral pterygoid muscle displaces the disc and again creates an obstruction to translatory movement back to the closed-joint position. The character of the reciprocal symptoms relates also to the extent of damage in the disc-condyle complex and gives clues as to the prognosis of therapy.

It should be noted that an important clinical feature that helps identify an anterior disc displacement is the variability of the closing symptoms. Also it should be noted that symptoms are more likely to occur when chewing on the symptomatic side. The incidence of disc interference relates intimately to changes in passive and active interarticular pressure. These features help distinguish disc displacement disorders from structural incompatibility disorders that induce similar clinical symptoms.

b) *Anteriorly thinned articular disc:* Loss of disc contour anteriorly predisposes to posterior displacement of the articular disc. In this case, the disc always occupies a normal position relative to the condyle in the resting closed-joint position, and no early opening symptoms occur as they do with anterior disc displacements. Following maximum intercuspation, however, the disc may remain stuck to the temporal articular surface as translatory movement begins, and it may remain until tugged loose by the discal ligaments. Following maximum intercuspation, early opening symptoms may occur which are similar to those of Class II interference. The difference is that with this type of disorder full rotatory opening (25 mm more or less) can take place before the symptoms occur, and the interference symptoms are usually less discrete.

As the condyle moves forward, the elastic traction of the superior retrodiscal lamina displaces the disc posteriorly. Symptoms at that time are largely subjective, and if an empty mouth closure is made, discrete symptoms may not occur at all as the disc is again replaced by the action of the superior lateral pterygoid muscle.

If a rapid closure or a power stroke is made, however, discrete interference symptoms may occur. A definite catching sensation just as closure begins is the usual symptom. An audible click or pop and sometimes an arrested closure occurs (so-called "open lock"). Such symptoms can usually be overcome by simply opening again and closing more cautiously. Most patients with this disorder have already learned how to do this.

Posterior displacements usually cause symptoms too mild to produce a complaint as far as empty-mouth functioning is concerned. Complaints usually have to do with symptoms that follow full maximum intercuspation (or bruxism), or that occur at mealtime. Some patients learn to create the closing interference (an audible click) at will by manipulating the jaw. Most patients with this disorder can identify the disc displacements subjectively even though no discrete symptoms are displayed.

2. Functional dislocation of the disc: If elongation, deterioration, or detachment of the discal collateral ligaments progresses until still greater displacement is permitted, and if deterioration of the articular disc is such as to permit it to be pulled through the articular disc space, functional dislocation of the disc can take place. There are different kinds of dislocation of the disc, namely, (1) spontaneous dislocation, which occurs with overextended opening and takes place in an anterior direction only, (2) traumatic dislocation, which results from direct external force (violence), and (3) functional dislocation, which occurs during the *normal* functioning of the joint and within the normal range of movement. Functional dislocation occurs as the result of a structural abnormality in the disc-condyle complex. When this happens, contact between condyle, disc, and articular eminence is lost, the articular disc space collapses, and the disc becomes trapped.

Anterior functional dislocation of the disc can occur when the inferior retrodiscal lamina becomes nonfunctional and when there is sufficient deterioration of the posterior portion of the articular disc to permit it to be pulled through the articular disc space anteriorly. The force that causes dislocation is the contraction of the superior lateral pterygoid muscle during a power stroke, rapid closure, or maximum intercuspation. *It is more likely to occur on the biting side.* When the articular disc space collapses, the disc is trapped anterior to the condyle, where it remains until reduced by posterior traction of the superior retrodiscal lamina as a full forward translatory movement is executed. It should be noted, however, that if the dislocated disc should block normal anterior movement of the condyle, then functional reduction is impossible, and the dislocated condition of the articular disc becomes protracted.

Posterior functional dislocation of the disc can occur when there is sufficient deterioration of the anterior portion of the articular disc to permit it to be pulled through the articular disc space posteriorly. The force that causes such dislocation is the posterior traction of the extended superior retrodiscal lamina during a full forward translatory cycle. When the articular disc space collapses, the disc is trapped posterior to the condyle until automatically reduced by the next closing effort, the reduction being accomplished by the contraction of the superior lateral pterygoid muscle as the result of a power stroke, rapid closure, or intercuspation. Protracted posterior functional dislocation does not occur.

The timing of the discal interference characteristic of functional dislocation depends on the actual mandibular movements made, as they relate to action of the superior lateral pterygoid muscle and the superior retrodiscal lamina, *for these are the forces that cause the dislocation and effect the reduction.* Between dislocation and reduction, movements are irregular in the absence of a functioning disc. An anteriorly dislocated disc displays a sensation of overstressed ipsilateral posterior teeth when clenched firmly.

It should be noted that, unless functional displacement follows acute trauma, the loss of disc contour and elongation of the discal collateral ligaments that permit such displacement of the articular disc are due to occlusal disharmony that displaces the condyle when the teeth are clenched. When such condylar displacement is directed posteriorly, encroachment on the posterior portion of the articular disc may cause appreciable loss of contour, thus predisposing to anterior displacement of the disc. When the condylar displacement is directed anteriorly, encroachment on the anterior part of the disc may cause sufficient loss of contour to predispose to posterior displacement of the articular disc. Therefore, when functional displacement is suspected, there should be either a history of external trauma or identifiable clinical evidence of present or former chronic occlusal disharmony that is gross enough to cause condylar displacement when the teeth are clenched. It should occur in the direction necessary to cause the disc-condyle complex damage that permits such discal displacement. Unless some other etiologically adequate traumatic incident can be established, the absence of such disharmony should serve to alert the examiner that the complaint may not be a true disc-displacement problem. Such determination has serious therapeutic implications.

Dysfunctional superior retrodiscal lamina. If the superior retrodiscal lamina is severed from the articular disc as a result of trauma, there is anterior prolapse of the disc to the extent permitted by the width of the articular disc space. This is manifested by discal interference during the forward turn-around phase of translatory cycles. The danger of spontaneous anterior dislocation is greatly increased, and if it should occur, it is permanent, because no other joint structure can be manipulated to exert posterior traction on the articular disc and thus bring about reduction. Likewise, if functional anterior dislocation should occur, it is irreversible except by surgical intervention.

Class IV Interference (Joint Hypermobility)

Subluxation refers to partial or incomplete dislocation of the articulating surfaces of a joint. In the temporomandibular joint, this can occur when translatory movement takes place without benefit of rotatory movement between the condyle and articular disc. Such arrested hinge action can occur if forward movement of the condyle exceeds that of the normal translatory cycle.

The forward limit of normal translatory movement is reached when the disc can no longer rotate posteriorly on the condyle, as determined by the condylar articular facet. As mouth opening takes place, the condyle rotates in the disc to separate the jaws, and the disc rotates on the condyle to maintain surface contact with the articular eminence. When these combined movements bring the posterior edge of the articular disc to the posterior margin of the condylar articular facet, hinge movement is arrested. Further opening effort causes partial dislocation between the disc and the articular eminence (see Fig 4–7). Such continued forward movement consists of a rough skid instead of smooth, silent, gliding, surface-to-surface movement of the disc-condyle complex along the temporal articular facet.

Class IV interference disorders occur *anterior to normal translation* due to excessive opening of the mouth, usually on a habitual level. Just prior to the typical skidding movement, a momentary pause usually is sensed. Then the condyle leaps forward to its full extent. The rough irregular movement is accompanied by noise and sometimes discomfort as well. It should be noted that a steeply inclined articular eminence predisposes to Class IV interference, which in turn predisposes to spontaneous anterior dislocation.

Class V Interference (Spontaneous Dislocation)

Normally, at the critical forward phase of the translatory cycle, sharp contact of the articulating parts is maintained by two conditions: (1) strong posteriorly directed rotatory traction on the articular disc exerted by the fully stretched superior retrodiscal lamina; and (2) relaxation of the superior lateral pterygoid muscle, so that no significant anteriorly directed counterforce is brought to bear on the disc. These conditions maintain a positive influence on the articular disc and, thus, preclude spontaneous dislocation. They keep it rotated as far posteriorly as the prevailing width of the articular disc space permits, thereby supplying continuing firm surface contact between the articulating parts.

Momentary muscular incoordination, however, can alter this protective relationship and induce dislocation. Normally, the superior lateral pterygoid muscle remains inactive throughout the translatory cycle, unless a power stroke ensues. Such strokes do not normally begin until after the forward turn-around phase of the cycle is completed and the return phase is well under way. Extremely precise timing of muscle action is required to accomplish this maneuver, especially when movements are rapid and when habitual hypermobility presents an added hazard. If premature contraction of the superior lateral pterygoid muscle takes place at the full forward (or overextended) position of the disc-condyle complex, such muscle action immediately overcomes the posterior traction force of the stretched superior retrodiscal lamina; the articular disc is rotated anteriorly on the condyle; and spontaneous dislocation occurs (Figs 7–1 and 7–2). No doubt, this mechanism accounts for the occasional acute spontaneous anterior dislocation of temporomandibular joints that occurs with yawning or when the muscles are fatigued by keeping the mouth open too long.

Another condition, however, is a more frequent cause of spontaneous dislocation. This has to do with the biomechanics of the posterior capsular ligament. As the condyle moves forward, the posterior wall of the capsular ligament opens up and straightens out. At full forward position, the posterior capsular ligament may become taut (see Fig 4–7). When this occurs, further forward movement of the condyle cannot take place. Instead, it simply rotates on itself. If the articular

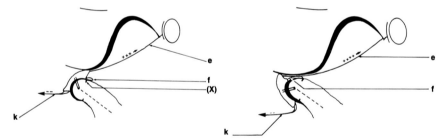

FIGURE 7–1   Spontaneous anterior dislocation of disc-condyle complex: *e*, superior retrodiscal lamina; *f*, inferior retrodiscal lamina; *k*, superior lateral pterygoid muscle; *x*, posterior margin of condylar articular facet. *Left*, subluxated disc-condyle complex prior to dislocation. Articular disc is fully rotated posteriorly. Dominant traction force on disc is that of the stretched superior retrodiscal lamina. Disc-condyle complex rotates bodily upon itself. Superior lateral pterygoid muscle is inactive. *Right*, dislocated disc-condyle complex. When articular disc loses contact with the articular eminence, the disc space collapses, the condyle moves superiorly against the articular eminence, and the disc is trapped in front. During dislocation, the posterior traction force of the superior retrodiscal lamina continues to act on the articular disc at all times except when the superior lateral pterygoid muscle contracts in conjunction with elevator muscles in attempts to close the mouth. Note that the extent of forward rotatory prolapse of the articular disc during dislocation is limited by the inferior retrodiscal lamina. An attempt to force closure against the trapped disc may cause strain on this ligament.

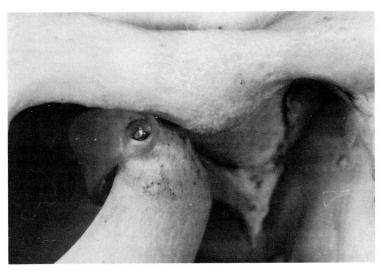

FIGURE 7–2 Photograph of dry skull with simulated articular disc hinged on condyle to illustrate the disc-condyle relationship that prevails during spontaneous anterior dislocation. Note that articular disc is prolapsed anteriorly, articular disc space is collapsed, condyle is in contact with the articular eminence, and the prolapsed disc is trapped in front of the condyle.

disc is already rotated posteriorly to its full limit as determined by the condylar articular facet, further rotation of the condyle moves the disc with it and, thus, may push it through the articular disc space. When this happens, spontaneous anterior dislocation takes place. This mechanism very likely accounts for dislocations that recur frequently and can be executed almost at will.

In spontaneous anterior dislocation, the articular disc prolapses on the condyle (see Fig 7–2). Contact between condyle, disc, and eminence is lost. The articular disc space collapses, and the condyle moves up against the eminence, thus trapping the disc anterior to the condyle. The amount of prolapse of the disc is limited by the inferior retrodiscal lamina, and attempts to close may cause undue strain on this ligamentous structure. Thus, forcing closure of the mouth without first reducing the dislocation may cause pain that emanates from the inferior retrodiscal lamina as well as the collateral discal ligaments.

It should be noted that the stretched superior retrodiscal lamina all the while is exerting positive posterior traction on the dislocated articular disc. This offers a ready means of spontaneous reduction, if only a sufficient width of articular disc space is provided. This should be remembered as the key factor in planning treatment for this condition. Many patients who dislocate frequently learn to effect reduction of the disc automatically and can do so at will.

Spontaneous anterior dislocation is characterized by sudden inability to close the mouth following a wide opening effort. Only the most posteriorly located teeth come into contact while the anteriors stand widely apart. No pain is induced unless force is used to reduce the dislocation. Force may strain the inferior retrodiscal lamina, thus inducing arthralgic pain. Forced efforts to close the mouth also may injure the discal ligaments, thus causing symptoms of capsulitis. Myospastic activity in the musculature may add to the discomfort and the problem of reduction. Myospasm of the superior lateral pterygoid muscle prevents reduction entirely, because it supercedes the ability of the superior retrodiscal lamina to reposition the disc, even if adequate disc space is provided. Contracture of this muscle causes chronic anterior dislocation. A nonfunctional superior retrodiscal lamina renders the dislocation permanent.

INFLAMMATORY DISORDERS OF THE JOINT

Inflammatory disorders of the joint have pain as their chief symptom— more or less continuous inflammatory arthralgic pain.[25] It tends to parallel the clinical course of the inflammatory process from which it emanates. Usually it is aggravated by the demands of function. Since it is usually continuous, secondary central excitatory effects are to be expected as part of the symptom complex.

Inflammatory disorders of the temporomandibular joint may be classified as (1) synovitis and capsulitis, (2) retrodiscitis, and (3) inflammatory arthritis.

Synovitis and Capsulitis

Inflammation of the synovial membrane and capsular ligament causes swelling and palpable tenderness over the involved joint. Synovitis proper characteristically causes fluctuating swelling due to effusion within the joint cavity, discomfort with movements, and alteration of the synovial fluid. It may result from localized trauma, abusive use, and specific infection. Inflammation of the capsular ligament may result from several causes, namely, (1) strain or injury due to forced excessive condylar movement, (2) inflammatory condition of the discal collateral ligaments or the temporomandibular ligament, (3) inflammatory arthritis, (4) excessive condylar movement in the presence of preexisting capsular fibrosis, and (5) direct extension from a periarticular inflammatory process.

It is difficult, and indeed clinically impractical, to distinguish between synovitis and capsulitis. The clinical symptoms by which synovitis and capsulitis may be recognized are:

Masticatory pain: The arthralgia is of capsular type. There is palpable tenderness over the joint proper, and the discomfort is increased by condylar movements that tend to stretch the capsule. (Note: If capsular pain increases in maximum intercuspation and is somewhat reduced by biting against a separator, the collateral ligaments and/or temporomandibular ligament should be suspected as the primary source of the inflammation.) Central excitatory effects may be seen also.

Restricted movement: Limitation of movement, if any, is due to capsular swelling. Limitation may range from slightly restricted extended translatory movements to almost complete immobilization of the joint.

Interference: Usually, no interference is present other than from a preexisting or coexisting condition. Sometimes gelation of the synovial fluid causes stiffness of the joint, especially after a period of inactivity. This may be accompanied by peculiar joint sounds. Such symptoms usually disappear rapidly as normal activity of the joint is resumed.

Acute malocclusion: Inflammatory effusion within the joint cavity may cause disclusion of the ipsilateral posterior teeth.

Retrodiscitis

Injury sustained by the retrodiscal tissue by direct external trauma may cause inflammatory swelling of the tissue which induces acute malocclusion and pain when the teeth are fully occluded. The clinical symptoms may simulate a mandibular fracture from which traumatic retrodiscitis must be differentiated. Possible hemarthrosis presents the hazard of adhesions between the disc and condyle or between the disc and articular eminence.

Insidious injury of the retrodiscal tissue may occur as the result of condylar encroachment due to occlusal disharmony that displaces the condyle posteriorly when the teeth are clenched.[26] Considerable deterioration must first take place in the disc and discal ligaments as well as in the inner horizontal portion of the temporomandibular ligament before repetitive condylar encroachment is possible. When degenerative elongation of the temporomandibular ligament is sufficient to permit such encroachment, the inital damage is sustained by the inferior retrodiscal lamina. It should be noted that this structure must become nonfunctional before displacement of the articular disc is sufficient to permit actual anterior dislocation. If such dislocation does occur, it subjects the entire retrodiscal tissue to trauma from the condyle. However, the highly essential superior retrodiscal lamina usually remains sufficiently functional to exert tractive force on the articular disc during the forward phase of the translatory cycle.

Since the clinical symptoms of acute retrodiscitis somewhat simulate those of Class I interference as well as those of inferior lateral pterygoid myospasm, accurate differentiation is needed. The clinical symptoms by which retrodiscitis may be recognized are:

Masticatory pain: Arthralgia of the retrodiscal type is initiated or aggravated by maximum intercuspation. It is usually reduced by biting against a tongue blade that prevents intercuspation. If the pain is clearly intermittent, no central excitatory effects are displayed.

Restricted movement: There is none, other than the inhibitory influence of pain.

Interference: None.

Acute malocclusion: Acute malocclusion may result from swelling of the retrodiscal tissue or from inflammatory effusion within the joint cavity. This causes a sensation of disclusion of the ipsilateral posterior teeth. Swelling of the retrodiscal tissue causes premature occlusion of the contralateral anterior teeth.

Inflammatory Arthritis

Ordinarily, the clinical identification of intracapsular inflammation is sufficient to make a diagnosis of inflammatory arthritis. The complex structure and functional intricacies of the temporomandibular joints offer exceptions to this rule, as indicated by inflammatory conditions of the collateral ligaments, the temporomandibular ligaments, and the retrodiscal tissue. It is important therapeutically that clinical differentiation be made. It should be noted that capsulitis is frequently a feature of inflammatory arthritis.

The different types of inflammatory arthritis may be indistinguishable on the basis of clinical symptoms. The initial step is to establish with certainty that such a condition is present. The particular type can later be determined on the basis of etiology, clinical response to therapy, and laboratory studies.

The clinical symptoms by which inflammatory arthritis may be recognized are:

Masticatory pain: The pain is arthralgic. Frequently, enough capsulitis is present to render the joint tender to manual palpation over the joint proper. Pain is more or less continuous but increases with functional demands. The symptom picture may be complicated by central excitatory effects. The speed and force of masticatory movements influence the discomfort.

Restricted movement: Limitation of movement may range from none to almost complete joint immobilization, due to capsulitis and secondary muscle effects.

Interference: Traumatic and degenerative arthritis may display a variety of disc-interference symptoms.

Acute malocclusion: Inflammatory effusion within the joint cavity or rapid osteolysis may cause acute malocclusion.

The pain level with different kinds of inflammatory arthritis is extremely variable. The same is true of functional interference. It may be surprising to see minimal pain and dysfunction when joint changes are great (e.g., some cases of degenerative arthritis). At other times, the discomfort may be wholly disproportionate to the structural change (e.g., hyperuricemia).

Different kinds of inflammatory arthritis afflict the temporomandibular joints, namely, traumatic arthritis, degenerative arthritis, infectious or septic arthritis, rheumatoid arthritis, and hyperuricemia.

Traumatic Arthritis. Inflammatory arthritis that results from extrinsic trauma usually is expressed initially as a synovitis, with or without hemarthrosis. Other structures of the joint may suffer injury, e.g., the articular disc, collateral ligaments, retrodiscal tissue, and the osseous supported articular surfaces of the joint. Localized pain and swelling over the joint proper, discomfort with and restriction of joint function, and interference during joint movements may occur, depending on the location and extent of injury. Usually, single joints are involved. An important diagnostic clue is a history of continuity of symptoms from the time of trauma to the joint. Coexisting muscle effects should be recognized, such as splinting, spasm, or inflammation. Secondary central excitatory effects may also develop if the acute symptoms persist.

Radiographic studies may give evidence of traumatized osseous structures. Chronic forms of traumatic arthritis may show radiographic evidence of previous injury to the articular surfaces that causes interference with normal functioning of the joint (Fig 7–3).

Degenerative Arthritis. Degenerative arthritis is the advanced inflammatory phase of disc-interference disorders, as previously described.[27] The history, therefore, is that of preexisting interference

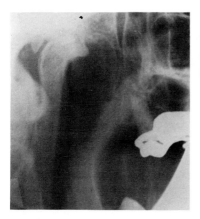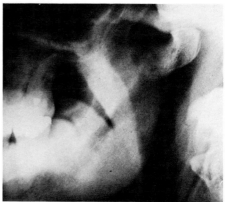

FIGURE 7–3   Radiographic confirmation of traumatic arthritis. *Left,* transfacial projection of left mandibular condyle deformed as result of former injury. *Right,* transfacial projection of a fractured mandibular condyloid process that has healed in malposition. (From Bell W.E.: *Orofacial Pains: Differential Diagnosis,* ed. 2. Chicago, Year Book Medical Publishers, 1979. Reproduced by permission.)

during mandibular movement. Although the examiner may not be able to discern the particular type of interference disorder represented, he may be able to identify etiologic factors that should be taken into consideration therapeutically. Chronic occlusal disharmony, especially aggravated by bruxism and activated by a high level of emotional tension, deserves careful consideration in all such conditions. The Class III disorders, especially those due to impaired disc-condyle complex function, predispose to inflammatory degenerative arthritis.

Although all sorts of functional abuse, including habitual excessive use of biting force, traumatic mannerisms and habits, nonphysiologic use of the mouth and jaws, bruxism, and occlusal interference of different kinds, are important etiologically in degenerative arthritis, one type of abusive force warrants special attention. That has to do with traumatic loading of the joint. Normally, joints are able to cope with considerable abuse and generally undergo various degrees and kinds of structural remodeling to compensate for conditions imposed on them. Overloading, however, tends to induce degenerative change in articular surfaces rather than physiologic remodeling.

When occlusal support in the posterior region of the mouth is insufficient, clenching causes the mandible to overclose in the posterior area—so-called *posterior overclosure.* If the remaining occluding teeth do not offer occlusal anchorage, the condyle slips posteriorly. But, if the remaining teeth do firmly hold the mandible and thus prevent posterior displacement, a fulcrum is formed at the location of the most posteriorly situated anchoring contact. Then as the teeth are fully occluded, the condyle rotates around this fulcrum, and the excessive force generated by the overclosure is directed upward and forward. Degenerative change is likely to take place in the impacted area since overloading occurs each time the teeth are brought into maximum intercuspation. Bruxism under these circumstances is especially abusive.

Radiographic confirmation of degenerative arthritis may include evidence of structural change in the subarticular bone (Fig 7–4). Evidence of occlusal disharmony also may be obtained if the disharmony is gross enough and takes place in the sagittal plane (see Figs 5–12 and 5–13).

Infectious Arthritis. Although synovitis may occur in conjunction with systemic infection as a nonspecific or immunologic response, ac-

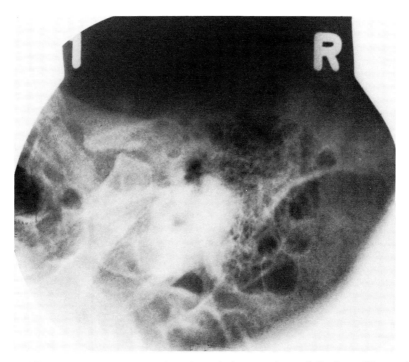

FIGURE 7–4 Radiographic confirmation of degenerative arthritis in a 65-year-old woman. Transparietal projection of right temporomandibular joint in closed position. There is visible loss of contour of the subarticular osseous surfaces and irregularity of the width of the articular disc space. (From Bell W.E.: Temporomandibular joint, in Goldman H.M., Forrest S.P., Byrd D.L., et al. (eds.): *Current Therapy in Dentistry.* St. Louis, C.V. Mosby Co., 1968, vol. 3. Reproduced with permission.)

tual purulent bacterial invasion of the joint may take place also. This may be due to penetrating wounds, trauma, or the spreading of infection from adjacent structures (e.g., otitis media). Occasionally, infectious arthritis may be the result of bacteremia from systemic infection (e.g., gonorrheal arthritis). The diagnosis is made from the history, clinical symptoms, examination of fluid aspirated from the joint cavity, and blood studies.[28]

Rheumatoid Arthritis.   The temporomandibular joints frequently are involved in rheumatoid arthritis. The symptoms may be mild and go unnoticed, but if other joints are involved, the diagnosis is usually obvious. Occasionally the temporomandibular joint is the initial joint of complaint. In that case, the diagnosis may be difficult indeed.

Rheumatoid arthritis is an inflammatory condition of unknown etiology in which the inflamed and hypertrophic synovial membrane grows onto the articulating surfaces. The presence of such vascularized and innervated tissue on pressure-bearing surfaces of the joint causes pain and inflammation with normal functioning of the joint. It may also predispose to fibrous ankylosis. Rheumatoid arthritis is extremely variable in incidence, severity, and clinical course. Severe forms may cause bizarre resorption of the supporting osseous structures. Loss of vertical height due to condylar resorption may induce a progressive open-bite relationship of the anterior teeth (see Fig 5–15). Diagnosis of rheumatoid arthritis requires medical confirmation.

Hyperuricemia.   An excessive level of serum uric acid causes a type of inflammatory arthritis in which pain with functional movements of the joint may be the chief complaint. This is also true of so-called subclinical gout, in which the serum uric acid level may run no higher than 6.0 mg/dl. As uric acid increases in concentration, the symptoms usually become greater. High levels may show deposits of urates in and about the joint. The symptoms are frequently polyarticular, episodic, and recurrent. It is seen more frequently in older persons. The diagnosis is confirmed by blood studies. The temporomandibular joints are involved with surprising frequency.

CHRONIC MANDIBULAR HYPOMOBILITIES

Another category of temporomandibular disorders has to do with painless restriction of mandibular movement. Such conditions may show signs of becoming progressively worse. When excessive force is used to move the mandible beyond the restraint imposed by such a condition, tethering adhesions may be injured and become inflamed, thus giving an element of pain to what otherwise is a painless disorder.

Depending on the location of the cause of restraint, these disorders are classified as (1) contracture of elevator muscles, (2) capsular fibrosis, and (3) ankylosis. They are to be differentiated from the extra-articular restrictions of mandibular movement.

The clinical symptoms by which the chronic mandibular hypomobilities may be recognized are:

Masticatory pain: There is none, unless the condition is injured by excessive movement or abusive use.

Restricted movement: Extracapsular limitation is due to contracture of an elevator muscle(s). Capsular limitation is due to capsular fibrosis. Intracapsular limitation is due to ankylosis.

Interference: There is none, unless the interference is preexistent.

Acute malocclusion: None.

Contracture of Elevator Muscle

Muscular contracture is regarded clinically as a reduction in the resting length of a muscle without seriously impairing its other functional capabilities. It is a painless condition unless injured by the application of forceful jaw opening, thus inducing myositis. Two types of muscle contracture are identifiable, namely, (1) *myostatic contracture,* which occurs as a result of failure to periodically stimulate the inverse stretch reflex, and (2) *myofibrotic contracture,* which occurs as a result of formation of excessive fibrous tissue within the muscle or its sheath. Myostatic contracture usually results from prolonged inability to open the mouth normally, the resting length of the elevator muscles decreasing until they conform to the degree of opening thus imposed. It may be reversible with proper therapy. Myofibrotic contracture is reactive to inflammation in and about the muscle and is not reversible.

Contracture of an elevator muscle restricts opening without appreciably limiting protrusion or contralateral excursion. The accompanying deflection of the midline path will be displayed with opening, but not with protrusion. This can be confirmed radiographically (see Fig 5–9).

Capsular Fibrosis

Fibrotic contracture of the capsular ligament is referred to as capsular fibrosis. It results from inflammation of the capsule, usually due to trauma. This includes surgery. The degree of restriction of mandibular movement depends on the resultant size of the capsule and thickness of the capsular wall. Capsular fibrosis restrains condylar movement in the outer ranges, imposing restriction on translatory movement of the condyle, whether for opening, protrusion, or lateral excursion. It is painless, unless force is used that causes injury to the capsule, thus inducing capsulitis. When this occurs, the true underlying condition may not become apparent until the acute symptoms subside. Then, evidence of preexisting capsular restriction of mandibular movement will remain. Radiographic confirmation is available (see Fig 5–10).

Ankylosis

Intracapsular adhesions or actual ossification that tether the condyle to the articular eminence is termed ankylosis. This results from trauma that causes hemarthrosis, which may organize and form a matrix for cicatrization. Although fibrous ankylosis is the usual type, occasionally ossification takes place (Fig 7–5). Ossification is more likely to occur when infection has been present. Ankylosis is usually unilateral because trauma is characteristically a single-joint affliction. It should be noted that when one joint is thus immobilized, degenerative change may take place in the opposite joint, due to the unnatural movements thus imposed.

Bilateral fibrous ankylosis may occur if the trauma is sufficient to cause hemarthrosis in both joints. This occurs with some frequency in small infants when the articular surfaces are still vascularized and vulnerable to injury that causes bleeding within the joints. A fall on the chin during the tottering stage may result in this condition. It may not be detected as a symptomatic disorder until many years later when restriction of opening and other movements are discovered, frequently as a result of dental treatment. Such patients chew vertically. When viewed in profile, they show no forward translation of the mandible with opening. Protrusive and lateral movements are nonexistent. Being a life-long condition, such abnormality in jaw function usually causes no subjective complaint because the individual has no knowledge of what normal mandibular movements are like. Only when strained by excessive opening or by forced lateral or protrusive movement—frequently by the dentist—does the condition become symptomatic. Pain results from injury to the tethering adhesions.

The degree to which fibrous ankylosis restricts jaw movement depends on the extent, location, and length of the fibrous adhesions. Tightly bound adhesions may restrict condylar movement to pure ro-

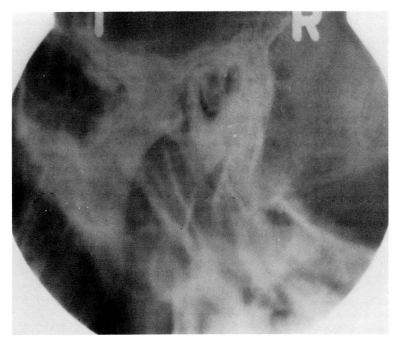

FIGURE 7–5 Radiographic confirmation of osseous ankylosis in a 41-year-old man. Transparietal projection of right temporomandibular joint in closed position. The entire articular disc space is obscured by diffuse radiopaque deposition of dense osseous tissue.

tation, thus limiting comfortable opening to about 25 mm. The midline deflects ipsilaterally with both opening and protrusion. Longer and more flexible adhesions permit greater movement. The condition remains quite painless unless injured by excessive jaw movements. Ankylosis may be complicated by myostatic contracture of the elevator muscles due to protracted inability to open properly.

Ankylosis must be differentiated from a contractured elevator muscle. Since the restriction of movement is intracapsular, protrusion and contralateral excursion will be limited as well as opening, and the incisal path will deflect with both opening and protrusion. This may be confirmed radiographically (Fig 7–6).

GROWTH DISORDERS OF THE JOINT

Disorders of growth that afflict the craniomandibular articulation are varied. Fortunately, growth disorders that are of sufficient importance

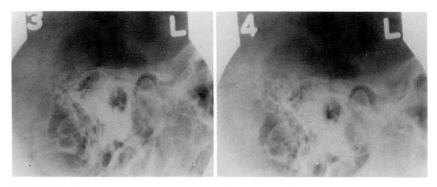

FIGURE 7–6   Radiographic confirmation of fibrous ankylosis in a 16-year-old girl. Transparietal projection of left temporomandibular joint. *Left,* lateral excursion to the opposite side. *Right,* maximum opening. Condylar movement in lateral position is minimal. There is similar restriction of condylar movement in open position.

to become symptomatic are low in incidence. They have several features that are similar enough to justify grouping them together, namely:

      1. The clinical symptoms occur directly from the structural changes that are present.

      2. Disturbance in function and the incidence of masticatory pain are secondary to those structural changes.

      3. Radiographic evidence is of primary importance in differential diagnosis.

    For sake of discussion, disorders of growth may be divided into three categories, namely, (1) aberrations related to the developmental process, (2) acquired changes in structural form, and (3) neoplasia. For more adequate discussion of disorders of this type, authoritative sources of information are available.[29–32]

Aberration of Development

A wide variation in size and shape of temporomandibular joint structure can be considered within normal limits. Even when structural variation exceeds what usually is considered normal, masticatory function may remain nonsymptomatic. It is when deficiency, hyperplasia, or asymmetry imposes a measure of dysfunction on the masticatory apparatus that symptoms become apparent. The cause of such aberration of development is either unknown or poorly understood. Deficiency problems are usually bilateral and symmetric. Some are associated with facial defects.

Bilateral hyperplasia results in mandibular prognathism; unilateral overgrowth causes facial asymmetry. When these conditions develop from an early age, quite satisfactory compensatory adjustment of the joints and dentition may take place, so that very little, if any, functional incompatibility (occlusal disharmony) is evident, even though improper articulation of the teeth may be obvious.

Dysplasia of the mandible as well as of the temporal bone is usually unilateral and asymmetric. Although the cause of such condition is not known precisely, experimental evidence indicates that a hematoma during the critical developmental period can cause similar defects.[30] Complete agenesis of the condyle may occur (Fig 7–7).

Acquired Change in Joint Structure

Some anomalies of growth occur after joint development and dentition are complete. Unilateral hyperplasia of the condyloid process in adults may cause marked malocclusion, such as cross-bite, thus creating structural incompatibility of the parts (Fig 7–8).

Perhaps the most frequently acquired change in joint structure occurs as a result of trauma. Actual alteration in the osseous relationship may result from fracture of the condyloid process. Traumatized bone may react by developing hypertrophic outgrowths that can become incompatible with normal joint function (see Fig 7–9).

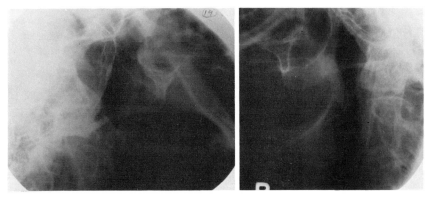

FIGURE 7–7 Mandibular dysplasia in a 60-year-old woman. Lateral oblique projection of left and right mandibular rami. Note that structural formation of the right side is normal. Left side shows agenesis of entire condylar process and most of the mandibular ramus.

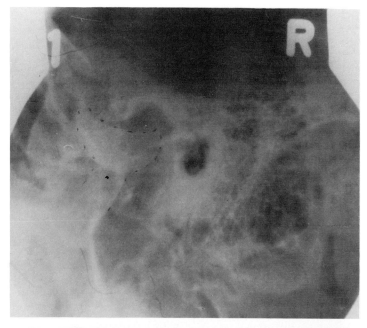

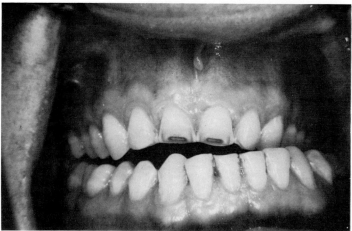

FIGURE 7–8   Radiographic confirmation of aberration of growth of the mandibular condyle in a 30-year-old man. *Top,* transparietal projection of right temporomandibular joint in closed position. Note the shape of condyle, with enlargement posteriorly as well as anteriorly. The posterior enlargement has shifted the position of the condyle anteriorly, thus causing gross malocclusion. *Bottom,* dentition occludes in cross-bite to the left side. (From Bell W.E.: Management of temporomandibular joint problems, in Goldman H.M., Gilmore H.W., Royer R.Q., et al. (eds.): *Current Therapy in Dentistry.* St. Louis, C.V. Mosby Co., 1970, vol. 4. Reproduced with permission.)

Ordinarily, all such aberrations of growth remain nonsymptomatic until the structural change interferes with normal functioning of the joint and/or dentition. The final symptomatology, therefore, is varied and depends on the particular situation at hand.

Neoplasia

Neoplastic involvement of a temporomandibular joint is relatively rare. Tumors of cartilage and osseous structure are reported most frequently. Osteoma of the condyle may be extremely difficult to distinguish from hyperplasia. Chondroma, osteochondroma,[33] giant cell granuloma, and hemangioma have been reported. All such tumors involving the mandibular condyle are extremely rare (Fig 7–9).

Although primary malignant disease of the temporomandibular joint proper has been reported, direct invasion from surrounding structures is considerably more frequent. When this occurs, the initial

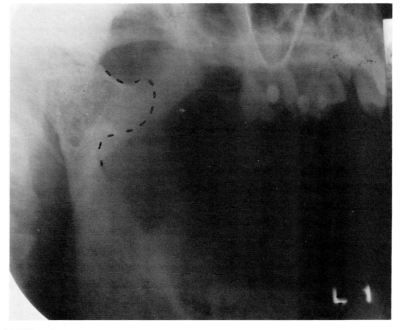

FIGURE 7–9 Radiographic confirmation of aberration of condylar growth due to benign neoplasia in a 41-year-old man. Transfacial projection of left mandibular condyle shows marked enlargement of the osseous structure anteriorly. Note that the superior surface of new growth conforms in shape to the fossa and articular eminence, evidence of slow, benign growth.

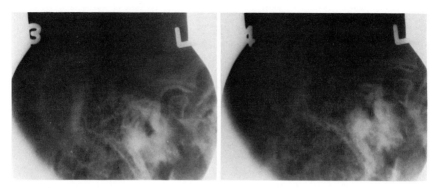

FIGURE 7–10   Radiographic confirmation of fixation of the temporomandibular joint due to extra-articular cause, later determined to be invasion by malignant neoplasm, in a 54-year-old woman. Transparietal projection of the left temporomandibular joint. *Left,* lateral excursion to the opposite side; *right,* maximum opening. Note that there is marked restriction of mandibular movement in both lateral excursion and opening, but not to exactly the same degree. The movement with opening slightly exceeds that of lateral excursion.

joint complaint is usually painless restriction of joint movement, which is highly suggestive of fibrous ankylosis. It is only when the disorder expresses itself as a progressively worsening condition with an increasing component of pain that malignancy may be suspected (Fig 7–10). Needle biopsy can help make a positive diagnosis.

REFERENCES

1. Costen J.B.: Syndrome of ear and sinus symptoms dependent upon disturbed function of the temporomandibular joint. *Ann. Otol. Rhinol. Laryngol.* 43:1, 1934.
2. *Dorland's Illustrated Medical Dictionary,* ed. 24. Philadelphia, W.B. Saunders Co., 1965.
3. Schwartz L.L.: A temporomandibular pain-dysfunction syndrome. *J. Chronic Dis.* 3:284, 1956.
4. Laskin D.M.: Etiology of the pain-dysfunction syndrome. *J. Am. Dent. Assoc.* 79:147, 1969.
5. *Dorland's Illustrated Medical Dictionary,* ed. 26. Philadelphia, W.B. Saunders Company, 1981.
6. Morgan D.H., Hall W.P., Vamvas S.J. (eds.): *Diseases of the Temporomandibular Apparatus.* St. Louis, C.V. Mosby Co., 1977.
7. Gelb H. (ed.): *Clinical Management of Head, Neck and TMJ Pain and Dysfunction.* Philadelphia, W.B. Saunders Co. 1977.
8. Sarnat B.G., Laskin D.M. (eds.): *The Temporomandibular Joint,* ed. 3. Springfield, Ill., Charles C Thomas, Publisher, 1979.

9. Zarb G.A., Carlsson G.E. (eds.): *Temporomandibular Joint Function and Dysfunction.* Copenhagen, Munksgaard, 1979.
10. Irby W.B. (ed.): *Current Advances in Oral Surgery,* Vol. 3. St. Louis, C.V. Mosby Co., 1980.
11. Bell W.E.: Management of temporomandibular joint problems, in Goldman H.M., Gilmore H.W., Royer R.Q., et al. (eds.): *Current Therapy in Dentistry,* Vol. 4. St. Louis, C.V. Mosby Co., 1970, pp. 398–415.
12. McNeill C., Danzig W.M., Farrar W.B., et al.: Craniomandibular (TMJ) disorders: The state of the art. *J. Prosthet. Dent.* 44:434, 1980.
13. Bell W.E.: Classification of TM disorders, in *The President's Conference on the Examination, Diagnosis and Management of Temporomandibular Disorders.* Chicago, American Dental Association, 1983, pp. 24–29.
14. Bell W.E.: *Clinical Management of Temporomandibular Disorders.* Chicago, Year Book Medical Publishers, 1982.
15. Laskin D.M., Greenfield W., Gale E., et al. (eds.): *The President's Conference on the Examination, Diagnosis, and Management of Temporomandibular Disorders.* Chicago, American Dental Association, 1983, pp. 182–184.
16. Bell W.E.: Clinical diagnosis of the pain-dysfunction syndrome. *J. Am. Dent. Assoc.* 79:154, 1969.
17. Sprinz R.: The role of the meniscus in the healing process following excision of the articular surfaces of the mandibular joint in rabbits. *J. Anat.* 97:345, 1963.
18. Nickerson J.W. Jr.: Letter to the editor. *J. Am. Dent. Assoc.* 103:382, 1981.
19. Moffett B.: Questions and Answers, Session 1, in Moffett B.C. (ed.): *Diagnosis of Internal Derangements of the Temporomandibular Joint,* Vol. 1. Seattle, University of Washington, 1984, p. 30.
20. Westesson P.: Diagnostic accuracy of double-contrast arthrography confirmed by dissection, in Moffett B.C. (ed.): *Diagnosis of Internal Derangements of the Temporomandibular Joint,* Vol. 1. Seattle, University of Washington, 1984, pp. 31–34.
21. Toller P.A.: Opaque arthrography of the temporomandibular joint. *Int. J. Oral Surg.* 3:17, 1974.
22. Nanthaviroj S., Omnell K., Randow K., et al.: Clicking and temporary "locking" in the temporomandibular joint. *Dentomaxillofac. Radiol.* 5:33, 1976.
23. Hellsing G., Holmlund A.: Development of anterior disc displacement in the temporomandibular joint: An autopsy study. *J. Prosthet. Dent.* 53: 397–401, 1985.
24. Zampese D.R., Photopoulos D.J., Manzione J.V.: Use of TMJ arthrotomography in the diagnosis and treatment of anterior disk dislocation. *J. Prosthet. Dent.* 50:821, 1983.
25. Bell W.E.: *Orofacial Pains,* ed. 3. Chicago, Year Book Medical Publishers, 1985.
26. Blackwood J.H.H.: Pathology of the temporomandibular joint. *J. Am. Dent. Assoc.* 79:118, 1969.

27. Toller P.A.: Temporomandibular arthropathy. *Proc. Roy. Soc. Lond.* 67:153, 1974.
28. Klinenberg J.R.: The arthritides, in Sarnat B.G., Laskin D.M. (eds.): *The Temporomandibular Joint,* ed. 3. Springfield, Ill., Charles C Thomas, Publisher, 1979, pp. 335–347.
29. Cherrick H.M.: Pathology, in Sarnat B.G., Laskin D.M. (eds.): *The Temporomandibular Joint,* ed. 3. Springfield, Ill., Charles C Thomas, Publisher, 1979, pp. 180–204.
30. Poswillo D.E.: Congenital malformations: Prenatal experimental studies, in Sarnat B.G., Laskin D.M. (eds.): *The Temporomandibular Joint,* ed. 3. Springfield, Ill., Charles C Thomas, Publisher, 1979, pp. 127–150.
31. Ross R.B.: Developmental anomalies and dysfunctions of the temporomandibular joint, in Zarb G.A., Carlsson G.E. (eds.): *Temporomandibular Joint Function and Dysfunction.* Copenhagen, Munksgaard, 1979, pp. 119–154.
32. Sarnat B.G., Laskin D.M. Surgical considerations, in Sarnat B.G., Laskin D.M. (eds.): *The Temporomandibular Joint,* ed. 3. Springfield, Ill., Charles C Thomas, Publisher, 1979, pp. 433–470.
33. Strickland R.D., Hirsch S.A., Goldberg J.S.: Osteochondroma of the mandibular condyle. *J. Craniomand. Pract.* 3:190–192, 1985.

8

Clinical Examination

The objective of a TM examination is to obtain the necessary data to make a proper diagnosis. This is a technical procedure that can be delegated to a trained technician, if necessary. The data needed to make a diagnosis consist of five parts:

1. Historical background of the complaint that may give clues to its etiology

2. Positive identification of the source(s) of masticatory pain

3. Identification of the location of any restriction of mandibular movement

4. Determination of the classification of disc-interference symptoms as they relate to the translatory cycle

5. Recognition of occlusal dysfunction, whether it be etiologic, symptomatic, or noncontributory

An examining procedure that effectively supplies this essential information without including extraneous data conserves both time and expense. Many TM disorders can be satisfactorily managed from a clinical diagnosis alone. If confirmation is needed before definitive therapy, additional diagnostic effort is warranted, such as analgesic blocking, radiography, special tests, and consultations. It is well to make a clinical diagnosis before committing the patient to what otherwise might be unnecessary examining procedures. Radiography should be for the purpose of confirming the clinical diagnosis. There is no substitute for a thorough evaluation of the patient and his problem at a clinical level.

CHIEF COMPLAINT

To initiate an examination of the craniomandibular articulation and masticatory musculature, one first should identify the patient's complaint which should be recorded in his own language, for this is going to be the final issue upon which he will judge the effectiveness of your management of his problem. It is important to keep in mind that this is *his complaint,* and what is chief to him is what it is all about.

Then, the complaint should be restated in the technical language of masticatory symptomatology. This statement of the problem should be the primary issue when the evaluation of the data is made and a diagnosis rendered. This should be the primary condition for which treatment is planned.

Identification of Masticatory Symptoms

The next step in data collection is the clear identification of all masticatory and concomitant symptoms, noting how they relate to the chief complaint and to each other. These should be divided into clinically recognizable conditions of (1) pain, (2) restriction of mandibular movement, (3) interference during mandibular movement, and (4) acute malocclusion.

Masticatory Pain.   Any complaint of pain should be classified according to its clinical characteristics as musculoskeletal pain of the deep somatic category.[1] Its true site should be located clinically by manual palpation and functional manipulation.

Restriction of Jaw Movement.   Any restriction of jaw movement should be noted in either joint as related to opening, protrusion, and lateral excursion. Restrictions that appear to relate to the inhibitory effects of pain rather than to structural causes should be noted.

Interference During Jaw Movement.   Abnormal sensations, noises, and movements during translatory cycles induced by opening-closing, protrusion-retrusion, and lateral excursion and return should be identified.

Acute Malocclusion. Malocclusion of which the patient is fully aware and which constitutes at least a part of his complaint should be identified. Any such acute malocclusion should be described in terms of overstressed or understressed teeth, premature striking or disclusion of teeth, cross-bite, or open-bite.

Concomitant Symptoms

Related headache, orofacial, auricular and cervical pains should be noted and described. Note should be taken of any obvious abnormality in the postural relationship between the mandible and the cervical structures.

HISTORY-TAKING

Obtaining an adequate history is essential because in it may usually be found the best clues as to the possible etiology of the patient's complaint. Etiologic factors may be divided into (1) those that are primarily of a predisposing nature, (2) those that may more actively initiate the symptoms, and (3) those that act as contributing influences that accentuate and perpetuate the complaint.

Personal History

Any previous symptoms or similar episodes should be recorded. Consideration should be given to anomalous development, acquired aberrations of growth, previous (even childhood) injuries, illnesses, joint complaints, muscle complaints, and emotional disturbances. The masticatory history should include chewing problems, malocclusion, abusive habits, and mannerisms; bruxism; dentition problems; and extensive dental, orthodontic, or surgical treatment involving the masticatory apparatus.

Specific History Relative to the Complaint

Note should be taken of any condition that took place immediately prior to the onset of symptoms. This would include such things as prior illness, physical fatigue, emotional crisis, injury, episode of pain about the head or neck, dental treatment, local or general anesthesia, or any alteration in the way the teeth, mouth, and jaws had been used. Any feeling of change in the bite; sensation of fatigue or muscle weakness in the jaws; or feeling of prior stiffness, catching, joint noise, or other unusual sensation should be recorded. Insomnia, restlessness, early morning fatigue, known increase in bruxism, or sensation of over-stressed teeth should be taken into account. Questions that tend to reveal the presence of unusually high emotional tension should be asked. All medications currently being used, and what they are prescribed for, should be reviewed. Such information may be obtained from the patient's physician, if the exact content of medications is not known.

Chronologic Record of Symptom Behavior

Each masticatory symptom, as identified above, should be traced chronologically from its inception to the present. It should be noted how the symptoms relate to each other in timing and how they relate to function, temporal patterns, known aggravating factors, and therapeutic efforts. Any previous diagnosis or treatment should be recorded along with the results obtained.

CLINICAL EXAMINATION

The clinical examination is for the purpose of accurately recording useful information about the masticatory symptoms that the patient displays. It should consist of four parts: (1) locating the source of pain; (2) determining the cause and location of any restriction of mandibular movement; (3) classifying disc-interference symptoms relative to the translatory cycle; and (4) identifying the presence of gross occlusal dysfunction and determining whether it is etiologic, symptomatic, or noncontributory.

Source of Masticatory Pain

Masticatory pain, like other musculoskeletal pains, relates intimately to the demands of function. It therefore will be initiated or accentuated by chewing movements as well as by opening, protruding the jaw, or moving it laterally. Like other musculoskeletal pains, it also responds rather proportionately to the degree of stimulation or provocation applied. Sites of masticatory pain may be accurately located by the patient's subjective description as verified by manual palpation and/or functional manipulation. Manual palpation is the best way to stimulate or provoke musculoskeletal pain, providing the structure is accessible. Inaccessible structures are examined by functional manipulation.

The joint proper is accessible for manual palpation directly over the lateral aspect of the condyle. This is best done by having the patient open, protrude, and move the jaw to the opposite side while pressing the finger against the condyle. Care should be taken to distinguish between true arthralgic pain and myalgic pain emanating from the deep portion of the masseter muscle which overlies the anterior portion of the joint capsule. Not only does this identify capsular pain and intensify disc-attachment pain, it also yields valuable information about joint movements and disc interferences. Retrodiscal pain can usually be initiated or accentuated by finger pressure through the external auditory canal. Care should be taken to distinguish between discomfort of auricular origin and that which emanates from the joint proper.

The masseter, temporalis, mylohyoid, and anterior digastric muscles are readily accessible for manual palpation to verify sites of pain. The temporalis muscle can be palpated by pressing it against the underlying cranial bone. Care should be taken to distinguish between muscle pain and that which may arise from the superficial temporal vessels or from the auriculotemporal nerve. The mylohyoid and anterior digastric muscles require bimanual palpation with one finger inside the mouth. The anterior border of the masseter muscle is best palpated bimanually with one finger inside the buccal vestibule. The remainder of the muscle can be pressed directly against the mandibular ramus. Care should be taken to distinguish between muscle pain and that which may emanate from the joint itself. The medial pterygoid muscle can be manually palpated intraorally if the mouth can be opened adequately. The finger is inserted deep to the pterygomandibular raphe, and the muscle is pressed laterally against the inner surface of the mandibular ramus.

Because of lack of accessibility[2] the pterygoid muscles are more accurately examined by functional manipulation. In the absence of pain emanating from the palpable structures, discomfort that is initiated or accentuated by both wide opening and hard biting identifies a painful site in the medial pterygoid muscle. Discomfort that is initiated or accentuated by both resisted protrusion and clenching and is reduced by biting against a tongue blade identifies inferior lateral pterygoid pain. Discomfort that occurs with hard biting whether against a tongue blade or not, but that does not occur with resisted protrusion or with opening widely, identifies a pain site in the superior lateral pterygoid muscle. Palatally located pain that increases with swallowing is indicative of discomfort in the tensor palati muscle.

Careful palpation of other orofacial structures should be done to locate extraneous pain sources. This should include the sternocleido-mastoid muscles as well as the other muscles of the head and neck. The neck should also be inspected for range of motion, noises, and posture.[3, 4]

It should be borne in mind that the recognition of sites of pain located by manual palpation and/or functional manipulation does not establish the true source of pain. It may emanate from a local source, such as inflammation or muscle spasm. Or it may be purely hetero-topic, with the primary source located elsewhere. If differentiation is needed to confirm the clinical diagnosis, then analgesic blocking should be done.[1] Other pitfalls of muscle palpation should be kept in mind, such as nearby tenderness in the parotid gland or lymph glands and the fact that some structures, like periosteum, are normally sensitive to pressure.[5]

Movements that either increase the length of the muscle or in-crease its isometric tension accentuate the patient's awareness of muscle pain. If passive movement is painful, one or more antagonist muscles should be suspected.[6] Therefore, it is well to test each muscle by (1) stretching, (2) active contraction, (3) resisted movement, and (4) passive movement.[7]

The following clinical characteristics of the pain should be noted:

1. Is the pain felt in a definite area, or is it more diffusely located?

2. Is the pain spontaneous and unrelated to jaw movements, or is it initiated or accentuated by mandibular function?

3. Does provocation increase the pain proportionately, or does it burst forth suddenly?

4. Does the pain clearly come and go, or is it persistent, with low and high levels of intensity?

5. Is the pain felt only at the site of provocation, or is it felt elsewhere as well?

6. Is the pain accentuated by light touch, or does it require deeper pressure?

7. When the jaw is immobilized with a small biteblock, can pain still be elicited by movement of the lips, tongue, or throat tissues?

8. Does the pain occur in conjunction with restricted movement or disc interference?

Restricted Mandibular Movement

Even though the patient may feel some discomfort, it is necessary to record jaw movements that reflect the jaw's true structural capability rather than restrictions that are the result of guarding or other inhibitory effects of pain or feelings of weakness.

The vertical opening path and the horizontal protrusive path should be plotted to show any deflection or deviation from straight, centered, midline movement. (Note: *Deflection* means discursive movement that does not return to the midline; *deviation* means discursive movement that does return to the midline.) Nondeflected opening and nondeflected protrusion should be measured *regardless of pain,* so that the point where deflection begins correctly marks where normal movement is arrested. Ipsilateral deflection is indicative of lateral movement in the opposite joint; contralateral deflection is indicative of lateral movement in the same joint. Note should be taken if any such deflection is coincident with muscle pain or with joint pain. Deviation of the midline is indicative of compensatory muscle patterns developed to maintain modified, but useful, joint movement in the presence of interference. Note should be taken of whether any such deviation is wholly unconscious or under some degree of volition.

Measurements of mandibular movement should be made with a millimeter gauge, as follows:

1. Nondeflected opening:
   Interincisal opening . . . . mm
   Overbite . . . . mm
   Total . . . . mm
2. Maximum opening:
   Total opening with deflection and overbite . . . . . . mm
   Deflection to the right side . . . . mm
   Deflection to the left side . . . . mm
3. Nondeflected protrusion:
   Forward interincisal movement. . . . . mm
   Overjet. . . . . mm
   Total . . . . mm
4. Maximum protrusion:
   Total protrusion with deflection and overjet . . . . . mm
   Deflection to the right side . . . . mm
   Deflection to the left side . . . . mm

5. Lateral movements:
    Maximum movement of the midline to the right . . .   mm
    Maximum movement of the midline to the left . . . .   mm

Disc-Interference Symptoms

Besides pain, the symptoms of disc-interference include (1) sensations of binding, rubbing, or catching that the patient can detect subjectively, (2) joint noises, such as clicking and grating, that the patient can hear and usually the examiner can hear also, if he uses a stethoscope, and (3) altered translation, such as rough or irregular movement, momentary locking, hard discrete locking, or soft locking that is sensed by the patient, observed clinically, or felt with the examiner's fingers. Deviation of the incisal path (as already plotted) should be noted. Care should be taken to observe symptoms that occur in conjunction with each other. A distinction should be made between discrete clicking noise, which is indicative of momentary obstruction of disc movement, and grating noise, which is indicative of degenerative change in articular surfaces or deterioration of the disc. A distinction should also be made between "hard locking," which is indicative of the disc being obstructed between the condyle and the eminence, and "soft locking," which is due to other causes, such as protracted functional dislocation, adhesions, capsular restrictions, and extracapsular restraints. When a stethoscope is used, extraneous sounds from the movement of the instrument on the skin should be distinguished from those emitted from the joint. An ultrasonic stethoscope is now available which may prove useful.[8]

The occurrence of disc-interference symptoms should be recorded in relation to the following maneuvers:

1. As the teeth are firmly clenched

2. Immediately upon release after clenching the teeth

3. Upon opening after clenching the teeth firmly

4. Upon opening after biting against a tongue blade

5. Upon opening normally

6. Upon opening rapidly

7. Upon opening while restraining translatory movement (rotatory opening)

8. Upon opening and closing from a three-tongue-blade separator

9. Upon closing normally

10. Upon closing rapidly

11. Upon biting firmly on a pencil or other separator just before closing

12. Upon unilateral chewing on resistant foods such as peanuts

13. Upon protruding the jaw

14. Upon lateral movement to the opposite side

Note should be taken if the closing symptoms remain constant, or if they vary in timing or intensity with the different maneuvers. It should also be recorded if the disc-interference symptoms relate to pain or to restricted movement.

Occlusal Dysfunction

The functional status of the dentition should be examined for the presence of gross malocclusion (disclusion, openbite, crossbite, mutilation, Class II Division 2 malocclusion, etc.), for adequacy of any prosthetic replacement, or for malformations. Note should be taken of any subjective awareness of malocclusion and, if so, whether it is recent or old. It should be noted if the malocclusion occurred following dental treatment, some unusual biting, trauma of some kind, or other known cause, and, particularly, if it constitutes a part of the present complaint. Occlusal interference that occurs prior to intercuspation of the teeth should be distinguished from that which occurs when the teeth are clenched from the unclenched, occluded position. Care should be taken to determine, if possible, how long any such interference has been present, and, particularly, if it occurred in relationship to the onset of the present complaint. Occlusal interference may sometimes be identified by tender or loose teeth, unusual wear facets, or an abnormal path of closure.

Any of the following deficiencies or abnormalities in occlusion of the teeth (natural or artificial) should be identified:

1. A sensation that teeth are overstressed when firmly clenched (anteriors or posteriors)

2. Insufficient occlusal contact between molar teeth (as indicated by tissue paper strips)

3. Missing or inadequately replaced molar teeth

4. Visible lateral shift of the mandibular midline when the teeth are firmly clenched from the unclenched, occluded position

5. Movement of the mandibular teeth when firmly clenched from the unclenched, occluded position as felt by the examiner's fingers placed along the buccal surfaces of the teeth. (The direction and extent of any such movement should be recorded.)

EXAMINATION FORM

As with all diagnostic efforts, a methodical examining technique does much to ensure completeness in obtaining the needed data without an unnecessary expenditure of time. A suitable examination form is needed for this purpose. Figure 8–1 illustrates such a form. (It should be noted that, although this particular examination form is copyrighted to prevent commercialization, it may be copied and used without further permission as long as it is for clinical diagnosis, research, or teaching purposes, and not for resale.) When properly used, this examination form will usually supply most of the essential data in each of the five categories needed to make a clinical diagnosis, namely:

1. Etiologic clues from the patient's history

2. Data by which masticatory pain can be identified and located

3. Location and extent of arrested mandibular movement

4. Data for determining the proper classification of disc interference as it relates to the translatory cycle

5. Identification of gross occlusal disharmony and data to help determine its etiologic and symptomatic implications

USING THE COLLECTED DATA

An examination does not automatically render a diagnosis. Examining the patient is for the purpose of obtaining usable data about the complaint. Making a diagnosis, however, is a different matter. This requires understanding of the meaning that may be attached to the data collected in the examining procedure. It is by the proper utilization of such data that a clinical diagnosis is made.

A

PATIENT'S NAME_____ Age_____

Date _____ Onset of complaint began _____

Patient's statement of the complaint:

> TM EXAMINATION FORM
> Copyright © 1985 By Welden E. Bell
> This form may be copied for
> clinical use but not for resale

Masticatory symptoms: Concomitant symptoms:

____Masticatory pain   ____Disc interference   ____Ear pain   ____Neck pain

____Restricted movement   ____Acute malocclusion   ____Headache   ____Posture problem

---

PART I. HISTORY

Prior symptoms or similar episodes: _____

Predisposing conditions: ____Dental problems   ____Abusive habits   ____Injuries   ____Illnesses

Activating factors: ____Dental Rx   ____Injury   ____Episode of pain   ____Unusual jaw use

    ____Emotional upset   ____Illness   ____Physical fatigue   ____Operation   ____Altered chewing

    ____Phenothiazine medication being used   ____Other possible factor: _____

Contributing factors: ____Illness   ____Emotional problems   ____Other head or neck pain or problem

    ____Awakes with jaws tired or teeth sore   ____Feeling of physical depletion   ____Nervousness

    ____Has sensation of weakness in the jaw muscles   ____Other possible factor: _____

Chronological account of the symptoms:

Masticatory pain _____

Restricted movement _____

Disc interference _____

Acute malocclusion_____

Previous diagnosis and treatment (with results):

PART II. SOURCE OF PAIN

Location of the pain _____

Pain behavior: ____Increased by chewing   ____opening   ____protruding   ____lateral excursions

    ____Is proportional to provocation   ____Bursts forth sporadically

    ____Is diffusely located   ____Is precisely located

    ____Felt at other than provoked site   ____Felt only at site of provocation

    ____Pain is continuous but variable   ____Pain is clearly intermittent

    ____Pain relates to restricted movement   ____Pain relates to disc interference

(R side)	PAIN INCREASED BY MANUAL PALPATION	(L side)
_____	Over condyle proper	_____
_____	Masseter muscle	_____
_____	Temporalis muscle	_____
_____	Mylohyoid muscle	_____
_____	Digastric muscle	_____
_____	Palpating elsewhere	_____

(R side)	EFFECT (up and down) ON PAIN OF MANIPULATION	(L side)
_____	Opening mouth widely	_____
_____	Clenching the teeth	_____
_____	Biting on a tongue blade	_____
_____	Protruding against resistance	_____
_____	Swallowing	_____
_____	Lip, tongue, throat movement	_____

PART III. RESTRICTED MOVEMENT

                OPENING PATH   PROTRUSIVE PATH

Plot deflection and/or
deviation of midline:
(Disregard pain or
sensation of muscle
weakness)   R |____| L   R |____| L

Arrested movement is
coincident with:

____Muscle pain

____Joint pain

FIGURE 8–1   A, examination chart, front side.

B Measured movements:
    Nondeflected opening ____mm plus overbite ____mm = total nondeflected opening ____mm
    Maximum opening (including overbite) ____mm. Deflection to R ____mm Deflection to L ____mm
    Nondeflected protrusion ____mm plus overjet ____mm = total ____mm
    Maximum protrusion (including overjet) ____mm. Deflection to R ____mm Deflection to L ____mm
    Maximum lateral movement to the right side ____mm. To the left side ____mm

---

PART IV. DISC INTERFERENCE
  Key to symptoms: A-1 binding, rubbing sensations
             A-2 catching sensations
             B-1 clicking or popping noise
             B-2 grating noise

                                        C-1 deviated midline with opening
                                        C-2 rough or irregular movement
                                        C-3 momentary locking
                                        C-4 hard locking
                                        C-5 soft locking

(R side)	INCIDENCE OF SYMPTOMS	(L side)
____	Clenching the teeth	____
____	Release after clenching	____
____	Clench before opening	____
	Biting on a tongue	
	blade before opening	____
____	Normal opening (at___mm)	____
____	Rapid opening	____
____	Rotatory opening	____
	Opening-closing from	
____	3 tongue blades	____

(R side)	INCIDENCE OF SYMPTOMS	(L side)
____	Normal closure (at ___mm)	____
____	Rapid closure (at___mm)	____
	Biting on a pencil prior	
____	to closure (at ___mm)	____
	Unilateral chewing	
____	(such as peanuts)	____
____	Protrusion (at ___mm)	____
	Lateral movement to	
____	the opposite side	____

____Closing symptoms are constant   ____Closing symptoms are variable
____Symptoms relate to pain   ____Symptoms relate to restricted movement

---

PART V. OCCLUSAL DYSFUNCTION

  Obvious malocclusion: ____Malformation ____Malposition ____Mutilation ____Poor replacement
    ____Patient is aware of malocclusion. ____Old ____Recent ____Part of present complaint
        It followed: ____Dental Rx ____Unusual biting ____Trauma ____Other known cause _____
  When clenched patient feels overstressed: ____Anteriors ____Right molars ____Left molars
  Deficient molar occlusal contact (natural or artificial): ____Right side ____Left side
  Missing or inadequately replaced molars: ____Right side ____Left side
  Visable shift of midline with clenching: ____To the right side ____To the left side
  During clenching, mandibular teeth move: On right side ____posteriorly ____anteriorly
        (as felt by examiner's fingers)   On left side ____posteriorly ____anteriorly

---

SUMMARY OF EXAMINATION DATA:

  (1) Clues to etiology (from history and occlusal dysfunction) _____
  (2) Structure from which the pain emanates _____
  (3) Location of restricted movement _____
  (4) Classification of disc interference _____
  (5) Muscle or joint-induced acute malocclusion _____

  CLINICAL DIAGNOSIS _____
      Confirmed by ____Radiography ____Anesthesia ____Other test ____Consultation ____Trial Rx
CONFIRMED WORKING DIAGNOSIS:

FIGURE 8–1 **B,** examination chart, back side.

REFERENCES

1. Bell W.E.: *Orofacial Pains,* ed. 3: Chicago, Year Book Medical Publishers, 1985.
2. Johnstone D.R., Templeton M.: The feasibility of palpating the lateral pterygoid muscle. *J. Prosthet. Dent.* 44:318, 1980.
3. Clark G.T.: Examining temporomandibular disorder patients for craniocervical dysfunction. *J. Craniomand. Pract.* 2(1):55, 1983.
4. Rocabado M.: Diagnosis and treatment of abnormal craniocervical and craniomandibular mechanics, in Solberg W.K., Clark G.T. (eds.): *Abnormal Jaw Mechanics.* Chicago, Quintessence Publishing Co., 1984, pp. 141–159.
5. Friedman M.H., Weisberg J.: Pitfalls of muscle palpation in TMJ diagnosis. *J. Prosthet. Dent.* 48:331, 1982.
6. MacDonald A.J.R.: Abnormally tender muscle regions and associated painful movements. *Pain* 8:197, 1980.
7. Frumker S.C.: Determining masticatory muscle spasm and TMJ capsulitis. *J. Craniomand. Pract.* 1(2):51, 1983.
8. Koskinen-Moffett L.: Mini-clinic demonstration: Ultrasonic stethoscope for temporomandibular joint sounds, in Moffett B.C. (ed.): *Diagnosis of Internal Derangements of the Temporomandibular Joint,* Vol. 1. Seattle, University of Washington, 1984, p. 113.

9

Making the Diagnosis

Making an accurate diagnosis is the most important single step in the management of TM disorders of all types. Without it, therapy is empirical at best and becomes little more than a trial-and-error procedure. This has been the weakest link in TM management since the beginning—and remains so. It is only with substantial improvement in diagnosis that more predictive treatment can be expected in the future.

Perhaps one reason for this deficiency has been too much reliance placed on tests, instruments, and diagnostic equipment rather than on the evaluation of the data thus obtained. An examination is not a diagnosis. This does not mean that such testing is any the less important or necessary, for it is essential in obtaining the data upon which a diagnosis is made. Rather, a diagnosis results from what such data mean to the doctor as indicative of departures from normal for that particular patient and as suggestive of what the abnormality likely is. So, it is prerequisite that the doctor understand normal structure and function as applied to the individual patient. Defective concepts of normal render the best collected data meaningless. The anatomically incorrect concepts that have been held by many in the past have no doubt contributed to poor diagnosis and equivocal therapy. If the goal of more successful management of TM disorders is to be attained, the need for a better educational foundation far exceeds the need for better examination facilities.

It goes without saying that accurate data are needed before evaluation is possible. But, data in themselves are useless facts until evaluated intelligently. The individual that makes the diagnosis does so by comparing the patient's symptoms with what he conceives to be normal.

The diagnostic conclusions can be no more accurate, however, than the correctness of his basic knowledge of what constitutes normal masticatory structure and function for that particular patient. In this there can be no compromise.

THE CLINICAL DIAGNOSIS

The data gleaned from the chief complaint, the masticatory and concomitant symptoms, the case history, and the functional manipulations of the joints should be summarized carefully and put into usable form. This is done best by arranging the summarized data into a standard sequence, as follows:

   1. Features in the history that are etiologically significant.

   2. Data relating to symptoms of masticatory pain, including (1) identifying the clinical characteristics that place the complaint into the deep musculoskeletal category, (2) establishing that the pain is either myogenous, arthralgic, or both, and (3) locating the structure(s) from which the pain emanates.[1]

   3. Data relating to the retriction of mandibular movement, including whether the location of such restriction is extracapsular, capsular, or intracapsular.

   4. Data relating to symptoms of interference during mandibular movements (abnormal sensations, noises, and/or movements), including (1) the classification of such interference as it relates to the translatory cycle, (2) whether it appears to relate to excessive passive interarticular pressure, lack of compatibility of the sliding surfaces, or impaired disc-condyle complex function (if such disorder is of the Class III category), and (3) whether it identifies arrested movement between the articular disc and condyle, damage to the articular disc proper, functional displacement of the disc, or dysfunction of the superior retrodiscal lamina (if impaired disc-condyle complex functioning is evident).

   5. Data relating to occlusal dysfunction to identify whether it is symptomatic (muscle induced or joint induced), etiologic, or irrelevant.

   With the summarized data thus arranged, it is much easier to make the necessary comparisons that effectuate a tentative clinical diagnosis.

Tentative Diagnosis

The development of a clinical diagnosis is best made in logical steps: determining first the main category represented by the complaint, then proceeding to subclassify the disorder to identify the particular condition (or conditions) that accounts for the patient's symptoms. These judgments usually can be made by comparing the data as summarized from the clinical examination with the characteristic features of the different manifestations of TM disorders.

It should be noted that the criteria for differential diagnosis throughout these clinical procedures use the same key numerals that were used in summarizing the collected data, namely: (1) designates the features that have etiologic significance as obtained from the patient's history; (2) designates data relative to the complaint of masticatory pain, especially its source; (3) designates information relevant to restrictions of mandibular movement, particularly the location of the cause of arrested movement; (4) designates disc-interference symptoms that occur with mandibular movements, especially as they relate to the translatory cycle and to causative factors; and (5) designates data concerning *acute* malocclusion, whether it is muscle-induced or joint-induced, as well as to the presence of clinically identifiable *chronic* occlusal discrepancies that may be etiologic.

Criteria for Identifying the Main TM Category

The following lists of criteria *(keyed numerically)* should help to identity the main category represented by the patient's complaint.

Muscle Disorders

1. Sudden onset; recurrence; variability; emotional upset; recent alteration in sensory or proprioceptive input from the mouth, teeth, muscles, or joints; prior muscle splinting-myospasm episode, prior deep pain episode, prior myofascial trigger point mechanism

2. Myalgia

3. Extracapsular restriction

4. *If any:* Interference due to excessive passive interarticular pressure

5. Muscle-induced symptomatic malocclusion. (Preexistent occlusal disharmony usually noncontributory unless recently induced)

Disc-Interference Disorders

1. Insidious onset, persistence, progressiveness, sudden onset or recurrence that follows myospastic activity or increased emotional tension, trauma, biting incident, prior dental treatment

2. Arthralgia of disc attachment type, intermittent and coincident with other disc-interference symptoms

3. *If any:* Intracapsular restriction due to obstructed or dislocated disc

4. Abnormal sensations, noises, and/or movements; deviated incisal path

5. *If any:* Joint-induced symptomatic malocclusion due to fracture or dislocation of the disc that causes a sensation of overstressed ipsilateral posterior teeth during clenching. (Etiologic disharmony consisting of inadequate occlusal contact of molar teeth or gross movement of mandibular teeth when clenched from the unclenched occluded position)

Inflammatory Disorders

1. Prior trauma, other arthritis, preexistent disc-interference disorder, illness

2. Arthralgia of inflammatory type. May induce central excitatory effects

3. *If any:* Restriction capsular; some possibly due to a preexistent condition, some possibly extracapsular due to secondary myospastic activity

4. *If any:* Due to disc-condyle complex dysfunction

5. *If any:* Due to retrodiscal swelling, inflammatory effusion, or rapid osteolysis. (Chronic malocclusion may be etiologic)

Chronic Mandibular Hypomobility

1. Protracted, slowly changing restricted movement; prior trauma, surgery, or infection

2. None, unless injured by abusive movement

3. Restriction may be extracapsular, capsular, or intracapsular depending on structure involved

4. None

5. None

Growth Disorders of the Joint

1. Insidious radiographically evident structural change

2. *If any:* Due to dysfunction imposed by growth aberration

3. *If any:* Due to growth aberration

4. *If any:* Due to disruption of disc-condyle complex function

5. *If any:* Due to rapid osseous change. (Chronic malocclusion may relate to growth aberration)

Criteria for Identifying the Disorder

Masticatory Muscle Disorders.   After the complaint has been properly categorized, the disorder represented should be identified. A masticatory muscle disorder can usually be classified as splinting, spasm, or inflammation by the following criteria *(keyed numerically)*:

Protective Muscle Splinting

1. May be recent change in sensory and/or proprioceptive input from the mouth, teeth, muscles, or joints due to dental treatment, injury, abusive use, emotional crisis, volitional chewing, or oral consciousness

2. Myalgia when muscles contract, sensation of weakness

3. None structurally, may be inhibited by pain and weakness

4. None

5. None. (Chronic malocclusion irrelevant unless recently altered)

Muscle Spasm Activity

1. May be (a) prior deep somatic pain input in trigeminal, facial, or cervical area, (b) prior muscle splinting from any cause (pro-

tracted by continued use or injudicious therapy), (c) prior nonspastic myofascial trigger point mechanism due to fatigue, emotional stress, illness, or central excitation, or (d) active phenothiazine therapy

2. Myalgia when muscle is stretched or contracted, little or no discomfort with muscle at rest

3. Extracapsular restriction due to contracted muscle

4. *If any:* Due to excessive passive interarticular pressure

5. Muscle-induced acute malocclusion. (Chronic malocclusion irrelevant unless recently induced or activated)

Muscle Inflammation

1. May be due to (a) prior local cause such as abusive use, strain, trauma, infection, or surgery, or (b) prior muscle spasm activity protracted by abusive use or injudicious therapy

2. Myalgia in resting muscle accentuated by all use; inflammatory signs

3. Extracapsular restriction due to swollen muscle

4. None

5. None. (Chronic disharmony irrelevant unless recently induced or altered)

Disc-Interference Disorders. If the complaint is categorized as a disc-interference disorder, its class can usually be identified by the following criteria:

Class I Interference

1. May be negative for etiologic clues

2. *If any:* Occurs as the teeth are clenched, prevented by biting on a tongue blade

3. None

4. A binding or rubbing sensation, sensed with clenching; clicking noise emitted as the biting pressure is released; both symptoms prevented by biting on a tongue blade

5. None. (Etiologic occlusal disharmony clinically evident)

Class II Interference

1. Prior Class I interference disorder, trauma sustained with the teeth occluded, habitual hard chewing, bruxism

2. *If any:* Occurs in conjunction with other symptoms, prevented by an occlusal stop that keeps condyle from returning to the fully occluded position

3. None

4. Click after clenching (or after an extended period of inactivity) just as the first jaw movement is made, prevented by an occlusal stop

5. None (If history yields prior Class I interference, chronic disharmony that shifts the mandible as the teeth are clenched should be present. If history is negative, inadequate molar occlusal contact may be identified.)

Class III Interference

1. May identify (a) an emotional or myospastic cause for excessive passive interarticular pressure, (b) abusive habits, trauma sustained with the teeth separated, hypomobility of the opposite joint, or structural anomaly, (c) joint trauma or surgery, (d) an unusual biting incident, or (e) prior Class I or Class II interference disorder

2. Disc attachment pain in conjunction with other interference symptoms

3. *If any:* Intracapsular restriction due to obstructed or dislocated articular disc

4. Interference symptoms (binding or catching sensation, clicking or grating noise, momentary locking, hard locking, or soft locking) may occur in different ways which indicate the underlying cause, as follows:
   (a) Sudden onset, recurrence, variability (indicative of excessive passive interarticular pressure)
   (b) Persistent, nonchanging, nonvariable symptoms accompanied by a nonvolitional deviation of the midline opening path (indicative of structural incompatibility of the sliding surfaces)
   (c) Noisy, irregular, skidding movement throughout the translatory cycle (indicative of adhesions between the disc and condyle)

(d) Grating noise that may be punctuated by discrete symptoms (indicative of degenerative joint disease)
(e) Recalcitrant, progressive, discrete symptoms that vary with the demands of function, and that may be accompanied by a volitional deviated incisal path (indicative of functional displacement of the articular disc)
(f) Soft locking near full opening (indicative of functional dislocation of the articular disc)

5. *If any:* Joint-induced acute disharmony sensed as over-stressed ipsilateral posterior teeth when clenched (indicative of fractured or dislocated articular disc). (Etiologic occlusal disharmony may be identified as shifting of the mandibular teeth when they are clenched)

Class IV Interference (Joint Hypermobility)

1. Habitual overextension of opening

2. *If any:* Disc attachment pain in conjunction with other symptoms

3. None

4. A momentary pause near wide opening followed by a rapid, skidding movement to full opening

5. None. (Chronic malocclusion irrelevant)

Class V Interference (Spontaneous Dislocation)

1. Many recurrent dislocations or a single instance of momentary excessive or prolonged opening

2. *If any:* Arthralgia associated with attempts to force the mouth closed

3. Inability to close the mouth

4. None

5. Joint-induced gross malocclusion with only the posterior teeth in contact. (Chronic malocclusion irrelevant)

Inflammatory Disorders. If the patient's complaint is categorized as an inflammatory disorder, it can usually be classified (a) as synovitis or capsulitis, (b) as retrodiscitis, or (c) as inflammatory arthritis by observing the following criteria:

Synovitis and Capsulitis

1. Trauma, arthritis, prior disc-interference disorder, or nearby inflammation that has involved the joint by direct extension

2. Arthralgia of capsular type with extended translatory movements that stretch the capsule, palpable tenderness over the condyle, central excitatory effects may be induced

3. *If any:* Capsular restriction due to inflamed, swollen capsule; symptoms of gelation

4. None, except preexistent or coexistent condition

5. *If any:* Joint-induced disharmony due to inflammatory effusion. (Chronic malocclusion possibly related to prior disc-interference disorder; otherwise noncontributory)

Retrodiscitis

1. Extrinsic trauma or functional anterior dislocation of the articular disc

2. Arthralgia of retrodiscal type accentuated when the teeth are clenched, reduced by biting on a tongue blade; central excitatory effects may be induced.

3. None

4. None

5. Joint-induced disharmony due to displacement of the condyle by swollen retrodiscal tissue or by inflammatory effusion. (Chronic malocclusion possibly related to prior functional anterior dislocation)

Inflammatory Arthritis

1. Trauma, infection, other arthritis, illness, or preexistent disc-interference disorder

2. Arthralgia of arthritic type (including capsular pain); central excitatory effects may be induced

3. *If any:* Restriction due to capsulitis and the inhibitory effects of pain; some may be extracapsular due to secondary myospastic activity

4. Interference due to degenerative change in the articular surfaces; preexistent disc-interference disorder

5. *If any:* Joint-induced disharmony due to inflammatory effusion. (Chronic malocclusion possibly related to prior disc-interference disorder)

Chronic Mandibular Hypomobility.   If the patient's complaint is categorized as a chronic mandibular hypomobility, the type can be determined by identifying its location. Chronic extracapsular hypomobility would be classified as elevator muscle contracture. Chronic capsular hypomobility is recognized as capsular fibrosis. Chronic intracapsular hypomobility is ankylosis.

Growth Disorders of the Joint.   If the patient's complaint is categorized as a growth disorder, determination of the type and significance of the disorder requires radiographic examination of the structures involved.

Clinical Diagnosis

A decision then should be made as to whether the tentative clinical diagnosis has sufficient merit and reasonableness to warrant initiating management procedures or whether further confirmation is needed. Ordinarily, if palliative therapy is expected to effectively manage the complaint, further confirmation, other than therapeutic trial, may be superfluous. But, if any question remains,' and especially if definitive therapy includes nonreversible dental or joint treatment measures, positive confirmation should be obtained.

CONFIRMATION OF THE CLINICAL DIAGNOSIS

There are several ways in which the clinical diagnosis can be confirmed. Of these, radiography, no doubt, is the most useful. That it furnishes permanent documentation that can be evaluated by others makes it especially desirable from both the consultative and medicolegal points of view.

RADIOGRAPHY

Radiographic visualization has essential confirming value.[2] The tissue injury induced by radiation is usually justified by the information gained. *It should not be used as a substitute for clinical diagnosis; it has too many limitations.* But its confirming value is great indeed.

Unfortunately, radiography compresses three-dimensional structures into a two-dimensional silhouette that represents the relative radiolucency of the tissues through which the x-rays are projected. In TM radiography only osseous tissue is recorded. With the rays passing through the cranium from the opposite side, superimposition of other structures presents a technical and interpretative problem. At best, the radiograph visualizes only the subarticular bone that supports the articular surfaces—not the articular surfaces themselves. Ordinary radiography does not display the location, shape, or condition of articular tissues. Only subarticular osseous changes can be visualized, which represents no more than a fraction of what we would like to see.

Most unfortunate of all, however, is that what the radiograph cannot show is what we need most to know about—the contents of the so-called "joint gap." It not only fails to disclose the articular surfaces of the condyle and eminence, it gives no information at all about the other two articular surfaces of the TM joint—the superior and inferior articular facets on the disc. So, even excellent radiographic visualization of the joint yields information about only two of the four articulating parts and nothing at all relative to the articular disc proper. In attempting to judge function (as from fluoroscopy), radiographic visualization shows only a fraction of the movements that actually take place within the joint during normal functioning—much less those that occur as a result of dysfunction. To utilize radiography for confirming, altering, or denying the clinical diagnosis, the examiner should always keep these serious limitations of the method in mind.

Regardless of the method used, certain criteria determine the accuracy and ultimate usefulness of radiography at a clinical level. Some methods require compromises, and, when this is necessary, the examiner should be aware of the consequences. To yield maximum diagnostic results, the radiographic method should provide for the following:

1. There should be reasonably clear visualization of the subarticular bone of both condyle and articular fossa with a minimum of distortion and superimposition.

2. Films should be made in the upright sitting position so as not to alter or inhibit mandibular movements.

3. The equipment and method used should not inhibit or alter normal joint function.

4. It should permit the making of serial radiographs in different mandibular positions with sufficient precision so that the images can be superimposed for reading.

5. It should permit the examining dentist to make or directly supervise the exposures so as to have full knowledge and control over the mandibular positions radiographed.

The radiographic methods applicable to TM diagnosis may be grouped into several categories, each having certain advantages and disadvantages. Frequently, more than one category is required to properly visualize the condition present.

1. Panoramic projection

2. Transcranial, transpharyngeal, transorbital projections

3. Tomography

4. Computed tomography (CT scanning)

5. Fluoroscopy and fluorography

6. Arthrotomography (contrast tomography)

7. Scintigraphy (nuclear scanning)

Panoramic Projection

Panoramic viewing of the teeth and facial bones, including the temporomandibular joints, provides a useful screening visualization of the masticatory structures. Since it is done in a single static position, its value is seriously limited. It often furnishes clues that justify more adequate radiographic examination of the joints.

Transcranial, Transpharyngeal, Transorbital Projections

No doubt the most frequent use of TM radiography is performed with ordinary dental x-ray equipment with the patient seated upright and by the dentist himself or under his direct supervision. With the addition of a suitable film holder, a proper series of exposures can be made with precision as well as with the minimum of radiation and expense to the patient. Current techniques produce excellent results with the minimum of distortion and superimposition. Such a method, therefore, quite satisfactorily fulfills the basic criteria for useful radiography of the TM joints.[3, 4] The marked advantages of availability and low cost to the patient make this method by far the most desirable for routine use. The more complex methods should be reserved for special application as the need arises. The limitations of this method, however, should be recognized, understood, and appreciated.

Through the years many workers have contributed to the original Lindbolm technique of transparietal radiography.[5–14] Currently, excellent techniques are available using ordinary dental x-ray equipment.[15, 16] A number of satisfactory film holders are marketed.

One technical problem has been that of properly directing the central ray down the mediolateral axis of the condyle without taking pilot films. This is needed to minimize distortion of the image. The long axis of the condyle in most subjects is perpendicular to the proximal portion of the mandibular ramus at a downward tilt from the opposite side of about 15 degrees.[17] Thus, by placing the film parallel to the central portion of the ramus anteroposteriorly, and by directing the central ray about 15 degrees downward at right angles to the film anteroposteriorly, a satisfactory projection of the condyle is obtained with a minimum of distortion.

It should be understood that the transcranial projection does not visualize the true subarticular osseous surfaces, but rather the outer lateral margins of the joint. Thus, the true articular disc space is not seen. If critical evaluation of the articular disc space or the subarticular osseous structures is needed, the tomographic method in the upright sitting position is required. Information concerning articular disc behavior must be *inferred from changes in width and position* of the so-called joint-gap space in the condyle-disc-eminence relationship as viewed in different functional positions of the joint.

This method yields a great deal of information in spite of its limitations. A fairly accurate estimate of the inclination of the articular eminence is available by comparing with the shadow of the supra-articular crest in the region of the eminence, the crest being nearly parallel to the Frankfort plane. (See Figs 3–6, 3–7.) The shape and gross structure of the subarticular bone are visualized. Films of the joints should be done in series so as to give information about joint functioning.[8, 18] Such a series should include at least four joint positions, namely, (1) closed unclenched position, (2) closed clenched position, (3) maximum unstrained lateral position (excursion to the opposite side), and (4) maximum unstrained open position. By comparing such radiographs with the known radiographic standards of normal,[9] departures from normal joint structure and function become obvious (Fig 9–1).

Normal TM joints should present the following radiographic features:

1. The subarticular osseous surfaces should be well defined, smooth, and rounded in contour.

2. The articular disc spaces should be of sufficient width to accommodate functioning articular discs.

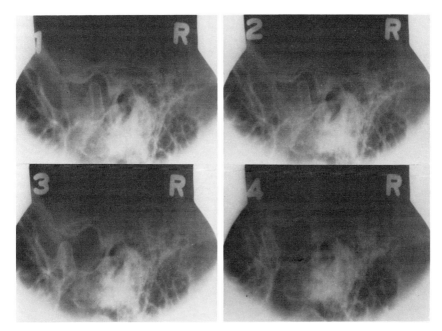

FIGURE 9–1 Transparietal radiographs of a structurally and functionally normal temporomandibular joint: *1,* unclenched, closed position of the joint; *2,* clenched, occluded position of the joint (maximum intercuspation); *3,* lateral excursion to the opposite side; *4,* maximum unstrained open position. Within the limitations imposed by flat-plate radiography, the osseous surfaces appear to be well defined, smooth, and rounded in contour; the articular disc space is of sufficient width to accommodate a functioning disc; the condyle in unclenched and clenched occluded positions exactly superimpose; in lateral excursion the condyle reaches the crest of the articular eminence; in open position the condyle movement exceeds that of lateral excursion.

3. The condyles in unclenched and clenched occluded positions should exactly superimpose. (Very flat joints may normally show slight discrepancy.)

4. The condyle position in lateral excursion to the opposite side should reach the crest of the articular eminence.

5. The condyle position in maximum open position should exceed that of lateral excursion to the opposite side.

6. The joints should present bilaterally symmetric condylar movements in opening and lateral excursion to the opposite side.

Interpretation of the relative condylar positions thus recorded can be made by superimposing the images of the articular fossa and eminence while directly observing the condylar outlines. A fine pencil tracing of the articular fossa and eminence upon which is superimposed tracings of the condyle in its various positions has the advantage of giving a permanent graphic record from which functional movements can be visualized and measurements made (Fig 9–2).[8]

Comparison of the unclenched and clenched occluded positions of the joint may disclose a gross condylar displacement if it occurs in the sagittal plane. It should be noted, however, that very flat joints with low-inclined articular eminences may normally display a minor lack of precise condylar superimposition. Otherwise, radiographically visible displacement represents gross occlusal disharmony (see Figs 5–12 and 5–13). This method has the advantage of identifying the extent and direction of condylar displacement, which should correlate with the clinical evidence of gross movement of the mandible when the teeth are firmly clenched. Such information has confirming value in the diagnosis of disc-interference disorders as well as that of degenerative arthritis. The precision serial radiography required to obtain this valuable information is well warranted.

Since the articular disc normally is not compressible to an extent that is radiographically visible, a decrease in the width of the articular disc space when the teeth are firmly clenched from the occluded, unclenched position may be indicative of deformation or deterioration of the disc from overloading (Fig 9–3). This should correlate with a clinical deficiency in molar occlusal contact and stands as confirming evidence of a disc-interference disorder, particularly that of the

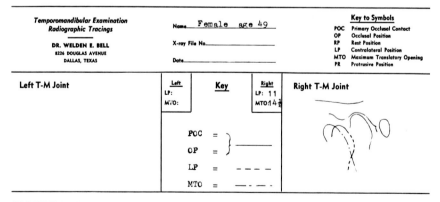

FIGURE 9–2 Radiographic tracings made from four transcranial films (Fig 9–1) of TM joints. Radiographically, joint displays normal structure and function. (From Bell W.E.: *Orofacial Pains: Classification, Diagnosis, Management,* ed. 3. Chicago, Year Book Medical Publishers, 1985. Reproduced with permission.)

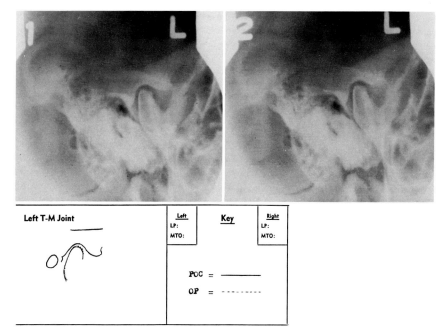

FIGURE 9–3 Illustration of radiographic evidence of deformation of articular disc due to lack of adequate occlusal contact of molar teeth. Note decrease in width of articular disc space when teeth are clenched *(OP)* compared with unclenched occluded position *(POC)*. (From Bell W.E.: *Orofacial Pains: Classification, Diagnosis, Management,* ed. 3. Chicago, Yea: Book Medical Publishers, 1985. Reproduced with permission.)

Class II category. Such evidence may also confirm intracapsular effusion.

Minor displacements cannot be visualized radiographically, nor can those that occur in other than the sagittal plane.

Comparison of the contralateral and open positions of the condyle gives information regarding the location of the cause of arrested mandibular movement. Normally, translatory movement in lateral excursion reaches well to the crest of the articular eminence while that of maximum opening exceeds contralateral excursive movement (see Fig 4–4). If the radiographic position of the condyle in lateral excursion is within normal limits, but that of opening is significantly less than normal, the restriction is extracapsular (see Fig 5–9). This would confirm restricted opening due to an extracapsular cause, such as myospasm of elevator muscles. It should correlate with clinically evident restriction of opening accompanied by deflection of the midline but with normal protrusive movement. If both lateral and open positions superimpose at a point somewhat less than normal for lateral movement, the restraint on condylar movement is capsular (see Fig 5–10). This would confirm a clinical diagnosis of capsulitis or capsular fibrosis and should correlate with restriction of movement in the outer ranges only. If the lateral and open condylar positions are similarly restricted, but fail to superimpose, it is suggestive of intracapsular arrested condylar movement at near full opening. If there is marked restriction of both lateral and opening movements, even though they do not exactly superimpose, the arrested movement is intracapsular (see Fig 5–11). This would confirm a clinical diagnosis of ankylosis or arrested movement by an obstructed articular disc. It should correlate with clinical evidence of restricted mandibular movement in which there is deflection of the midline with both opening and protrusive movements.

The transcranial visualization of the TM joint compares favorably with other methods. Lindvall[19] found that in grossly sectioned joints tomography was superior in the detection of bony defects but that transcranial radiography nevertheless gave a satisfactory demonstration of the actual condition. Dixon et al.[20] found that transcranial radiography lacked validity for diagnosing anterior disc displacements. In contrast, Farrar and McCarty[15] considered it to be a practical method in this regard. Van Sickels et al.[21] confirmed the usefulness of transcranial radiography in the evaluation of craniomandibular disorders that involve the lateral aspect of the joint. Mongini[22] found that transcranial radiographs were similar to tomograms for observing the lateral aspect of the joint but that tomograms were needed to evaluate osseous changes. Eckerdal and Lundberg[23] found that there was concordance in structural diagnosis between transcranial radiography and direct morphologic inspection in 78% of the defects found in autopsy specimens.

The transpharyngeal (transfacial) projection of the TM joint gives an excellent profile view of the condyle but does not show the upper structures of the joint clearly. It, therefore, cannot be used to examine relationships between the condyle and articular eminence, thus drastically restricting its usefulness. It serves best as an auxiliary film to a transcranial series.

The transorbital projection gives a very satisfactory frontal view of the condyle. Although it has limited usefulness in confirming TM joint dysfunction, it does show structural deviations in the condyle that cannot be discerned in the sagittal plane. Its value is largely to supplement tomographic films that show osseous defects in the condyle.

Tomography

Tomography affords the most accurate radiographic visualization of the temporomandibular joint. If the patient is positioned in the upright sitting posture, films made by this method *in properly controlled series* are an excellent means of measuring accurately the articular disc space during functional movements of the joint. This offers a good chance of radiographically discerning abnormalities of articular disc function, even though the disc itself is not visible.

Ricketts[24] pioneered the adaptation of the laminographic method to TM diagnosis. Equipment especially designed for this purpose has made it available as an office procedure, thus making it a practical, cost-effective technique. This method provides for visualization of the medial and central portions of the joint which cannot be examined by transcranial radiography. It reduces the chance of erroneous assumptions concerning the overall condition of the joint that can result from viewing the lateral structures only.[25] Eckerdal,[26] however, found that tomography was wholly satisfactory for only the central two thirds of the joint.

Although tomography in the erect sitting position is admittedly a superior method for visualizing the subarticular osseous structures of the joint and for measuring the width of the articular disc space, it does not reduce the inherent limitations of radiography relative to articular disc function. In addition, it presents very real problems in accomplishing a satisfactory serial examination that is so indispensable in the evaluation of functional relationships. It offers little, if any, advantage over transcranial radiography as far as the lateral portion of the joint is concerned—the part of the joint that sustains the greatest compressive force, where most problems develop anyway. To confirm the clinical diagnosis, a proper series of well-made transcranial films continues to remain the most practical overall method of joint examination. Tomography is valuable to supplement such an examination, especially when structural defects need further evaluation and when conditions in the central and medial portions of the joint require visualization.

Computed Tomography (CT Scanning)

Utilizing computer technology, tomographic data can be displayed to reflect tissue radiolucency bilaterally or in either the sagittal or the frontal planes without additional radiation. It can be manipulated for either soft tissue or bone. It is comparable to arthrography rather than to transcranial or tomographic radiography.

Compared with arthrography, the advantages of CT scanning are that (1) it is a noninvasive technique, (2) both joints can be examined simultaneously without additional radiation, (3) it can evaluate different densities of tissue, and (4) less total radiation is required for the information obtained. The disadvantages are very real, however: (1) the cost, (2) the lack of availability, (3) the total absence of functional information because of the necessary static open-mouth posture, and (4) its inability to disclose perforations of the disc or retrodiscal tissue.[27, 28] Blaschke[25] reported good structural correlation between arthrograms and CT scans but an absence of information regarding joint function. On the assumption that a joint click is indicative of the "reduction of a displaced articular disc," Helms et al.[29] suggested that the open-mouth posture be set at a point just short of where the click occurs, so as to visualize the "displaced disc." Helms et al.[30] reported that, of 92 CT scanned patients who subsequently underwent either arthrography or surgery, there was agreement with the scan 96% of the time; 3 of the scans were false positives, and 1 was false negative. Wilkinson and Maryniuk[31] reported that (1) soft-tissue-mode CT scans distorted the osseous image, (2) CT scans failed to reveal all the anatomic structures seen in dissection, (3) the difference between normal and displaced articular discs was slight, (4) the disc appearance varied with the depth of the scan, and (5) the disc and the muscle tendon appeared similar.

Computed tomography scanning on the whole appears to compare favorably with arthrography, with the marked advantage of being noninvasive but with the serious disadvantage of disclosing no information on joint function. The results at this stage of development are not impressive. Although CT scanning has an important place in TM research, it has very little applicability at a clinical practice level.

Fluoroscopy and Fluorography

The only method of examining the TM joint during functional movements is fluoroscopy. Permanent recording by means of video or cinefluorography enhances its value in that frame-by-frame examination is possible. Additional information is obtained by injecting a contrast medium which discloses the synovial fluid movements during the translatory cycle. Fluoroscopic studies have contributed significantly to our knowledge of joint function.[32–34] It is an excellent research and teaching technique. Except for its use in conjunction with arthrotomography, it has little usefulness in the clinical management of TM disorders. It embodies all the limitations inherent in transcranial radiography.

Arthrotomography

Injecting the joint with a contrast medium renders the synovial fluid radiopaque. This method of TM examination was introduced in 1944 by Norgaard[35, 36] but was soon discarded. It was reintroduced in 1978 by Wilkes,[37] and has since been used extensively in conjunction with the management of disc-interference disorders, especially those due to displacement or dislocation of the articular disc. Simple arthrography using the transcranial projection has very limited value, because the overlapping of the synovial sacs laterally obscures the articular disc space.[38] Arthrotomography is needed to visualize the disc space. Unfortunately, the tomographic method is fully satisfactory only in the central two thirds of the joint, which reduces the overall usefulness of the method.[26]

Arthrography was once used rather extensively to examine the synovial cavity of the knee joint. The technique provided for the withdrawal of a quantity of synovial fluid that exactly equaled the amount of contrast medium to be injected. In this way the internal pressure of the joint was not altered. Unfortunately, this technique could not be applied to TM arthrography, because no appreciable quantity of synovial fluid can be aspirated from the TM joint.[39] Therefore, the injection of the contrast medium renders the joint hyperbaric, which seriously alters normal joint function. The added pressure within the joint increases the articular disc space. In the resting joint, muscle tonus in the superior lateral pterygoid muscle rotates the disc forward as far as this increased width of disc space permits. *In a normal joint* the contour of the disc prevents displacement; only rotatory movement of the disc on the condyle takes place. But, if there is already enough deterioration in disc contour and elongation of the discal collateral ligaments to permit displacement of the disc, the hyperbaric condition produced by the addition of contrast medium *exaggerates that displacement to the extent of the widened articular disc space.* Therefore, when the arthrogram discloses anterior displacement of the articular disc, it should be assumed that the actual displacement is somewhat less than the radiograph suggests. The extent of the artifact thus created can be judged by measuring the thickness of any radiopaque material seen between the articular surfaces of the joint. In a center-cut tomogram there normally is apposition of these surfaces because of muscle tonus in the elevator muscles. Any thickness of radiopaque material, therefore, is indicative of hyperbaric separation of the articulating parts and, consequently, a similar widening of the articular disc space. To the degree that this space is artificially widened, the disc is also artificially shifted anteriorly. This principle does not apply, however, to discs that are completely dislocated in front of the condyle, because additional widening of the articular disc space would have no effect. The overall value of arthrotomography for confirming the displacement or dislocation of articular discs in disc-interference disorders is well established.[40–44]

The method is not without certain hazards, however. Salon and Ross[45] have listed several, namely, (1) joint infection, (2) needle damage to joint structures, (3) hypersensitivity to the contrast material, and (4) unpleasant postinjection sequelae, such as pain, swelling, and temporary acute malocclusion.

Although Blaschke et al.[42] advised the opacification of both synovial cavities, Dolwick et al.[46] found that upper joint examination by arthrography was considerably less dependable than that of the lower joint. Usually, the lower joint only is injected. The resulting radiograph shows the synovial fluid as a radiopaque mass, thus outlining the confines of the synovial sac. Posteriorly, the sac is confined by the inferior retrodiscal lamina, which attaches from the condylar articular facet to the lower posterior part of the articular disc. Anteriorly, the sac is confined by the inferior portion of the anterior wall of the articular capsule, which attaches from the condylar articular facet to the lower anterior portion of the articular disc. Since the disc proper is invisible because of its radiolucency, its position can be determined by identifying the attachment of the inferior retrodiscal lamina posteriorly and that of the anterior capsular wall at the front of the disc. The difficulty that arises, however, is that the retrodiscal tissue posteriorly and the superior lateral pterygoid muscle anteriorly are also radiolucent like the disc, and no demarcation is seen to identify exactly where the disc begins and ends. It is not accurately done by examining disc contour, because *loss of contour is required before displacement is possible.* By identifying the attachments of the synovial sac to the disc, its limits can be discerned, but the distention by the increased intracapsular pressure may distort the appearance of these attachments. The exact identification of disc position in arthrograms is not easy.

In the closed joint position, the distended synovial sacs permit rather equal distribution of the fluid in front of and behind the condyle. But, as translation takes place and the disc rotates posteriorly, the anterior capsular wall becomes increasingly taut while the inferior retrodiscal lamina relaxes. The shape of the opacified synovial fluid conforms to the distended synovial sac. As the condyle moves forward, the fluid anterior to the condyle decreases and that posterior to it increases. In full forward position, almost all the fluid will be found posterior to the disc, and the shape of the opacified fluid will reflect this. When displacement of the disc is permitted, however, its forward position keeps the inferior retrodiscal lamina taut and reduces the posterior flow of fluid. A completely dislocated disc holds most of the fluid forward in the closed joint position, and this does not change appreciably as the condyle translates. Thus, the shape of the opacified synovial fluid does correlate with the position of the disc. These criteria have excellent confirming value in disc-interference disorders that entail displacement or dislocation of the articular disc.

Bronstein[47] found that of 21 patients examined postsurgically 4 displayed arthrograms that were nondiagnostic. Westesson[48] reported that arthrography had been only 85% accurate as correlated with dissection findings. The most dependable arthrographic data have to do with perforations of the disc or retrodiscal tissue,[43] especially if accompanied by palpable crepitus.[44] It is also dependable with protracted functional anterior dislocations of the disc.

Double-Contrast Arthrotomography.   An excellent refinement of arthrotomography was introduced in 1980 by Westesson et al.[49] This has come to be known as double-contrast arthrotomography. Both upper and lower compartments are cannulated and injected with contrast medium, which is then aspirated, and air injected.[50] This leaves a thin radiopaque film on the articular surfaces and on the walls of both the upper and the lower synovial sacs. Thus, for the first time, the articular surfaces of the condyle, disc, and articular eminence have been visualized radiographically. Unfortunately, the retrodiscal tissue and the superior lateral pterygoid muscle still display the same radiolucency as the articular disc. So, locating the anterior and posterior limits of the disc proper remains dependent on identifying the attachments of the synovial sacs.

Double-contrast arthrotomography is a superior technique. For the first time, torqued, displaced articular discs have been seen radiographically,[51] a condition that has been only presumed since 1918.[52] Also, posterior displacements of the articular disc have been demonstrated radiographically—a condition that heretofore has been only presumed. This new method has contributed materially to our knowledge of disc-interference disorders of the TM joint.[53] It is a valuable research tool, but has little application to the clinical management of TM disorders.

Arthrograms do not give information that affects the surgery.[54] Since disc-interference disorders (including anterior displacements and dislocations of the articular disc) may be diagnosed with a high degree of precision by a proper clinical examination and confirmed by transcranial radiography,[15] the *diagnostic* use of arthrotomography is largely superfluous. For medicolegal reasons, however, it is wise to document the justification for surgery. For teaching and research purposes, arthrotomography and especially the double-contrast method are indispensable.

Scintigraphy (Nuclear Scanning)

While the structural definition of osseous tissue is examined by transmission x-ray techniques, bone reactivity is seen by emission techniques using an isotope medium. So-called nuclear scanning is done by injecting a radioisotope intravenously and detecting the resultant gamma ray emission with a scintillation camera. This yields a planar radionuclide image that is indicative of increased osseous reactivity. Single proton emission computed tomography (SPECT) is a modification whereby the scintillation camera is moved so as to make "slices," and then reconstructed by computer technology.[55]

Corrected tomographic nuclear scanning is useful in confirming osteoarthritic changes in the TM joint.[56] Radionuclide imaging is extremely sensitive but lacks specificity in assessing osseous changes. Simple active remodeling cannot be distinguished from overt degenerative joint disease. It has very limited usefulness as an isolated modality. Since it has the propensity to detect changes in osseous tissue long before they become evident radiographically, it may furnish confirming evidence of active bone change, if that is an issue in TM diagnosis.

ANALGESIC BLOCKING

When positive confirmation of the true source of pain is needed, especially when it is necessary to distinguish between primary pain and referred pain or secondary hyperalgesia, skillful use of local anesthesia is dependable and accurate.[1] The following general rules should be followed:

1. Actively inflamed structures should be avoided.

2. Acceptable aseptic technique should be followed routinely.

3. One should be thoroughly familiar with all anatomical structures through which the needle is to pass.

4. One should be thoroughly familiar with the solution to be used, especially its proper dosage, contraindications, and possible side effects.

5. Invariably, one should aspirate prior to injecting the solution.

6. One should be prepared by training as well as by the availability of needed equipment to meet any related emergency that may arise.

It should be noted that good local anesthesia of skeletal muscle requires that the solution contain no epinephrine-like substance. Plain aqueous procaine should be used in muscle tissue. Also, it usually requires somewhat more time for anesthesia to become effective (5 minutes or more).

As a general rule, muscle injections are preferred to those for anesthesia of the joint proper. To obtain satisfactory anesthesia of the joint, two injections are needed: (1) an infiltration of solution at a point just posterior to the neck of the condyloid process to anesthetize the auriculotemporal nerve; and (2) a small infiltration just anterior to the joint proper to anesthetize the anterior third of the capsular ligament. A modified auriculotemporal block has been described.[57]

The local anesthetic injections for the main masticatory muscles by the extraoral route are illustrated in Figures 9–4 through 9–7. It should be understood that injections about the temporomandibular area may include motor fibers of the facial nerve. This may induce paralysis of the eyelid for the duration of anesthesia. Patients should be forewarned.

Every practitioner who is serious about temporomandibular disorders should make himself especially proficient in the use of local analgesic blocking techniques. When they are needed, there is no substi-

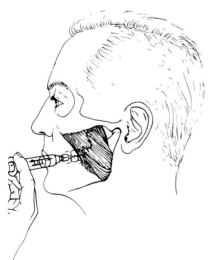

FIGURE 9–4 Technique for external injection of masseter muscle. The needle enters the muscle at the anterior border about midbody and is passed through the muscle at several angles and depths to reach the deep and superficial layers. With each pass of the needle, after aspirating it, the solution is deposited slowly as the needle is withdrawn. (From Bell W.E.: Management of masticatory pain, in Alling C.C., Mahan P.E. (eds.): *Facial Pain,* ed. 2. Philadelphia, Lea & Febiger, 1977. Reproduced with permission.)

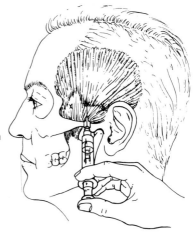

FIGURE 9–5 Technique for injection of temporalis muscle. Needle penetrates the muscle at several points *(X)* just above the zygomatic arch to reach most of the fibers. With each penetration, after aspirating the needle, solution is deposited slowly. (From Bell W.E.: Management of masticatory pain, in Alling C.C., Mahan P.E. (eds.): *Facial Pain,* ed. 2. Philadelphia, Lea & Febiger, 1977. Reproduced with permission.)

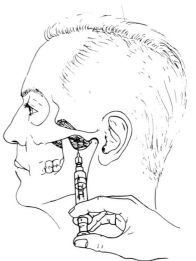

FIGURE 9–6 Technique for external injection of lateral pterygoid muscle. After the needle is passed through the mandibular sigmoid notch, it is directed slightly upward and inward to a total depth of 35 to 40 mm. After aspiration of the needle, the solution is deposited slowly. Do not deposit any solution as needle is inserted or withdrawn. Motor fibers of the facial nerve also may be anesthetized. (From Bell W.E.: Management of masticatory pain, in Alling C.C., Mahan P.E. (eds.): *Facial Pain,* ed. 2. Philadelphia, Lea & Febiger, 1977. Reproduced with permission.)

tute. This method is extremely useful both diagnostically and therapeutically. The minor injury such injections may cause is more than justified by the benefit obtained.

ARTHROSCOPY

Perhaps the most promising of future examining aids in TM diagnosis is arthroscopy.[58] Microfiberoptic technology has made fine-needle arthroscopy adaptable for use in the TM joint. Westesson[59] has demon-

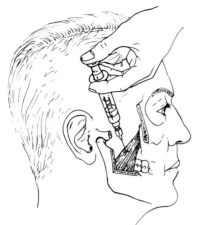

FIGURE 9–7 Technique for external injection of medial pterygoid muscle. After the needle is passed through the mandibular sigmoid notch, it is directed boldly downward and inward to a total depth of about 40 mm. After aspiration of the needle, the solution is deposited slowly. Do not deposit any solution as needle is inserted or withdrawn. Motor fibers of the facial nerve also may be anesthetized. (From Bell W.E.: Management of masticatory pain, in Alling C.C., Mahan P.E. (eds.): *Facial Pain,* ed. 2. Philadelphia, Lea & Febiger, 1977. Reproduced with permission.)

strated its practicality in cadaver studies. McCarty is working with the instrument. If it proves as successful in TM diagnosis as with the knee joint, it may likely render TM arthrography obsolete. Although invasive, the fine needle-like instrument is much less so than arthrography, and, more importantly, it does not alter the structural relationship of the articular disc by changing the intracapsular pressure unless air or saline pressure is used for better visualization.

ELECTROMYOGRAPHY

Electromyographic examination of masticatory muscles may have confirming value for a clinical diagnosis of myospasm which characteristically shows a marked increase in EMG activity when the muscle is at rest.[60] Electromyographic activity is known to be increased as a result of pain generated within the muscle.[61]

The masseteric EMG silent period has been found to be prolonged in patients with myofascial pain-dysfunction symptoms.[62–64] Due to the remarkable variability and inconsistency of silent periods, criteria for pathologic levels have not been established. Useful as such testing may be at a research level, there is currently little or no practical application for it in the clinical management of TM disorders.[65]

SONOGRAPHY

By utilizing electronic auscultation and sonographic audiospectral analysis of the TM joint, it has been determined that most individuals have a reproducible TM joint sound print. Nonsymptomatic groups display long, smooth bursts of sound, while symptomatic patients yield shorter, coarser, irregular bursts of sound during opening-closing movements.[66] Whether such testing can be used to confirm the source of noise heard with the stethoscope is conjectural.

OCCLUSION

It has long been recognized that a conflict between the mandibular position prescribed by the temporomandibular joints as the result of muscle action and that prescribed by the occlusion of the teeth must be resolved to assure normal masticatory function.[67] Interference that occurs during mandibular movements may affect muscle action. Recent changes that are registered by altered signals to the CNS may induce muscle splinting which, if not quickly resolved, may terminate in myospastic activity. Typical pantographic tracings are said to result from muscle spasm as well as from internal derangements.[68] Occlusal interference that alters condylar position when the teeth are clenched may predispose to articular changes in the joint.

Study Casts

If occlusion is an issue, either etiologically or symptomatically, study casts help to visualize the relationship that exists. Although hand-held casts may be useful, face-bow mounting enhances their value. The rigidity of plaster and metal, the lack of sensory and proprioceptive feedback, and the absence of neuromuscular action impose serious limitations on the information that can be obtained concerning masticatory function. The gross structural relationship, however, particularly as viewed from the lingual side, may be demonstrated by this method. Thus, confirmation of occlusal disharmony may be established.

Condyle Path Registration

It has been established that when the articular disc is displaced anteriorly the resultant protrusive and retrusive inferior deflections of the condyle path do not superimpose, but the retrusive deflection remains below that of the protrusive path during closure.[69] However, reciprocal clicking due to structural incompatibility of the sliding surfaces displays good superimposition of these deflections of the condylar path. This can be confirming evidence to distinguish between these two common

types of Class III disc interference. It correlates with the clinical finding that interference symptoms during closing movements due to disc
displacement may be varied according to the demands of function,
while those due to structural incompatibility occur at exactly the same
point during opening-closing movements of the mandible and remain
constant regardless of function.

BEHAVIORAL EXAMINATIONS

Olson[70] found that psychologic tests administered to individual patients
with myofascial pain-dysfunction symptoms (1) yielded no information
of diagnostic significance, (2) shed no light on etiology, and (3) offered
no help in the selection of treatment. He recommended against the use
of such testing in the routine clinical management of TM disorders.

NUCLEAR MAGNETIC RESONANCE IMAGING (NMR)

When a patient is placed in a magnetic field, the atomic nuclei polarize.
Then, when bombarded with a high-frequency energy source, the nuclei resonate. When the radiowave is turned off, they emit their own
radiowaves, which are recorded by sensitive antennae surrounding the
patient. Computer analysis of these signals produces a cross-sectional
anatomical image similar to CT imaging. The NMR image shows a map
of tissue proton density differences which are primarily due to differences in tissue water density. Fluid-containing tissue appears white
while bone appears black.

Although NMR imaging is still in its infancy relative to TM diagnosis, it may prove to be better than CT scanning and arthrography. It
utilizes no radiation and is wholly noninvasive, thus eliminating the
hazards of radiation and tissue damage.[71] Presently, it is expensive and
not readily available. It holds good promise for the future, especially
as a research tool.

THERMOGRAPHY

Thermography is a technique for recording variations in the surface
temperature of the skin. It is reported that skin temperature changes
correlate with pain. It is known that a noticeable temperature gradient
exists at myofascial trigger points.[60] Fischer[72] reported that thermo-

grams of skin overlying active trigger points have shown areas of increased skin temperature from 5 to 10 cm in diameter. Travell[60] witnessed decreased temperature changes in areas of pain reference when the etiologic trigger points were stimulated by compression. A determination of the usefulness of thermography to confirm the source of pain in TM disorders requires further investigation and documentation.

LABORATORY TESTS

Several laboratory tests may help confirm specific disorders of the temporomandibular joints. The serum uric acid test is essential to the diagnosis of hyperuricemia. Sedimentation rate and latex fixation test, a serologic test for rheumatoid factor, are useful in making a diagnosis of rheumatoid arthritis. Negative findings, however, do not preclude the disease. Synovial fluid examination and blood studies may be needed to confirm synovitis and infectious inflammatory arthritis.

Catecholamine Level

A high level of urinary catecholamines, which usually is taken as evidence of psychologic stress, has been reported in patients with myofascial pain-dysfunction symptoms.[73] Urinary catecholamines are also increased with nocturnal masseter activity, expecially with active bruxing.[74] So, whether the increase is a manifestation of stress, as generally assumed, or due to muscle activity, has not been decided. The value of the test at this time is equivocal.

CONSULTATIONS

Some conditions may require the opinion of other practitioners, both dental and medical. Dental specialists may be needed to help settle questions about occlusion, oral rehabilitation, and surgical considerations. Medical specialists who may help resolve certain questions include otolaryngologists, neurologists, orthopedists, anesthesiologists, internists, psychologists, and physiotherapists.

CLINICAL TRIAL

Response to therapy is not to be ignored for its confirming value. To ascertain the correctness of a diagnosis, one should be familiar with placebo effect, which may account for up to about 35% of the effectiveness of any treatment. If benefit from initial therapy well exceeds placebo effect, it is presumptive evidence that the diagnosis is correct and the treatment proper.

It is wise, however, to use only reversible palliative therapy for its confirming value. All serious definitive and especially irreversible therapy should await a confirmed working diagnosis. It should be understood, however, that effective results indicate only the acceptability of the treatment used; they cannot be taken as scientific evidence to prove or disprove anything.[75]

CONFIRMED WORKING DIAGNOSIS

A confirmed working diagnosis should be the objective of every examination. Only when positive confirmation is established can one really plan and embark on definitive therapy with predictive effectiveness.

Final Evaluation of Data

It should be the rule to judge the effectiveness of therapy on a continuing basis. At any time that serious inconsistency in the management of a temporomandibular disorder becomes evident, it is well to suspend further treatment until such is reasonably resolved. *Relapse soon after treatment, recurrence or persistence of symptoms, and chronicity without organic justification are warning signals that should be heeded.* Caution should always be exercised, especially when irreversible therapeutic measures are undertaken.

REFERENCES

1. Bell W.E.: *Orofacial Pains*, ed. 3. Chicago, Year Book Medical Publishers, 1985.
2. Hansson L., Hansson T., Petersson A.: A comparison between clinical and radiographic findings in 259 temporomandibular joint patients. *J. Prosthet. Dent.* 50:89, 1983.
3. Weinberg L.A.: Practical evaluation of the lateral temporomandibular joint radiograph. *J. Prosthet. Dent.* 51:676, 1984.
4. Rieder C.E., Martinoff J.T.: Comparison of the multiphasic dysfunction profile with lateral transcranial radiographs. *J. Prosthet. Dent.* 52:572–580, 1984.
5. Updegrave W.J.: Temporomandibular articulation x-ray examination. *Dent. Radiogr. Photogr.* 26:41, 1953.

6. Richards A.G., Alling C.C.: Extraoral radiography, mandible and tempo-romandibular articulation. *Dent. Radiogr. Photogr.* 28:1, 1955.
7. Updegrave W.J.: Roentgenographic observations of functioning temporo-mandibular joints. *J. Am. Dent. Assoc.* 54:488, 1957.
8. Bell W.E.: *Temporomandibular Joint Disease.* Dallas, Egan Company Press, 1960.
9. Bell W.E.: Standards of normal for temporomandibular diagnosis. *Proc. Inst. Med. Chic.* 23:168, 1960.
10. Updegrave W.J.: Practical evaluation of the techniques and interpretation in the roentgenographic examination of temporomandibular joints. *Dent. Clin. North Am.* July 1961, p. 421.
11. Schier M.B.A.: Temporomandibular joint roentgenography: Controlled erect technics. *J. Am. Dent. Assoc.* 65:456, 1962.
12. Robinson M., Lytle J.: Simplified method for office roentgenograms of the temporomandibular joint. *J. Oral Surg.* 20:217, 1962.
13. Updegrave W.J.: Interpretation of temporomandibular joint radiographs. *Dent. Clin. North Am.* Nov. 1966, p. 567.
14. Yale S.H.: Radiographic evaluation of the temporomandibular joint. *J. Am. Dent. Assoc.* 79:102, 1969.
15. Farrar W.B., McCarty W.L.: *A Clinical Outline of Temporomandibular Joint Diagnosis and Treatment,* ed. 7. Montgomery, Ala., Normandie Publications, 1982.
16. Preti G., Arduino A., Pera P.: Consistency of performance of a new cran-iostat for oblique lateral transcranial radiographs of the temporomandib-ular joint. *J. Prosthet. Dent.* 52:270, 1984.
17. Vogler J.B. III, Helms C.A.: Conventional radiography, in Helms C.A., Katzberg R.W., Dolwick M.F. (eds.): *Internal Derangements of the Temporo-mandibular Joint.* San Francisco, Radiology Research and Education Foun-dation, 1983, pp. 43–61.
18. Donovan R.W.: Method of temporomandibular joint roentgenography for serial or multiple records. *J. Am. Dent. Assoc.* 49:401, 1954.
19. Lindvall A.M.: Radiographic examination of the temporomandibular joint. *Dentomax. Radiol.* 5:24, 1976.
20. Dixon D.C., Graham G.S., Mayhow R.B., et al.: The validity of transcran-ial radiography in diagnosing TMJ anterior disc displacement. *J. Am. Dent. Assoc.* 108:615, 1984.
21. Van Sickels J.E., Bianco H.J. Jr., Pifer R.G.: Transcranial radiographs in the evaluation of craniomandibular (TMJ) disorders. *J. Prosthet. Dent.* 49:244, 1983.
22. Mongini F.: The importance of radiography in the diagnosis of TMJ dys-functions: A comparative evaluation of transcranial radiographs and serial tomography. *J. Prosthet. Dent.* 45:186, 1981.
23. Eckerdal O., Lundberg M.: The structural situation in temporomandibu-lar joints: A comparison between conventional oblique transcranial radio-graphs, tomograms, and histologic sections. *Dentomax. Radiol.* 8:42, 1979.

24. Ricketts R.M.: Laminography in the diagnosis of temporomandibular joint disorders. *J. Am. Dent. Assoc.* 46:620, 1953.

25. Blaschke D.D.: Radiology of the temporomandibular joint: Current status of transcranial, tomographic, and arthrographic procedures, in *The President's Conference on the Examination, Diagnosis and Management of Temporomandibular Disorders.* Chicago, American Dental Association, 1983, pp. 64–74.

26. Eckerdal O.: Tomography of the temporomandibular joint: Correlation between tomographic image and histologic sections in a three-dimensional system. *Acta Radiol.* [Suppl.] (Stockh.) 329:1, 1973.

27. Helms C.A., Katzberg R.W., Manzione J.V.: Computed tomography, in Helms C.A., Katzberg R.W., Dolwick M.F. (eds.): *Internal Derangements of the Temporomandibular Joint.* San Francisco, Radiology Research and Education Foundation, 1983, pp. 135–166.

28. Helms C.A., Vogler J.B. III, Moorish R.B. Jr.: Diagnosis by computed tomography of temporomandibular joint meniscus displacement. *J. Prosthet. Dent.* 51:544, 1984.

29. Helms C.A., Katzberg R.W., Moorish R., et al.: Computed tomography of the temporomandibular meniscus. *J. Oral Maxillofac. Surg.* 41:512, 1983.

30. Helms C.A., Richardson M.L., Vogler J.B. III, et al.: Computed tomography for diagnosing temporomandibular joint disc displacement. *J. Craniomand. Pract.* 3:24–26, 1984.

31. Wilkinson T., Maryniuk G.: The correlation between sagittal anatomic sections and computerized tomography of the TMJ. *J.Craniomand. Pract.* 1(3):37, 1983.

32. Berry H.M. Jr., Hofmann F.A.: Cinefluorography with image intensification for observing temporomandibular joint movements. *J. Am. Dent. Assoc.* 53:517, 1956.

33. Scully J.J.: *Cinefluorographic Studies of the Masticatory Movements of the Human Mandible.* Thesis, University of Illinois, 1959.

34. McLeran J.H., Montgomery J.C., Hale M.L.: A cinefluorographic analysis of the temporomandibular joint. *J. Am. Dent. Assoc.* 75:1394, 1967.

35. Norgaard F.: Arthrography of the mandibular joint. *Acta Radiol.* 25:679–685, 1944.

36. Norgaard F.: *Temporomandibular Arthrography.* Copenhagen, Munksgaard, 1947.

37. Wilkes C.H.: Structural and functional situations of the temporomandibular joint. *Northwest Dent.* 57:287, 1978.

38. Westesson P.: Development and clinical use of double-contrast arthrography of the temporomandibular joint, in Moffett B.C. (ed.): *Diagnosis of Internal Derangements of the Temporomandibular Joint,* Vol. 1. Seattle, University of Washington, 1984, pp. 21–26.

39. Mahan P.E.: Anatomic, histologic, and physiologic features of TMJ, in Irby W.B. (ed.): *Current Advances in Oral Surgery,* Vol. III. St. Louis, C.V. Mosby Co., 1980, pp. 3–9.

40. Wilkes C.H.: Arthrography of the temporomandibular joint. *Minn. Med.* 61:645, 1978.

41. Farrar W.B., McCarty W.L.: Inferior joint space arthrography and characteristics of condylar paths in internal derangements of the TMJ. *J. Prosthet. Dent.* 41:548, 1979.

42. Blaschke D.D., Solberg W.K., Sanders B.: Arthrography of the temporomandibular joint: Review of current status. *J. Am. Dent. Assoc.* 100:388, 1980.

43. Oberg T.: Radiology of the temporomandibular joint, in Solberg W.K., Clark G.T. (eds.): *Temporomandibular Joint Problems.* Chicago, Quintessence Publishing Company, 1980, pp. 49–68.

44. Graham G.S., Ferraro N.F., Simms D.A.: Perforations of the temporomandibular joint meniscus: Arthrographic, surgical, and clinical findings. *J. Oral Maxillofac. Surg.* 42:35, 1984.

45. Salon J.M., Ross R.J.: Computerized tomography with multiplanar reconstruction for examining the TMJ. *J. Craniomand. Pract.* 1(4):27, 1983.

46. Dolwick M.F., Lipton J.S., Warner M.R., et al.: Sagittal anatomy of the human temporomandibular joint spaces. *J. Oral Maxillofac. Surg.* 41:86, 1983.

47. Bronstein S.L.: Postsurgical TMJ arthrography. *J. Craniomand. Pract.* 2(2):165, 1984.

48. Westesson P.: Arthrography of the temporomandibular joint. *J. Prosthet. Dent.* 51:535, 1984.

49. Westesson P., Omnell K., Rohlin M.: Double-contrast tomography of the temporomandibular joint: A new technique based on autopsy specimen examinations. *Acta Radiol.* [*Diagn.*] *(Stock.)* 21:777–785, 1980.

50. Westesson P.: Double-contrast arthrotomography of the temporomandibular joint: Introduction of an arthrographic technique for visualization of the disc and articular surfaces. *J. Oral Maxillofac. Surg.* 41:163, 1983.

51. Westesson P.: Diagnostic accuracy of double-contrast arthrotomography confirmed by dissection, in Moffett B.C. (ed.): *Diagnosis of Internal Derangements of the Temporomandibular Joint,* Vol. 1. Seattle, University of Washington, 1984, pp. 31–34.

52. Pringle J.H.: Displacement of the mandibular meniscus and its treatment. *Br. J. Surg.* 6:385–389, 1918.

53. Moffett B.C. (ed.): *Diagnosis of Internal Derangements of the Temporomandibular Joint,* Vol. 1. Seattle, University of Washington, 1984.

54. Dolwick M.F.: Diagnosis and etiology of internal derangements of the temporomandibular joint, in *The President's Conference on the Examination, Diagnosis, and Management of Temporomandibular Disorders.* Chicago, American Dental Association, 1983, pp. 112–117.

55. Katzberg R.W., O'Mara R.E., Tallents R.H., et al.: Radionuclide skeletal imaging and single proton emission computed tomography in suspected internal derangements of the temporomandibular joint. *J. Oral Maxillofac. Surg.* 42:782–787, 1984.

56. Goldman S.M., Taylor R.: Radiographic examination of the abnormal temporomandibular joint. *J. Prosthet. Dent.* 49:711, 1983.

57. Donlon W.C., Truta M.P., Eversole L.R.: A modified auriculotemporal nerve block for regional anesthesia of the temporomandibular joint. *J. Oral Maxillofac. Surg.* 42:544, 1984.

58. Burke R.H.: Temporomandibular joint diagnosis: Arthroscopy. *J. Craniomand. Pract.* 3:234–236, 1985.

59. Westesson P.: Clinical and arthrographic findings in patients with TMJ disorders, in Moffett B.C. (ed.): *Diagnosis of Internal Derangements of the Temporomandibular Joint*, Vol. 1. Seattle, University of Washington, 1984, pp. 59–71.

60. Travell J.G., Simons D.G.: *Myofascial Pain and Dysfunction*. Baltimore, Williams & Wilkins Co., 1983.

61. Cobb C.R., DeVries H.A., Urban R.T., et al.: Electrical activity in muscle pain. *Am. J. Phys. Med.* 54:80, 1975.

62. Bessette R., Bishop B., Mohl N.: Duration of masseteric silent period in patients with TMJ syndrome. *J. Appl. Physiol.* 30:864, 1971.

63. Bessette R.W., Mohl N.D., DiCosimo C.J. II.: Comparison of results of electromyographic and radiographic examination in patients with myofascial pain-dysfunction syndrome. *J. Am. Dent. Assoc.* 89:1358, 1974.

64. Skiba T.J., Laskin D.M.: Masticatory muscle silent periods in patients with MPD syndrome before and after treatment. *J. Dent. Res.* 60:699, 1981.

65. Hellsing G., Klineberg L.: The masseter muscle: The silent period and its clinical implications. *J. Prosthet. Dent.* 49:106, 1983.

66. Quellette P.L.: TMJ sound prints: Electronic auscultation and sonographic audiospectral analysis of the temporomandibular joint. *J. Am. Dent. Assoc.* 89:623, 1974.

67. Jeffreys F.E.: The temporomandibular joint and occlusion. *J. Am. Dent. Assoc.* 57:801, 1958.

68. Mongini F., Capurso U.: Factors influencing the pantographic tracings of mandibular border movements. *J. Prosthet. Dent.* 48:585, 1982.

69. Isberg-Holm A., Westesson P.L.: Movement of disc and condyle in temporomandibular joints with clicking, in *Temporomandibular Joint Clicking* (thesis). Malmo, 1980.

70. Olson R.E.: Behavioral examinations in MPD, in *The President's Conference on the Examination, Diagnosis and Management of Temporomandibular Disorders*. Chicago, American Dental Association, 1983, pp. 104–105.

71. Helms C.A., Richardson M.L., Moon K.L., et al.: Nuclear magnetic resonance imaging of the temporomandibular joint: Preliminary observations. *J. Craniomand. Pract.* 2(3):219, 1984.

72. Fischer A.A.: Thermography and pain. *Arch. Phys. Med. Rehabil.* 62:542, 1981.

73. Evaskus D.S., Laskin D.M.: A biochemical measure of stress in patients with myofascial pain-dysfunction syndrome. *J. Dent. Res.* 51:1464, 1972.

74. Clark G.T., Rugh J.D., Handelman S.L.: Nocturnal masseter muscle activity and urinary catecholamine levels in bruxers. *J. Dent. Res.* 59:1571, 1980.

75. Sicher H.: Positions and movements of the mandible. *J. Am. Dent. Assoc.* 48:620, 1954.

10 | Therapeutic Guidelines

The successful management of a patient with a TM complaint, like the treatment of other bodily ailments, consists of seven general principles, namely:

1. *Diagnosis:* Know what is wrong, where, and, if possible, why.

2. *The helping process:* Treat the patient, not the complaint.

3. *Palliative therapy:* Provide for the patient's immediate concerns—his pain, his disability, his anxiety about the cause and consequences, his panic and fear.

4. *Natural resolution:* Enlist the patient's cooperation to reduce adverse activities and to foster natural healing.

5. *Cause-related therapy:* Eliminate, reduce, or neutralize the factors and conditions that predispose to, that activate, and that perpetuate the disorder.

6. *Specific therapy:* Institute rational therapy to arrest the progress of the condition, to resolve the disorder, and to forestall its relapse or recurrence.

7. *Rehabilitation:* Help the patient regain his former state of health and help him to cope with any part of the disorder that cannot be so resolved.

Good therapy suggests that these principles be followed in the proper order. To apply specific therapy by jumping over the first five steps is to invite failure. And to ignore the last step is to leave the patient only partially treated.

DIAGNOSIS

The most important step in therapy is an accurate diagnosis. Nothing can take its place. Diagnosis should always precede therapy. Assuming that a diagnosis has been made, including what is wrong, where, and why, one should be able to make a reasonably accurate prognosis as to how the future will unfold. One should be able to predict to what degree therapy can be expected to produce favorable results, something of the time factor involved, what treatment modalities may be required, and what residual or progressive symptoms or conditions may remain for future consideration.

The importance of diagnosis should not be underestimated. The most perfectly executed treatment can hardly prove effective if it is for the wrong thing.

THE HELPING PROCESS

In this scientific age it is easy to become so preoccupied with the patient's complaint that one may forget the patient. So great and spectacular are the feats of modern medical science that there is a tendency for doctors to become "little gods." In dental practice one who successfully manages painful dysfunctions of the masticatory system may become more concerned about the disorder he manages than with the patient who presents it—especially if he utilizes rather heroic forms of therapy. The helping process, however, is a highly personalized cooperative effort that involves two *people*. In medical situations, these are the patient and the doctor. It is not a matter of the patient's disorder and the doctor's treatment; it, rather, is a relationship between two human beings—each with his own particular capabilities and limitations and needs.

The helping process begins with one person seeking aid from another who presumably is able and willing to render it. The one who seeks aid must trust his helper and be willing to cooperate with him. The helper should accept the unique personhood of the one needing aid and enter honestly into a helping relationship with him. Honesty on the helper's part comprises not only his willingness to help, but also his ability to do so. In a doctor-patient relationship this implies competence on the doctor's part—his ability to understand the person, to diagnose his ailment properly, and to treat it competently. Good professional rapport is essential to effective therapy, and such rapport depends on an honest helping relationship between patient and doctor.

If one proposes to care for a patient's complaint, he should first care about the person who has the complaint. It is only by entering into a helping relationship with an open mind that one can discover the person who has the complaint. "For human beings are more than patients that have to be treated. They are persons who are threatened in their existence and are crying for help."[1]

PALLIATIVE THERAPY

Palliative therapy includes measures that can be taken to give the patient some comfort while more serious efforts are underway to find out the facts in the case and plan more definitive treatment.

Control of Pain

It is important that pain be controlled with dispatch. But one should not underestimate the value of pain as a diagnostic symptom, as a deterrent to restrain abusive joint use, and as a means of judging progress in the resolution of a complaint. Certainly no effort should be made to eliminate pain entirely, and the patient should be so informed. If pain is eliminated completely, the patient loses his number-one signal to stop doing whatever it is that hurts.

Analgesic medications may be needed. If the patient is persuaded to restrict jaw use within painless limits, enough benefit usually accrues that simple household pain remedies may suffice. Narcotic analgesics should be avoided as much as possible because of their undesirable effects: nausea, constipation, respiratory depression, hypotension, and possible dependence. They should be used with caution, preferably under active medical supervision, for patients with head injuries, patients suffering from asthma, patients recently treated with monoamine oxidase inhibitors, and patients that are pregnant or nursing. All analgesics should be restricted to dosage that will make the pain tolerable without eliminating it completely.

Other useful palliative measures are available for the control of pain, such as (1) stimulation of superficial cutaneous receptors by light massage, thermal applications, hydrotherapy, vapocoolants, vibration, electroanalgesia, and transcutaneous nerve stimulators, and (2) suggestion, distraction, and good rapport.[2]

NATURAL RESOLUTION

It is a widely reported clinical observation that upwards of 70% of TM complaints become nonsymptomatic regardless of the type of treatment employed.[3–10] This, no doubt, accounts for the variety of treatment programs that have been used in the past. The reasonable conclusion that should be drawn is that natural resolution is an important element in the eradication of masticatory symptoms. The second conclusion, however, is that the 25% to 30% who do not respond so favorably are in need of better diagnostic understanding of their complaints and of more rational application of therapy.

There are two features of TM disorders in which natural resolution by way of full active patient cooperation may be the determinant of success, namely, (1) pains of muscle origin, and (2) excessive loading of the joint. It is expedient, therefore, that the patient's cooperation be enlisted at the earliest possible time. This can be done by giving him proper insight into his problem and into the important role that he must play in his recovery.

Myogenous Pain

Pain of muscle origin frequently displays a cycling mechanism, whereby the pain of use accentuates the patient's problem. The normal biologic response to pain is—or should be—a marked reduction in the functional activity of the painful part. If this inhibitory influence is heeded, resolution begins promptly. If it is ignored—and it so frequently is, due to the variety of uses civilization has placed on the mouth—the condition tends to be aggravated and perpetuated. This should be explained to the patient, with the admonition to voluntarily restrain mandibular function within painless limits. Thus, by natural resolution is accomplished the same benefits that may otherwise be obtained through therapeutic efforts such as occlusal disengagement with interocclusal devices, biofeedback training, and relaxation techniques.

Excessive Loading

Deterioration of the articular discs, degenerative change in the articular tissues of the condyle and eminence, and elongation of the discal collateral ligaments may result from overloading forces within the joint. This may take the form of static overloading, impact loading, or frictional movement. Although the disc and discal ligaments have little, if any, propensity for recovery from such damage, the articular tissues of the TM joints do, since they are composed of fibrous tissue rather than hyaline cartilage. Natural resolution of the damage sustained by these articular tissues is an essential factor in the elimination of joint symptoms. Abusive loading occurs from clenching, bruxism, or excessively hard biting, and from abusive habits or mannerisms. It therefore is highly beneficial to persuade the patient to avoid clenching and excessively hard chewing, to eliminate abusive habits and mannerisms, and to modify chewing toward softer foods, smaller bites, and slower jaw movements. Thus, the voluntary cooperation of the patient ensures the termination of abusive loading and institutes the benefits of natural resolution at the earliest possible moment.

In all planning for the correction of temporomandibular complaints, the patient should be brought actively into the program so that he may assume his burden of responsibility for the effectiveness of therapy. Being musculoskeletal in type, all such complaints of the masticatory system have an interlocking relationship with masticatory function. This is where the patient comes into the problem: *he is the source and determination of function.* He cannot avoid sharing responsibility for the effectiveness of therapy, and he must know this.

CAUSE-RELATED THERAPY

The first step in definitive treatment is to eliminate or neutralize the cause of the condition. This may apply to predisposing factors, activating factors, and prepetuating influences.

Predisposing Factors

Chronic occlusal disharmony may be a predisposing factor in many temporomandibular disorders. Slight disharmony may initiate sensory and proprioceptive input that is answered by acute muscle disorders. More severe disharmony that causes gross displacement of the disc-condyle complex during maximum intercuspation predisposes to interference disorders of the joint. Such changes may involve the osseous-supported articular surfaces, the articular discs, the structures of the disc-condyle complex (especially the discal ligaments), the temporomandibular ligament, and the retrodiscal tissue. Elimination of such chronic occlusal disharmony is mandatory. The timing of correction, however, may vary, depending on the type of disorder present and whether a component of acute malocclusion is to be taken into account.

Skeletal and craniofacial disharmony as well as former trauma to the facial structures are important factors that influence functioning of the masticatory apparatus, particularly the disc-condyle complex. The elimination of such causes is not a practical consideration. Rather, it should be an objective of therapy to minimize, if not eliminate entirely, the effects of such factors.

Very important predisposing factors are abnormal or excessive functional demands, such as habitual excessive use of chewing force, abusive mannerisms, using the teeth and jaws for nonmasticatory purposes, and bruxism. Usually, habit training can be successfully employed to minimize such conditions, including bruxism, which no doubt is the most difficult of all to manage. Daytime bruxism may be controlled by habit training to voluntarily leave the teeth separated or ajar. The use of reminders, such as a small piece of chewing gum patted along the occlusal surfaces of the molar teeth, may be helpful. Nighttime bruxism may be reduced by sleeping flat on the back without a pillow, by autosuggestion that "I will not clench my teeth while asleep!," or by positive posthypnotic suggestion. A night-guard device that separates the teeth helps to control the condition.

Activating Factors

The most important activating cause of temporomandibular disorders is emotional tension. It is thought to be a major cause of bruxism, of excessive passive interarticular pressure, and of many acute muscle disorders. Tension control programs may include (1) medicinal therapy in the form of tranquilizers and muscle relaxants; (2) psychological care in the form of counseling, autosuggestion, hypnotherapy, or psychotherapy; (3) biofeedback techniques; and (4) genuine understanding and empathy by which the burden of being human is made more tolerable.

An important activator of acute muscle spasm is the continuous input of deep-pain impulses that initiate central excitatory effects. To eliminate this important and frequent cause requires the skillful identification and eradication of the primary pain source—which may not be related to the masticatory system, or even to dentistry. Very careful differential diagnosis of orofacial pain syndromes is prerequisite to success.[2]

Perpetuating Influences

Constitutional factors may have a real influence on the continuation of symptoms. Such conditions as diabetes, rheumatoid arthritis, hyperuricemia, and other systemic illness should be explored on a medical level by the patient's physician. Emotional influences may also bear importantly on the outcome of therapy, and there are occasions when some professional aid should be obtained. Coexisting symptoms of almost any type should alert the dentist to the need for determining whether they may be related to the patient's masticatory disorder.

SPECIFIC THERAPY

Structural changes in the musculature and joints do not go away simply because etiologic factors are eliminated. Natural resolution may occur, is always desirable, and should be taken into consideration in treatment planning.[11, 12] Indeed, the temporomandibular joints are constructed favorably for this. As a rule, however, special measures are required for damaged parts to be brought within the limit of tolerability for the patient. Absolute return to normal may not be accomplished. The patient should understand this.

In addition to palliative therapy and measures to eliminate cause, appropriate treatment guidelines for the various disorders identified and classified in chapter 7 will be listed. It should be recognized that the individual case may not respond to all the principles proposed. It requires the special attention of the therapist to adapt the principles outlined to meet the circumstances of a particular problem.

If a particular complaint represents more than a single temporomandibular disorder (and many of them do), it is necessary to modify and combine suggestions in the various guidelines to meet the requirements of the case. Also to be considered are transitional phases in masticatory conditions, which require clinical judgment for the selection of the most appropriate course of therapeutic action.

Serious workers in this field should be well informed on all philosophies of management, all concepts of function and dysfunction, and all modalities of treatment, for something is to be learned from each, with perhaps something to be utilized. It should be obvious that the more rational the therapy, the more effective it likely will be. Rational therapy reflects an understanding of basics: functional anatomy, critical standards for judging abnormality, dependable criteria for evaluating symptoms, and techniques for establishing a confirmed diagnosis. Fortunately, the dental literature now has a wealth of source material which can be drawn upon to supply this important information.

Many temporomandibular disorders are related etiologically to occlusal disharmony. Many are not. Occlusal disharmony may be a predisposing factor that requires activation by other factors before it becomes a decisive cause. The mere identification of disharmony in the dentition is no assurance that such abnormality is etiologic. It may be irrelevant: It may be symptomatic. Before definitive treatment of the dentition is undertaken, care should be exercised to determine whether malocclusion is acute (symptomatic) or chronic (preexistent and possibly etiologic), or both. *The safe guideline is to postpone all definitive measures, such as equilibration, alteration, restoration, or reconstruction, until normalization of the muscles and, if possible, the joints.* In the meantime, if correction of the occlusion is needed, it is better to use temporary reversible measures, such as occlusal splinting. When the component of acute malocclusion has been eliminated, it is possible to determine with greater accuracy what needs to be done on a definitive level.

If the dentition is at fault, it has its chief effect during power strokes and/or maximum intercuspation, which may be either functional for masticatory purposes or parafunctional due to bruxism. Muscle action is influenced by the dentition from the beginning of a power stroke until intercuspation is achieved and released. The joint proper is influenced by changes in interarticular pressure induced by power strokes and maximum intercuspation. Finally, the decisive effect of tooth form and position on the joints and musculature is greatest during maximum intercuspation—clenching the teeth in closed position. It is important that discrepancies be identified and taken into account therapeutically. *In these guidelines only temporary occlusal splinting will be suggested when occlusal therapy is indicated. The manner of definitive occlusal therapy will be left to the judgment of the dentist.*

Masticatory Muscle Splinting

In addition to the elimination of cause, the proper treatment for muscle splinting is restriction of use and institution of muscle-relaxant therapy. Chewing should be minimized, for that is what muscle splinting is trying to say: "Stop using me!" Exercises and physiotherapy are contraindicated. All forms of active therapy for protective muscle splinting may accentuate the condition rather than relieve it. Abusive use, injudicious therapy, or extended duration may induce myospastic activity in the splinted muscle.

Masticatory Muscle Spasm

If etiologic factors have been eliminated (or no longer exist), the following principles should resolve a masticatory muscle spasm quickly:

1. *Voluntary restriction of all jaw use within painless limits.* Whatever hurts, don't do! Since it is the pain of use (contracting or stretching the spastic muscle) that has so much to do with perpetuating the spasm, this is an essential first step toward resolving it. This requires understanding and complete cooperation on the part of the patient. Restriction of jaw use must be voluntary; it cannot be imposed by such measures as ligation of the teeth, because that does not prevent contraction of elevator muscles or stretching of lateral pterygoids.

2. *The muscles should be used to the maximum painless limit.* This may seem paradoxical and conflictory, but it is not. Normal use and painless stretching stimulate muscle spindles and Golgi tendon organs, thus reducing activity in the muscle.[13] The continuance of normal painless use is essential to normalization of the muscle. The trick is to properly combine these two principles, both of which are voluntary and require good insight and complete cooperation on the part of the patient. The muscles should not be exercised so much as be put to normal, but painless, use. As the pain disappears, the amount of use should be increased gradually until full normal functioning is reestablished. This occurs as spastic activity disappears.

3. *Muscle relaxation should be induced.* An excellent result can be obtained by occlusal disengagement. Disengagement means that the tooth surfaces should not be brought into full occlusion. This is to reduce sensory input initiated by the teeth, whether there is occlusal disharmony or not, because it is this input that has much to do with initiating splinting and spastic activity in the first place. It also temporarily arrests all conflicts between the dentition and musculature, whether chronic or acute. Again, it is necessary to have the full cooperation of the patient. This usually can be accomplished voluntarily by simply leaving the teeth apart or ajar. At least, this is true during the waking hours.

If bruxing takes place during the sleeping hours, additional help likely will be needed. Such support is available in the form of nighttime muscle-relaxant therapy. This is done best by starting at bedtime with a small dose of commonly used relaxant (such as diazepam, 2½ mg) and then estimating its effect the following morning. None is used in the daytime. Then, each night add to the dose until enough effect is obtained that the patient still is able to arouse himself and attend to his duties, *but does so reluctantly.* This should be his maximum dose without interfering with daytime activities also. If such measures fail to eliminate nighttime bruxism, an interocclusal appliance should be used.

(a) *Disengaging occlusal splints:* It is well established that occlusal splinting decreases the EMG activity in contracted elevator muscles.[14-17] Many different types of interocclusal devices have been advocated for this purpose, but all seem to yield about the same benefit as long as they are acceptable to the patient. Sometimes, they aggravate the problem.[17] This is presumed to be due either to increasing the patient's emotional tension by the unacceptability of the appliance or to violation of the patient's interocclusal clearance. It is not yet fully understood how splinting accomplishes its relaxing effects.[18]

Thompson[19] introduced occlusal splinting in 1951. The Thompson-type splint, modified to give it full coverage (see Appendix for the technique of construction), may be utilized for occlusal disengagement or for the temporary correction of occlusal disharmony that relates to overloading. It can also serve as the basic foundation for a mandibular repositioning device. Easy to make and to modify, it is exceptionally versatile and effective—yet quite inexpensive. Other more elaborately designed and constructed types of interocclusal devices may be used. Some add a deprogramming anterior jig which aids in muscle therapy.[20] Other devices in common use include Lucia jigs, anterior bite plates, soft or resilient night guards, Shore mandibular autorepositioning appliances, mandibular orthopedic repositioning appliances (MORAs), and other splinting devices with and without pulsing with the Jankelson Myo-Monitor.[21]

Carraro and Caffesse[22] found that full arch stabilized splints gave total relief of muscle pain in 59% and substantial improvement in another 26% of their reported patient group. Clark[23] reported that, when used in conjunction with occlusal adjustment and prosthetic care, interocclusal appliance therapy was 70% to 90% effective. Clark[24] found that such therapy was more effective for muscle pain than for other masticatory symptoms. Lerman[25, 26] reported the successful use of a hydrostatic interocclusal appliance in the treatment of refractory muscle pain-dysfunction symptoms.

If a full coverage Thompson-type splint is used, as muscle normalization occurs and the acute malocclusion disappears, the device will need to be adjusted by grinding off the occlusal matrix and replacing it in the new occlusal relationship. A disengaging splint should be checked for correctness every 2 to 3 days and altered as needed. When the muscles normalize, it will be noted that further occlusal change ceases.

(b) *Other relaxation techniques:* Some patients can accomplish satisfactory relaxation of contracted elevator muscles by a variety of relaxation techniques[27] with and without the benefit of biofeedback training.[28, 29] Massed practice therapy for bruxism[30] has been recommended. This consists of a series of six periods of sustained clenching for 1 minute alternated with 1 minute of relaxation repeated 6 times daily for 2 weeks. Schwartz[31] proposed the use of exercises that reflexly induce relaxation of muscles. This was based on the principle of reciprocal inhibition: As a muscle is actively contracted, its antagonists are reflexly relaxed. Therefore, exercises that consist of opening the mouth against resistance in alternating rhythmic movements tend to relax contracted elevator muscles. Rocabado[32] advocated "joint distraction" with an appliance that incorporated a clothespin-like spring that separated the teeth posteriorly. The resultant stimulation of proprioceptors in the joint ligaments exerted inhibitory influence on the elevator muscles. Ultrasonic therapy has been reported to be helpful in recalcitrant muscle complaints.[33–35] The usefulness of "spray and stretch" therapy as advocated by Travell and Simons[36] is well established. Greene and Laskin[37] reported a 58% improvement with meprobamate therapy as against a 31% improvement with placebo. They noted, however, that such improvement appeared to be more subjective than objective. Active psychotherapy has been reported to be helpful, especially in recalcitrant muscle disorders.[38–40.]

It should be particularly interesting to note that a large group of patients with myogenous masticatory pain were treated randomly by (1) physiotherapy, (2) occlusal splinting, (3) biofeedback assisted relaxation, and (4) relaxation training without biofeedback assistance.[3] The results obtained by the four methods were not significantly different. The conclusion that should be drawn, therefore, is that patients are benefitted by any method that accomplishes relaxation of the muscles, and no one method is superior. The therapeutic option that is selected should be individualized, depending on the particular patient, the duration of the complaint, the type of symptoms displayed, the circumstances that prevail, and particularly on the results of prior therapy, if any.

4. *Interrupt the cycling myospastic activity by analgesic blocking.* The offending muscle(s) should be infiltrated with plain aqueous procaine according to the technique suggested in chapter 9, unless there is some specific contraindication. During the period of anesthesia, pain input is shut off, and the muscle can be *massaged gently and manipulated* by stretching and contracting against resistance. This has an excellent normalizing effect without causing pain which would otherwise attend such therapy. The duration of benefit from this treatment should be compared with the known time of anesthesia. If the benefit is of considerably longer duration than the time of anesthesia, then it should be repeated after 5 to 7 days. If no benefit occurs, repetition is not indi-

cated. If such therapy noticeably increases the symptoms (pain and dysfunction), it may be assumed that inflammatory changes are under way. The diagnosis should then be changed to *myositis,* and the treatment altered accordingly.

When analgesic blocking cannot be done due to specific contraindication or refusal on the patient's part, an alternative method may be substituted. This consists of the use of a vapocoolant, such as Fluori-Methane Spray (Gebauer Chemical Company, Cleveland, Ohio), combined with massage and manipulation.[36] While the offending muscle is under moderate stretch, the overlying skin is streaked with the vapocoolant, holding the nozzle about 12 to 14 inches away. This is repeated several times at intervals of a minute or so. Then, while the pain of spasm is obtunded by the intermittent stimulation of the cutaneous receptors, the muscle is massaged gently and manipulated by stretching and contracting against resistance. This kind of therapy may be repeated as the benefit justifies. It should be understood that the value of vapocoolant therapy is not that of topical anesthesia, and the surface skin should not be frosted.

5. *Postpone definitive therapy until spastic activity is eliminated.* Permanent correction of the occlusion and definitive measures directed toward the muscles or joints should be withheld until the pain and dysfunction symptoms caused by muscle spasm activity have been relieved.

A correctly diagnosed and treated masticatory muscle spasm should resolve quickly and completely in a few days because nothing irreversible is wrong with the muscle. As soon as the CNS impulses that cause the contraction are shut off, the muscle relaxes and the symptoms disappear.

If Class III disc-interference symptoms are part of the complaint and are initiated by increased passive interarticular pressure due to continued contraction of elevator muscles, such interference also will disappear as the spastic activity is relieved. If there is persistent interference after the spasm is resolved, it likely *(a)* is preexistent, *(b)* represents the activation of an otherwise dormant, nonsymptomatic interference disorder of the joint, or *(c)* represents damage to the joint as a result of the muscle spasm. *Interference that persists after resolution of the muscle spasm requires a revision of the diagnosis and therapy planned accordingly.*

If the spasm resolves with proper therapy and then promptly recurs when therapy ceases, it should be evident that the etiologic factors responsible for it are still active. This indicates that the diagnosis is incomplete or inaccurate in that it does not properly identify the cause. Two likely possibilities should be investigated: *(a)* continued input of sensory and/or proprioceptive impulses from the dentition, muscles, or joints due to functional disharmony, and *(b)* continued input of deep-pain impulses somewhere in the head and neck that is inducing secondary central excitatory effects. Until such cause is located and eliminated, continued therapy for the myospasm will produce only temporary results.

If the spasm fails to respond quickly, there is something wrong with the diagnosis or treatment, or both. It may be that myositis, rather than myospasm, is present. It may be that the condition is really an inflammatory disorder of the joint, and the muscle symptoms are only central excitatory effects. It may be that the treatment has not shut off the central impulses that provoke the spasm. It may be that injudicious treatment is perpetuating the spasm.

The crux of the matter is that if a masticatory myospasm cannot be resolved completely and without relapse within a few days, something is wrong with the diagnosis or the treatment, and further efforts are needed to determine what is wrong. All continued therapy should be palliative until the cause for failure has been identified and corrected.

Masticatory Muscle Inflammation

When a masticatory muscle becomes inflamed, a different regimen of therapy is needed. What quickly normalizes a myospasm may aggravate myositis. The principles of therapy for masticatory myositis, in addition to the elimination of cause, include the following:

1. Jaw use should be restricted until pain and acute inflammatory symptoms subside. Exercises, stretching the muscle, and injections of the muscle with a local anesthetic are *contraindicated.*

2. Antibiotic therapy and other medical and surgical supportive care are indicated if infection is the chief cause of the inflammation.

3. Nonsteroid anti-inflammatory medications may help resolve the inflammation. These should be employed with medical consent or supervision, especially when used for an extended period of time.

4. The judicious use of deep-heat therapy, such as diathermy or ultrasound, is usually beneficial. *Judicious use* means that such therapy should be initiated cautiously, utilizing a minimal dose at first and waiting to judge the benefit, if any. If such therapy produces negative re-

sults, further application should be delayed. If there is improvement, however, the treatment may become more aggressive as the symptoms subside.

5. As pain and the acute inflammatory symptoms subside, exercises should be instituted, care being taken to *keep them below a painful level.* If such therapy seems to aggravate the condition, it should be minimized or postponed for a while. Such exercises should gradually be increased in frequency and vigor as resolution takes place. Eventually, this should become the dominant feature of therapy.

6. Toward the end of resolution, two considerations warrant attention: *(a)* frequent *momentary* stretching of the muscle should be done to reverse myostatic contracture that may have occurred during the extended time when the muscle was immobilized by inflammation, and *(b)* added isometric exercises consisting of muscle contraction against resistance should be done to rebuild the strength of the muscle lost through atrophic change that results from disuse.

All exercise therapy should be employed with judgment, taking care that it is not excessive or injurious to the healing muscle. *Muscle fatigue must be avoided.* Injudicious physiotherapy may perpetuate and worsen the condition. Perhaps the most important feature of treating myositis is a good understanding on the part of the patient concerning its cause, expected behavior, and treatment problems that exist. No shortcuts are available. *Overzealous therapy may be harmful.* Resolution follows an inflammatory curve. Patience is required because the process may be slow—weeks and months, compared with days for myospasm. The muscular dysfunction usually outlasts the pain.

The most serious residual problem after resolution of the inflammation is muscular contracture. If it is myostatic, it usually can be reversed. Myofibrotic contracture, however, may be lasting.

Class I Disc-Interference Disorders

Careful diagnosis is required to classify properly the interference that occurs during jaw movements—the chief symptom of such disorders of the joint. *Etiology should be identified and eliminated if possible.*

Interference disorders may occur as painless, dormant, nonsymptomatic conditions of which the patient may be quite unaware. Many times such conditions are noticed by the dentist first. They may represent various types of discrete complaints, with and without an element of pain. They suddenly may become activated or seriously aggravated by trauma, emotional stress, or spastic activity in elevator masticatory muscles. They may complicate other joint complaints, such as acute muscle disorders and inflammatory joint conditions. They may develop into inflammatory degenerative arthritis.

After acute muscle conditions, interference disorders of the joint are the most frequent temporomandibular complaint. Interference during jaw movements includes (1) *abnormal sensations,* such as a feeling of rubbing, binding, or catching, (2) *abnormal sounds,* such as clicking, popping, snapping, or grating noise, (3) *abnormal movements,* such as rough, irregular, slipping, catching, or jumping movements, or deviations of the incisal path, and (4) *pain* that relates in timing to the other symptoms of interference. The ultimate in interference is locking of the joint due to obstruction of the disc or to blockage by an anteriorly dislocated disc.

Class I interference disorders cause symptoms in the closed-joint relationship. They occur with clenching the teeth firmly from the unclenched closed-joint position. The primary etiologic factor is occlusal disharmony that induces or permits movement of the disc-condyle complex during maximum intercuspation. Bruxism and habitual excessively hard biting are activating factors. The symptoms can be prevented temporarily by biting against a separator between the teeth.

Treatment for this disorder is correction of the occlusion. This should be done temporarily by using an occlusal splint. When it has been properly confirmed that such correction does eliminate the symptoms, definitive correction of the occlusion is needed.

Class I disc-interference disorders occur with a high degree of frequency and represent the earliest pathologic change in joint conditions that can be identified clinically. It is at this stage that interceptive therapy on a dental level can be so important to the patient. This condition is due to occlusal disharmony and is correctable by occlusal therapy. But, the type of disharmony and the type of correction must be understood. Interference during jaw movements[41] may contribute to the problem in the form of muscle effects, but neither such interference, nor its elimination, is the real issue in Class I disorders. This condition is due to condylar displacement when the teeth are clenched, and only the elimination of the disharmony that causes such displacement is corrective. Williamson and Lundquist[42] reported that activity in the temporal and masseter muscles was reduced when posterior disclusion is obtained by an appropriate anterior guidance. This beneficial effect on the musculature is helpful, but it does not arrest the displacement of the condyle, which may exhaust the weeping lubrication.[43] Nonrigid concepts of occlusal function are needed to cope with such conditions.[44-46] Weinberg[47] has proposed that prosthetic therapy for anterior displacement of the condyle should consist of the removal of centric relation deflective contacts while that for posterior condylar displacement needs an overlay to alter the vertical dimension of occlusion and reposition the mandible. Ordinarily, an occlusion-correcting splint offers quite satisfactory temporary therapy in either case.

The definitive occlusal therapy should be such as to arrest the condylar movement that occurs after full contact of the teeth and during clenching efforts. The correction of other occlusal interference may be helpful, but will not be decisive therapeutically.

Class II Disc-Interference Disorders

The symptoms of Class II disc interference occur following maximum intercuspation of the teeth, just as the translatory cycle begins. They also may occur with the first movement after a period of jaw inactivity. (Some modified repeat of symptoms may occur if a power stroke ends in maximum intercuspation.) The symptoms are timed to the first few millimeters of opening. The primary etiologic factor is occlusal disharmony. Trauma sustained while the teeth are occluded, bruxism, and habitual excessive biting force are other etiologic factors. The symptoms are averted by an occlusal stop that prevents return of the disc-condyle complex to the closed position.

In addition to the elimination of etiologic factors, treatment consists of preventing the disc-condyle complex from returning to the closed position for a period long enough for natural resolution to repair the damaged surfaces that cause sticking of the articular disc after maximum intercuspation. This is done best by an occlusal splint. Usually, it is necessary only to increase the vertical dimension a few millimeters. Occasionally, however, slight protrusion is required to keep vertical dimension within tolerable limits. A properly constructed splint will prevent the symptoms, yet establish a secure, comfortable, stable occlusal matrix that is satisfactory for chewing purposes. *It must be used 24 hours a day for an extended period.* When the patient has been symptom-free for 3 to 4 months, it is well to start adjusting the splint at about 30-day intervals for the purpose of reducing its artificial influence on the patient's occlusion, but without relapse of the complaint. To do this, grind down the occlusal matrix portion of the splint until the symptoms return. Then, add a thin layer of rapid-curing acrylic *sufficient to arrest the symptoms* and create a new occlusal matrix. This step-by-step procedure should continue monthly as long as progress is made in reducing the thickness of the occlusal stop or until the splint is eliminated entirely, which is the ideal objective of therapy. If after several months a plateau of improvement is reached and no further reduction in thickness of the splint can be made without return of the symptoms, permanent alteration of the occlusion in the splinted relationship is indicated. This can be done by permanent splinting (metallic), occlusal onlays, occlusal reconstruction, or orthodontic treatment. One method that warrants consideration is to make a metallic splint and use it long enough to test for correctness. Then, cut off a posterior segment on one side to permit drifting together of two molar teeth. When these come into occlusion and are equilibrated for good contact, cut off a similar segment on the other side and follow the same procedure. This step-by-step removal of the splint should continue until a new occlusal relationship is established in the splinted closed position, and the splint is eliminated completely. Whatever method is used for permanent alteration of the occluded relationship of the teeth should duplicate the splinted position.

The types of occlusal disharmony that can induce Class II disc interference should be understood, identified, and eliminated. This condition can result from frictional movement due to condylar displacement as a progression from a Class I interference disorder. When this is the case, the same type of occlusal correction is required. More frequently, however, this disorder results from static overloading due to a slight, but identifiable, lack of adequate occlusal contact between the opposing ipsilateral molar teeth. This is associated especially with dental restorations and with partial dentures that replace missing teeth by means of a posterior extension saddle. If bruxism is a contributing factor, it should be controlled. Careful habit training should be instituted to eliminate abusive movements, mannerisms, and excessively hard chewing forces.

Class III Disc-Interference Disorders

The symptoms of Class III disc interference occur during the course of normal translatory cycles. (This interference does not include symptoms that occur as a result of excessive opening of the mouth or strained movements.) Three basic etiologic situations account for disorders of this type, namely, excessive passive interarticular pressure, structural incompatibility of the sliding surfaces of the joint, and impairment of disc-condyle complex function. Guidelines for the treatment of each of these groups will be considered.

Symptoms Due to Excessive Passive Pressure. The best indication that the Class III symptoms are activated by excessive passive interarticular pressure is the timing of the complaint: Sudden onset, variability, episodial behavior, and recurrence. If the symptoms follow increased emotional tension, measures to reduce such tension should be instituted. This may be by way of counseling, medicinal therapy by the patient's physician, or by psychotherapy. If the symptoms follow spastic activity in elevator muscles, the therapy for myospasm should resolve the disc-interference symptoms also. Otherwise, relaxation therapy for the elevator muscles as previously discussed should be instituted.

During such periods of interference, the patient should voluntarily reduce the speed and force of jaw movements and modify his diet to minimize the interference and prevent more serious damage to the joint. A disengaging occlusal splint is usually quite effective. Biofeedback training and relaxation techniques as well as muscle relaxant therapy may be indicated, especially if the symptoms persist.

Symptoms Due to Structural Incompatibility. The best indication that the Class III interference symptoms are due to structural defects in the sliding surfaces is the pattern of sameness: The symptoms occur each time the same jaw movement is executed, and they persist and change very slowly. Although the severity and character of the symptoms may be altered by variation in the speed of movement, the timing is not. If the symptoms are reciprocal, the timing of the closing symptoms does not vary with alterations in power stroking, and the reciprocal symptoms maintain a similar relationship to the translatory cycle. A deviated opening pattern, if any, is wholly unconscious. It may also be noted that the patient usually chews habitually on the symptomatic side.

For treatment of Class III symptoms from this cause:

1. Jaw use should be modified by habit training. This should include *(a)* the elimination of abusive habits, mannerisms, and nonessential jaw use, *(b)* more deliberate, slower, and less forceful chewing strokes, and *(c)* chewing mainly on the symptomatic side.

2. Habit training should be used to find and develop a purposely deviated path of opening-closing that averts the interference. This is a very useful form of therapy, if properly done. One way is to have the patient slowly open until he begins to *feel* the interference, then stop and move laterally one way and then the other until he can "feel" his

way around the interference. If some such deviated path can be found, then have the patient watch himself make these movements in a mirror until he understands what he is doing. Instruct the patient to practice these deviated opening-closing paths for 15 to 20 minutes several times each day, using the mirror as needed. As time goes on and habit patterns slowly are built up to guide the muscles, the movements should become faster, until he develops enough speed to make chewing efforts with these newly acquired compensatory jaw movements practical. With the interference thus eliminated or minimized, natural resolution at the site of obstruction may reduce further the structural incompatibility that causes it.

3. If the condition becomes intolerable and definitive therapy is required, surgical intervention may be necessary. The most promising operation is an eminectomy. It not only eliminates the structural interference but also reduces the required amount of rotatory movement in the disc-condyle complex during translatory cycles by decreasing the inclination of the articular eminence.

Symptoms Due to Disc-Condyle Complex Damage.   The best indications that the Class III interference symptoms stem from structural impairment of the disc-condyle complex are: (1) more or less continuous interference throughout translatory cycles, punctuated by catching, clicking, or locking, (2) variation in the timing of symptoms according to the demands of function, (3) sensations of overstressed ipsilateral posterior teeth when clenched, and (4) accentuation of symptoms by chewing on the symptomatic side.

Conservative therapeutic efforts for Class III disorders due to impaired disc-condyle complex functioning may not be rewarding. Many times the best that can be done, short of surgical intervention, is to minimize abusive use in order to retard or arrest progressive deterioration and help the patient accept and tolerate an undesirable situation. The patient should be given full insight into the problem and its cause so that he can understand the symptoms better and do his part to help retard progress toward degenerative arthritis. Habit training to make chewing less stressful should be encouraged. This means softer foods, smaller bites, slower and less vigorous chewing movements. It is necessary to eliminate as much as possible all abusive joint use, minimize functional demands, and learn to sense and avoid discrete instances of disc obstruction. Palliative treatment to control pain and careful elimination of etiologic factors, *especially chronic occlusal disharmony,* are definitely indicated. Rational definitive therapy depends chiefly on the accuracy of diagnosis.

Disc-condyle adhesions. Fibrous adhesions may unite the disc with the articular surface of the condyle in such a manner as to eliminate normal rotatory movement in the lower joint. Thus, as the condyle translates, the disc-condyle complex must skid bodily along the articular eminence instead of gliding smoothly. This causes irregular, noisy movements and predisposes to degenerative joint disease. There is no nonsurgical treatment for this condition. If the symptoms become intolerable, definitive therapy requires surgical intervention.

Damaged articular disc. Abusive overloading and frictional movement are not modified by cellular remodeling in the articular disc. Such abuse causes deterioration of the disc that is evidenced by a grating sound that may be punctuated by a catching sensation or clicking noise at a point of greater interference. This is usually accompanied by degenerative change in the condylar and eminence articular surfaces— degenerative joint disease. Fracture of the disc causes a sensation of overstressed ipsilateral posterior teeth when clenched, if the fragments are separated. There is no nonsurgical therapy for a damaged articular disc. Nor is there any regenerative capability. If the symptoms become intolerable, definitive treatment requires surgical intervention.

Displaced articular disc. When the damage to the disc-condyle complex consists of loss of contour and elongation of the discal collateral ligaments, linear sliding movement can take place between disc and condyle. This is termed *disc displacement.* The displaced (and usually torqued) disc may obstruct condylar translation, and symptoms of interference result.

The *direction of displacement* depends on the location of the lost contour: Lost contour posteriorly permits anterior displacement; lost contour anteriorly permits posterior displacement. The *extent of displacement* depends on the extent of lost contour and the elongation of collateral discal ligaments. The degree of displacement alters the clinical symptoms: *Minor displacement* causes early symptoms that are discrete, painful, and sometimes accompanied by muscle effects; *moderate displacement* causes later symptoms that are less discrete, less painful, and without muscle effects; *severe displacement* may permit dislocation of the disc with collapse of the disc space, entrapment, and no discrete symptoms at all.

Such Class III symptoms may occur suddenly as the direct result of external trauma, or they may occur insidiously as a progression from Class I and Class II disc-interference disorders. *This constitutes the noninflammatory phase of degenerative joint disease and predisposes to inflammatory degenerative arthritis.*

Insidious disc displacement due to occlusal disharmony should display clinical evidence of that disharmony: An anteriorly displaced disc should display evidence of posterior condylar displacement when clenched; a posteriorly displaced disc should display anterior condylar displacement when clenched. *It is mandatory in the treatment of such displacements to identify and correct the etiologic occlusal disharmony in order to arrest further damage to the disc-condyle complex.* It goes without saying, however, that such occlusal correction does not arrest the symptoms, because the damage to the complex is already done.

Anterior displacement of the disc.   Anteriorly displaced articular discs have been successfully managed by surgery since 1887.[48] Pringle[49] in 1918 reported excision of the disc for such conditions. Through the years, anterior displacements have been identified surgically[50-55] with excision of the disc being the usual treatment. In 1951 Ireland[56] recommended condylectomy for the condition. The recent renewed interest in disc-interference disorders has been led by Farrar[57, 58] and McCarty and Farrar.[59]

It is necessary to distinguish the Class III reciprocal symptoms that result from discal displacements from those caused by structural incompatibility as previously discussed, because the treatment is not the same. Since disc displacements are due to muscle action anteriorly and retrodiscal elasticity posteriorly, rather than from structural incompatibility, the closing symptoms can be varied by alterations in power stroking. Since deviation of jaw movement can minimize the symptoms, the patient is aware of a deviated incisal path if one is present. And patients with this disorder usually avoid chewing on the symptomatic side.

Since the manner of use has much to do with the patient's complaint, the closing symptoms can be minimized by slower chewing movements, smaller bites, softer foods, and biting on the nonsymptomatic side. Such habit training is important therapeutically, regardless of what else is done.

Although surgery has been the predominant treatment through the years, Farrar pioneered the management of disc displacements by nonsurgical therapy. This consisted of mandibular repositioning that moved the condyle into the displaced disc so that translation could begin from a more normal disc-condyle relationship and therefore reduce the chance of obstructing the opening movement. Such management is a practical solution to the problem, as long as it can be done without excessive forward movement of the mandible. If it is retained forward for several months, there appears to be sufficient resolution and new muscle patterning to permit some stepping back of the condyle to a more natural position. At some point, however, the occlusion needs to be stabilized and reconstructed at the position required to arrest the opening symptoms. This can be accomplished by whatever means are feasible in the individual case. The closing symptoms are controlled chiefly by habit training.

An undocumented auxiliary aid that holds promise of benefit in these cases is reinforcement of the lateral capsular wall by artificially induced fibrosis. The strengthening of this tissue should do much to stabilize the disc and therefore improve the nonsurgical treatment of anterior disc displacements. It also should permit an occlusal position that is more favorable. Chemical agents that stimulate the proliferation of fibrous tissue were used in the treatment of joint hypermobility many years ago.[60] Through the years such agents have been used in the treatment of superficial hemangiomas and venous varicosities. Lately, radiofrequency coagulation has been used in the retrodiscal area.[61] It may be found useful to promote fibrous tissue in the capsular wall also.

Of the nonsurgical regimens, different splinting devices have been offered.[62–66] Also, alternative methods of repositioning the mandible have been suggested.[67, 68] In evaluation reports, pain appears to be controlled better than disc noise.[69, 70] Manzione et al.[71] reported that about half the patients who had been treated by clinically satisfactory mandibular repositioning splints still had an anteriorly displaced disc when examined by lower joint arthrography. Further long-term studies are needed to properly evaluate the effectiveness of nonsurgical management.

Anteriorly displaced discs that require a forward positioning of the mandible much in excess of 3 mm and functionally dislocated discs are two clinical indications for surgical intervention if the symptoms become intolerable and a more definitive type of treatment is needed. The surgical management of Class III disc-interference symptoms calls for either excision or plication of the disc. Excision of the disc eliminates the symptoms of pain and noise. Having been used for many years, its record is quite good subjectively—except for difficulties involving the occlusion.[72] The objective results, however, are not that satisfactory. Eriksson and Westesson[73] reported on a long-term evaluation (mean follow-up 29 years) in which it was found that all such joints operated on displayed radiographic evidence of degenerative joint disease. Fibrous adhesions appeared not to be too much of a problem, however.

Plication of the disc to reposition and hold it on the condyle has a much shorter historic record. The operation as currently done usually entails the excision of a portion of the retrodiscal tissue,[59, 72] presumably on the theory that the superior retrodiscal lamina "holds the disc on the condyle." Actually, it is the *inferior* lamina that serves that particular function. Normal elasticity of the superior lamina is required for free forward translation of the disc-condyle complex. The highly vascularized retrodiscal tissue comprises an extremely important source of synovial fluid to the joint. It therefore is essential to the normal nutrition and metabolism of the nonvascularized parts of the joint as well as to the lubrication of the moving articular surfaces. Being vascularized, it is the chief source of surgical hemarthrosis, which constitutes a serious hazard to lower joint surgery due to the possible formation of adhesions between the disc and condyle. The unique structure and function of the retrodiscal tissue in the TM joint raises the question of the wisdom of subjecting it to surgical trauma, unless it has already been metaplastically converted into nonvascularized fibrous tissue as a result of abusive condylar encroachment. In spite of the possible complications that such surgery entails, the short-term control of joint pain and noise has been quite good.

The plication operation is sometimes augmented by shaping the disc, smoothing the condyle, and excising the articular eminence. Other operations have been used, such as meniscoplasty and eminectomy without entering the lower joint,[74] plication of both superior and inferior retrodiscal laminae,[75] and plastic repair of perforations of the articular disc.[76]

Early reports on disc plication were euphoric, with success rates ranging as high as 94%.[59] The American Association of Oral and Maxillofacial Surgeons lists the short-term failure rate at 10% to 20%.[77] An evaluation of over 1,000 TM patients, of whom 2.7% required surgery, reported that 41% of the patients who were operated on did not consider the benefit worth the surgery.[78] An evaluation of 132 joints operated on (including both excision and plication) reported that 80% of the patients were better and would repeat the operation if needed, while 20% considered their disorder to be worse as a result of the surgery.[79] Long-term evaluations of disc plication surgery have not yet been reported.

The conclusion that should be drawn regarding surgical management of disc-interference disorders is that surgery is beneficial in carefully selected cases, but it should not be considered an option simply because less than satisfactory results accrue to nonsurgical management. In spite of the early successful control of pain and disc noise, surgical intervention is not without possible long-term complications and hazards. Excision of the disc converts the compound TM joint into a simple one that fundamentally changes its functional capabilities and eliminates the important stabilizing mechanism—thus predisposing the joint to degenerative arthritis. Plication of the disc compromises the vital retrodiscal tissue, jeopardizes both the nutritive and lubricative functions of the joint, and risks the formation of adhesions between the disc and condyle. Both types of surgery may invite serious difficulties with the occlusion, and both entail the hazard of painful traumatic neuroma formation in the capsular scar tissue. Adequate provision for all such postsurgical sequelae should be included in the treatment plan, and the informed consent for surgery should clearly identify them.

In spite of the possible complications and hazards, there are specific indications for joint surgery in the management of anterior disc displacements and dislocations. The indications for such surgery have been established by the American Association of Oral and Maxillofacial Surgeons, as follows:[77]

1. Accurate diagnosis should document the disorder as a bona fide articular disc derangement.

2. The disorder should constitute a physical disability.

3. The patient should be involved in the decision to operate after full disclosure.

Westesson[80] has suggested the following criteria for surgical intervention in the management of derangements of the temporomandibular joint:

1. All forms of nonsurgical therapy should be attempted before surgery is advised.

2. Arthrograms should document pathologic changes in the joint.

3. The patient should have pain or considerable dysfunction.

4. The pain should emanate from the joint proper.

The decision to advise surgery should be based on the *intolerability of the patient's complaint*. Surgery should not be expected to make a good joint out of a bad one but, rather, to make a tolerable situation out of an otherwise intolerable one.

Posterior displacement of the disc. Posterior displacement of the articular disc occurs as the result of elastic traction of the superior retrodiscal lamina during forward translatory movement, when such displacement is made possible by the loss of disc contour anteriorly and elongation of the discal collateral ligaments. Since the disc-condyle relationship remains normal in the closed-joint position, early symptoms due to obstruction of the condyle against a displaced disc do not occur. There may be no early opening symptoms at all unless preceded by firm maximum intercuspation that causes the disc to stick against the articular fossa. Symptoms may occur reciprocally, being very slight usually in the late opening phase and more marked during the closing phase, depending on the type of stroke. The closing symptoms occur due to obstruction of the condyle against a displaced disc that is suddenly drawn forward and likely torqued by contraction of the superior lateral pterygoid muscle during a power stroke. This frequently is displayed as a catching sensation, a momentary locking, or a loud, cracking noise just as a biting stroke begins. Otherwise, the symptoms may consist of nothing more than subjective sensations.

The treatment for posterior displacement of the disc is restriction of opening at a point just short of the displacement. Habit training with or without a training device (as used in the treatment of Class IV interferences) usually suffices. *Correction of the causative occlusal disharmony, however, is mandatory.* This can be done temporarily by utilizing an occlusion-correcting splint. Permanent correction should be based on what is feasible for the individual case.

Although posterior dislocation of the disc is possible when such gross displacement is permitted by the loss of contour and elongation of discal ligaments, it is automatically reduced by the next closing movement. Protracted posterior dislocation, therefore, does not occur.

In all disc displacement disorders of the TM joint, the patient should be taught how to best avoid such displacement or dislocation. Anterior displacements can be minimized by chewing on the nonsymptomatic side, by avoiding foods that require hard biting or large bites, and by habitually using slow, deliberate jaw movements. Posterior displacements can be minimized by avoiding full opening or extended protrusive jaw movements.

Dysfunctional superior retrodiscal lamina. A nonfunctional superior retrodiscal lamina eliminates the only intracapsular source of posterior traction on the articular disc. In such case, anterior dislocation of the articular disc, whether it be traumatic, spontaneous, or functional, is *permanent.* Surgical intervention is the only form of effective therapy.

Class IV Disc-Interference Disorders

The symptoms of Class IV interference occur during overextension of opening beyond the limits of normal rotation in the disc-condyle complex. This condition is referred to usually as joint hypermobility. The cause is habitual overextension of mouth opening.

The treatment for Class IV disorders is habit training to restrict mouth opening within normal limits. This usually can be accomplished by voluntary restraint on the part of the patient. Sometimes a training device is very helpful. This consists of placing Ivy eyelets or ligating jeweler loops at each of the four first bicuspid teeth. Then tie a piece of 6-pound monofilament nylon fishing cord to the right mandibular loop and pass it up through the right maxillary loop, across and down through the left maxillary loop, and through the left mandibular loop. Then open the mouth to a point just short of the symptoms and tie off the nylon cord at the left mandibular loop (Fig 10–1). This device does not interfere with normal opening and chewing. When excessive opening is attempted, however, the cord arrests it. The device should be used for several weeks, until the restricted opening becomes habitual. The patient should be taught how to replace the nylon cord to the measured opening proper for his case, because it is chewed through in a few days.

If such habit training fails and the condition becomes intolerable, sclerosing therapy may be tried.[60] True definitive treatment, however, is surgical. This is best done by eminectomy.[81–83] The operation flattens the articular eminence and reduces the amount of posterior rotation required for a full forward translatory movement. By so doing, the rotatory movement in the disc-condyle complex no longer exceeds normal limits, and arrested movement of the disc on the condyle does not take place.

Class V Disc-Interference Disorders

Class V disc interference is known as *spontaneous anterior dislocation.* If, at the moment of full or extended opening, the articular disc is forced through the articular disc space by an overextended opening, or if there is premature contraction of the superior lateral pterygoid muscle, the disc loses contact with the articular eminence; the disc space collapses; the condyle moves up against the articular eminence; and the disc is trapped in front of the condyle. With the articular disc space collapsed, the superior retrodiscal lamina cannot rotate the trapped disc posteriorly. When an effort is made to close, the superior lateral

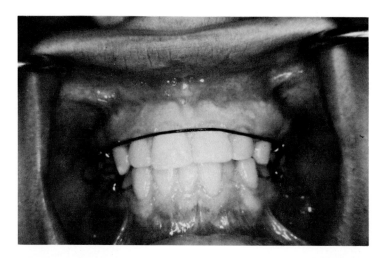

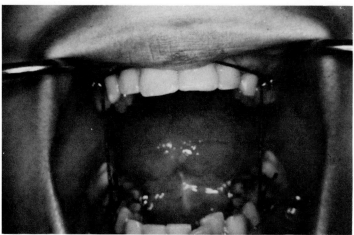

FIGURE 10–1. Simple restraining device limits the extent of mouth opening for the purpose of training the musculature to control habitual excessive opening of the mouth. *Top,* an Ivy eyelet or jeweler loop is placed at the mesial of the maxillary first bicuspid teeth and between the mandibular bicuspid teeth. A nylon cord (6-pound monofilament nylon fishing cord) is tied to the right mandibular loop, passed up through the right maxillary, across and down through the left maxillary, and on through the left mandibular loop. The mouth is opened to the desired point of restraint and the cord drawn tight and tied off at the left mandibular loop. *Bottom,* mouth opened to the maximum permitted by the restraining device. Within the imposed limit there is satisfactory freedom of mandibular movement.

pterygoid muscle contracts simultaneously with the elevator muscles, thus prolapsing the disc forward on the condyle. The dislocated disc remains anterior to the condyle and normal closure is blocked. The posterior teeth strike, while the anteriors stand widely apart.

To reduce a spontaneously dislocated articular disc, all that is needed is to widen the collapsed articular disc space just enough to permit the stretched superior retrodiscal lamina to rotate the disc back into position on the condyle. When such space is provided, reduction is automatic. Contraction of the superior lateral pterygoid muscle prevents reduction. Since this muscle contracts simultaneously with elevator muscles, any maneuver that entails contraction of elevator muscles (biting force) also prevents reduction; the contracted superior lateral pterygoid muscle nullifies the elastic traction of the stretched superior retrodiscal lamina that is essential to such reduction. Any such maneuver, therefore, is contraindicated.

Acute Spontaneous Anterior Dislocation. To reduce acute spontaneous dislocation, relaxation of the elevator and superior lateral pterygoid muscles is needed to widen the collapsed articular disc space. This is done best by having the patient yawn as widely as he can. At that moment, slight posterior pressure on the chin is usually enough to accomplish reduction. If a little more space is needed, pressing the mandible downward with the thumbs on the external oblique ridges *while the patient yawns* will suffice. A patient can be taught this maneuver to reduce his own dislocations. Forced attempts at reduction by the patient or the doctor may complicate the situation considerably. Forced reduction tends to initiate myospasm activity in the elevator muscles, making widening of the collapsed articular disc space all the more difficult. If this should take place, local anesthesia of the spastic muscles usually will facilitate reduction. Myospasm of the lateral pterygoid muscle renders reduction impossible. If this should occur, local anesthesia of that muscle is mandatory, or a general anesthetic with succinylcholine chloride muscle relaxant may become necessary.

Recurrent Spontaneous Anterior Dislocation. When spontaneous anterior dislocation occurs frequently, the patient should be taught how to reduce it effectively without introducing complications caused by the use of force. It is better, however, that it be prevented. This condition is the result of habitually opening the mouth too widely and almost always is a complication of chronic hypermobility. Most such patients can be trained to open less widely and, therefore, eliminate both Class IV interference and occasional spontaneous dislocation.

This can be done by utilizing the habit-training device described for the management of hypermobility. If the condition is not controlled by habit training and becomes intolerable, thus requiring definitive therapy, surgical intervention is needed. The operation best suited to eliminate this condition is an eminectomy, because it flattens the articular eminence and thus reduces the amount of posterior rotation of the articular disc during forward translatory movements.[84] When the amount of discal rotation is reduced, normal forward limits of the translatory cycle are extended, and spontaneous anterior dislocation does not take place with full opening movements.

Chronic Anterior Dislocation.   Chronic anterior dislocation of the temporomandibular joint is due to (1) contracture of the lateral pterygoid muscle, (2) permanent prolapse of the articular disc from a nonfunctional superior retrodiscal lamina, or (3) healed fracture-dislocation following trauma. Correction of this condition calls for surgical intervention. Several operations are used depending on the particular problem at hand, namely, myotomy of the lateral pterygoid muscle,[85] eminectomy, arthroplasty,[83] and reconstructive surgery.

Capsulitis and Synovitis

Capsulitis occurring as a separate entity usually is due to trauma. The majority of cases displaying symptoms of capsulitis are secondary to other inflammatory conditions arising as the result of injury to the discal collateral ligaments or the temporomandibular ligament. Some are secondary to inflammatory arthritis, periarticular conditions, or injury to a preexistent capsular fibrosis. Etiology usually entails the identification of other types of disorders. Consequently, therapy may be directed toward conditions besides the capsulitis per se.

In general, for treating capsulitis and synovitis:

1. Condylar movements that tend to stretch the capsule should be restricted.

2. Deep-heat therapy using diathermy or ultrasound should be instituted.

3. Anti-inflammatory medications should be given.[86] If the capsulitis is due to trauma and not likely to be repeated, a single injection of corticosteroid made laterally to the capsular ligament is usually effective.

4. Special considerations are needed if the capsulitis is secondary to other disorders: *(a)* If the capsulitis accompanies pain that is reduced by biting against a separator, it likely relates to inflamed discal ligaments or temporomandibular ligament. Occlusal correction with a temporary occlusal splint is indicated. Permanent correction may be planned when the capsulitis has subsided. *(b)* If the capsulitis is due to periarticular inflammation, active treatment of the primary condition, including antibiotics and supportive medical and surgical care, may be needed. *(c)* If the capsulitis is a manifestation of inflammatory arthritis, treatment should be directed primarily toward the arthritic condition.

Retrodiscitis

Some inflammatory conditions of the retrodiscal tissue result from extrinsic trauma of a type that could have caused a mandibular fracture. The diagnosis usually is made only after a futile radiographic search for a fracture line. Since hemarthrosis may be present, treatment should take into account the prevention of ankylosis. For treatment of this kind of retrodiscitis:

1. Normal occlusal relations should be established through intermaxillary fixation.

2. The fixation should be periodically released and the joint actively moved for 5 to 10 minutes at least twice daily.

3. As soon as the occlusion will remain stabilized without the aid of intermaxillary fixation, active movement of the joint should be encouraged until resolution is complete.

Retrodiscitis may occur as a complication of anterior functional dislocation of the articular disc, accompanying the other symptoms of that condition as previously described. This has sometimes been called a "posterior capsulitis." The condition usually diminishes with chronicity of the dislocation and becomes essentially nonsymptomatic as the tissue is converted metaplastically into dense avascular fibrous tissue somewhat similar to that of the articular disc.[87]

Inflammatory Arthritis

The symptoms of generalized inflammation of the joint are much the same, regardless of cause. Therefore, certain general principles of treatment may apply to all types.[88] As the particular kind of arthritis becomes evident, special considerations are needed. The following therapeutic principles are usually indicated:

1. Functional demands should be reduced voluntarily to bring them well within the capabilities of the inflamed joint.

2. Nonpainful movements of the joint should be maintained on a periodic schedule of 5 to 10 minutes 2 to 3 times daily to keep the joint mobile. This should not be carried to the point of pain or other sign of aggravation of the inflammatory condition.

3. Acute malocclusion and other obvious discrepancies in occlusal function should be neutralized by occlusal disengagement. If a disengaging splint is used, it should be corrected periodically as resolution or further deterioration takes place.

4. Medically supervised anti-inflammatory medications and other supportive medical treatment usually are indicated.

5. Judicious physiotherapy in the form of deep heat (diathermy or ultrasound) should be used, unless it seems to aggravate the condition.

6. Since inflammatory arthritis frequently causes arthralgic pain of a more or less continuous type, some secondary central excitatory effects may accompany the disorder and complicate the symptom picture. Secondary referred pains and muscle spasm activity should be identified. The referred pain will remain dependent on the arthralgia, but muscle spasm activity may display independent cycling pain-dysfunction symptoms that require separate management. It should be understood that, until the arthralgia is eliminated or at least brought to the stage of intermittency, lasting resolution of such muscle spasm activity cannot be expected.

7. Some special considerations depend on the kind of arthritis present. *Degenerative arthritis* requires special management of the preexistent disc-interference disorder. Surgical intervention may be required, such as closed condylotomy[89] or arthroplasty.[82, 83, 90–94] Good postsurgical care and follow-up are essential to satisfactory management of the case. *Rheumatoid arthritis* is essentially a medical problem. The dentist's responsibility rests largely with adjusting the occlusion as necessary. Progressive loss of contact of the anterior teeth may require occlusal splinting, adjusted periodically as further change takes place. Reconstructive arthroplasty may be needed. *Traumatic and infectious arthritis* may require antibiotic therapy as well as general supportive med-

ical and surgical care. Caution should be exercised to minimize undesirable sequelae, if possible. *Hyperuricemia* is a medical problem requiring active treatment and follow-up. Since it follows a recurring pattern, continuing medical supervision is needed.

8. Corticosteroid therapy may have a place in the treatment program, but considerable judgment should be exercised in its use. It is frequently part of rheumatoid arthritis treatment.[95] Injections of corticosteroid substances into the joint proper may be justified at times. It is known to predispose to further deterioration[96] and encourages excessive use of the joint during the time that it suppresses the inflammation. When it has been established that a surgical approach to degenerative arthritis is to be made, periodic injections of corticosteroid into the joint may be used to keep the patient comfortable pending surgery.

Contractured Elevator Muscle

Usually, no treatment of any kind is needed for chronic mandibular hypomobilities, unless they are injured by movements that exceed the limitations imposed and, thus, cause inflammatory symptoms. Good management of all chronic hypomobilities includes adequate insight into the problem on the patient's part, so he may be able to avoid abusive use of the joint. Careful habit training to keep all joint functioning well within the structural capabilities of the joint is needed. Care should be exercised by the dentist to avoid opening the mouth too widely. It should be understood that the opposite joint should be kept under observation, because the restricted movements in the hypomobile joint may cause destructive changes in the mobile joint.

Extracapsular chronic mandibular hypomobility due to muscular contracture may become inflamed due to excessive opening efforts. As such, it should be treated as *myositis,* until the acute symptoms subside.

Myostatic Contracture. If contracture is due to protracted restriction of opening, it may usually be reversed with proper therapy. This consists of *gentle momentary stretching* of the muscle many times each day. Stretching should not be great enough to cause pain or forceful enough to cause muscle inflammation. It should be just enough to stimulate the inverse stretch reflex. Many weeks are required for the resting length of the muscle to be increased.

It should be noted that myostatic contracture may complicate other kinds of chronic mandibular hypomobility, especially myofibrotic contracture and ankylosis. This is to be considered when other forms are under treatment. Even though correction of such other disorders is properly planned and executed, provision should be made in the post-surgical treatment regimen for the reversal of any accompanying myostatic contracture that may be present.

Myofibrotic Contracture.   If the contracture is due to the formation of cicatricial tissue in and about the muscle, the shortening is permanent. Mild but continuous elastic traction to lengthen the muscle by linear growth may accomplish some degree of benefit. If definitive treatment is required, surgical detachment and reattachment is necessary.

Capsular Fibrosis

Capsular fibrosis restricts movement in the outer ranges only and usually poses no intolerable condition that requires definitive treatment. The usual problem is merely that of injury induced by excessive force used to extend condylar movement. As such, the injured capsule becomes inflamed, and the condition should be treated as a *capsulitis*.

Ankylosis

The usual form of ankylosis is fibrous, in which adhesions join the disc-condyle complex to the articular eminence-fossa surface. Forceful movements may injure the adhesions, thus causing pain and inflammation. Treatment consists of voluntary restraint of joint use until the inflammatory condition subsides. Anti-inflammatory medications and deep-heat therapy (diathermy or ultrasound) are usually beneficial. Exercises are contraindicated.

Ordinarily a 25-mm opening can be made, whether the condition is fibrous or osseous. If a larger opening is required and the complaint becomes intolerable, surgery is necessary.[82, 83, 91, 92, 94, 96–99] Good postsurgical care and follow-up are essential to satisfactory final results.

Ankylosis may be complicated by myostatic contracture of several or all elevator muscles due to the protracted inability to open the mouth normally. This complicates the diagnosis as well as the treatment. When it is determined that such contracture exists, provision for the normalization of the contractured muscles should be included in the treatment plan.

Growth Disorders

Disorders of growth involving the craniomandibular articulation usually occur insidiously. Compensatory changes occur in such a manner that little or no pain or dysfunction becomes evident until the condition is well developed. Such disorders are usually apparent radiographically before symptoms develop enough to require definitive therapy.

Aberrations related to the developmental process, acquired changes in structural form, and benign neoplasia usually require interdisciplinary planning and corrective treatment that embraces surgery, orthodontics, rehabilitation efforts, and cosmetic procedures.[82, 92, 100, 101] Malignancy involving the joint requires the services of a consulting oncologist.

LONG-TERM RESULTS OF TREATMENT

Although occlusal splint therapy is by far the most frequently used modality in the management of TM disorders generally, its effectiveness has not been tested by scientific methods. Reports are generally of a testimonial character. Okeson et al.[102] have suggested a design for more accurate evaluation of this method of treatment. Howard[103] reported on 400 disorders, of which 87% were found in female patients; the mean age of patients was 29 years. He reported that only symptoms were managed, that splinting seldom provided a cure, and that clicking joints treated by repositioning appliances usually resumed clicking. He concluded that the objective of therapy should be to control the symptoms and to arrest the progress of the disorder. Agerberg and Carlsson[104] reported on the long-term results (3–5 years) of the treatment of 81 patients with TM disorders for which occlusal splinting was used on 54%. They reported that while 80% showed some overall improvement, only 33% displayed improvement in the clicking symptoms, and 25% reported no improvement in joint pain. Greene and Laskin[105] reported on the long-term (average 3 years) evaluation of 100 "successfully treated" myofascial pain-dysfunction (MPD) syndrome patients. Of these, 51 had no recurrence of symptoms, 41 had minor episodes of symptoms, 6 were failures, 2 required other therapy. Magnusson and Carlsson[106] reported the findings on 80 consecutive TM patients for which occlusal splinting comprised at least part of the therapy for 78%. They reported significant decrease in muscle pain but little specific effect on joint noise. Greene et al.[107] reported on the long-term outcome of TM clicking in 100 MPD patients. They found that, although many did not have a change in their clicking patterns as the result of treatment, few had progressed to more severe dysfunction symptoms—suggesting that the feature of disc noise may not be a progressive symptom. Bronstein[108] examined 21 surgically treated joints arthrographically and found only 4 that were "normal." As previously cited,[72, 73, 77–79] the objective results of disc plication operations are not impressive, and, although excision of the disc gives excellent long-term *subjective* benefit, the radiographic evidence of degenerative joint disease thus displayed causes one to withhold favorable judgment. It is interesting to note that Graham[10] reported the data on 3 patients with "displaced discs" confirmed by arthrography who were unsuccessfully treated nonsurgically and were recommended for surgery—but refused the treatment. In all 3 cases the symptoms subsided with the passage of time, and no further treatment was required.

The conclusion that should be drawn from the record of management of TM disorders in general is that the present "state-of-the-art" leaves much to be desired. In the face of several nonanatomical concepts of joint structure and function, failure to differentiate between the different types of TM disorders, and somewhat empirical application of therapy, there should be little wonder that the long-term effectiveness of efforts in this field of dental practice is not impressive. However, with full utilization of the basic knowledge that is currently available, the future outlook for more effective management of TM disorders should be improved considerably.

REHABILITATION

Most acute muscle disorders can be expected to return to normal with little or no continuing disability. A chronic muscle disorder such as contracture may present therapeutic problems. Myostatic contracture can usually be improved with proper therapy. Myofibrotic contracture, however, usually requires surgical intervention, and some residual disability may continue.

Disorders of the joint proper present a different outlook. Although the condylar and eminence articular surfaces do have some regenerative capability, it is far from adequate. The articular disc has none. The discal ligaments may "heal," but they remain loose and elongated. A damaged joint, therefore, remains so: some residual disability must be expected.

The treatment of joint disorders is largely to control the symptoms and make the condition more tolerable. "Cure" should not be expected.

Depending on what the disorder consists of, some continuing disability will remain even if the symptoms are rendered acceptable.

It is necessary that the patient understand from the outset that marked limitations stand imposed on the results of TM therapy—both surgical and nonsurgical. These consequences must be accepted and coped with. Considerable judgment may be required when therapy is recommended, whether a proposed treatment can reasonably be justified as expected benefits are weighed against possible complications.

A good treatment program, therefore, should include giving the patient proper insight concerning the true nature of the disorder and the limitations that exist relative to recovery. He should be instructed on how he can contribute to his recovery by modification not only of the foods he chooses but also of his manner of jaw use. He must be prepared to accept the residual disability that likely will remain after therapy, and to cope with a less-than-ideal situation.

The doctor can help in a patient's rehabilitation—but only the patient himself can do it.

MEDICOLEGAL CONSIDERATIONS

The diagnosis and management of TM disorders is an emerging area of dental practice. Fundamentally an orthopedic problem, its position in medical science has yet to be clearly defined. Its relationship to masticatory function has placed it in the field of dentistry. Yet, interprofessional treatment is required at times, and intraprofessional efforts are frequently needed to produce effective results. The medicolegal considerations, therefore, should be understood. Caution in management is advised.

Zinman[109] provided an excellent review of these aspects of practice. He pointed out that successful malpractice litigation requires:

1. A bona fide doctor-patient relationship

2. A breach of the doctor's duty owed to the patient

3. Injury sustained by the patient as a result of such breach of duty

Honest errors in judgment do not entail liability, but the burden of proof rests on the doctor. The following are legal causes of action for professional malpractice:

1. Breach of warranty and/or contract

2. Battery

3. Negligence from lack of informed consent

4. Experimental or unorthodox therapy

5. Invalid consent

6. Professional negligence

Breach of Warranty and/or Contract

Breach of warranty entails failure to deliver *promised* results. The citing of any specific result that may be expected from either diagnosis or therapy should be avoided. Positive statements of the diagnosis or prognosis should rest on diagnostic data that are properly evaluated and confirmed. Statements of the therapeutic results that are to be expected should be tempered and qualified.

Battery

Unconsented therapy of any type constitutes battery and is a legal cause of action.

Negligence from Lack of Informed Consent

Failure to obtain proper informed consent may constitute negligence.

Experimental or Unorthodox Therapy

Liability for any unorthodox or experimental procedure should be absolved by special legal documentation over and above ordinary informed consent.

Invalid Consent

A signed consent form may not be valid unless it clearly states the complications and hazards that can reasonably result from the treatment. It must be couched in language that the patient can understand. It must be fully comprehended by the patient or his legal guardian. Unconscious, sick, emotionally disturbed, medicated, or sedated patients require special consideration to establish the validity of informed consent.

Professional Negligence

A doctor has the right to refuse to accept a patient, but he must not abandon the patient once a doctor-patient relationship has been established. The patient has the obligation to be cooperative within reasonable limits. The doctor-patient relationship may be terminated by mutual consent. Service rendered without charge does not alter the doctor's responsibility. Negligence includes such things as the failure to obtain the proper data for a diagnosis, the failure to use reasonable diligence in the management of the patient, permitting complications and hazards to occur that could reasonably have been prevented, the failure to care for complications that do arise, and the failure to attend the patient at reasonable intervals. Incorrect diagnosis has increasingly become a cause of action. In malpractice litigation, damage must be established by the patient.

Prophylaxis Against Litigation

1. Maintain good records
2. Adequately document the diagnosis and treatment
3. Maintain good professional rapport
4. Avoid disparaging remarks
5. Practice the Golden Rule

REFERENCES

1. Degenaar J.J.: Some philosophical considerations on pain. *Pain* 7:281–304, 1979.
2. Bell W.E.: *Orofacial Pains*, ed. 3. Chicago, Year Book Medical Publishers, 1985.
3. Brooke R.I., Stenn P.G.: Myofascial pain dysfunction syndrome: How effective is biofeedback-assisted relaxation training? in Bonica J.J., Lindblom U., Iggo A. (eds.): *Advances in Pain Research and Therapy*, Vol. 5. New York, Raven Press, 1983, pp. 809–812.
4. King E.: Kinesiology, in Morgan D.H., House L.R., Hall W.P., et al. (eds.): *Diseases of the Temporomandibular Apparatus*, ed. 2. St. Louis, C.V. Mosby Co., 1982, pp. 497–499.
5. Lay E.M.: The osteopathic management of temporomandibular joint dysfunction, in Gelb H. (ed.): *Clinical Management of Head, Neck and TMJ*

Pain and Dysfunction. Philadelphia, W.B. Saunders Co., 1977, pp. 507–532.

6. Goodman P., Greene C.S., Laskin D.M.: Response of patients with myofascial pain-dysfunction syndrome to mock equilibration. *J. Am. Dent. Assoc.* 92:755, 1976.

7. Greene C.S., Laskin D.M.: Long-term evaluation of treatment for myofascial pain-dysfunction syndrome: A comparative analysis. *J. Am. Dent. Assoc.* 107:235, 1983.

8. Cohen S.R.: Follow-up evaluation of 105 patients with myofascial pain-dysfunction syndrome. *J. Am. Dent. Assoc.* 97:825, 1978.

9. Mejersjo C., Carlsson G.E.: Long-term results of treatment for temporomandibular joint pain-dysfunction. *J. Prosthet. Dent.* 49:809, 1983.

10. Graham G.S.: Nonsurgical management of internal derangement: A report of three cases. *J. Craniomand. Pract.* 2:253, 1984.

11. Blackwood H.J.J.: Pathology of the temporomandibular joint. *J. Am. Dent. Assoc.* 79:118, 1969.

12. Mongini F.: Condylar remodeling after occlusal therapy. *J. Prosthet. Dent.* 43:568, 1980.

13. De Steno C.V.: The pathophysiology of TMJ dysfunction and related pain, in Gelb H. (ed.): *Clinical Management of Head, Neck and TMJ Pain and Dysfunction.* Philadelphia, W.B. Saunders Co., 1977, pp. 1–31.

14. Ingersoll W.B., Kerens E.G.: A treatment for excessive occlusal trauma or bruxism. *J. Am. Dent. Assoc.* 44:22, 1952.

15. Solberg W.K., Clark G.T., Rugh J.D.: Nocturnal electromyographic evaluation of bruxing patients undergoing short-term splint therapy. *J. Oral Rehabil.* 2(3):215, 1975.

16. Kovaleski W.C., DeBoever J.: Influence of occlusal splints on jaw position and musculature in patients with temporomandibular joint dysfunction. *J. Prosthet. Dent.* 35:321–327, 1975.

17. Clark G.T., Beemsterboer P.L., Solberg W.K., et al.: Nocturnal electromyographic evaluation of myofascial pain-dysfunction in patients undergoing occlusal splint therapy. *J. Am. Dent. Assoc.* 99:607, 1979.

18. Clark G.T.: Occlusal therapy: Occlusal appliances, in *The President's Conference on the Examination, Diagnosis, and Management of Temporomandibular Disorders.* Chicago, American Dental Association, 1983, pp. 137–146.

19. Thompson J.R.: Temporomandibular disorders: Diagnosis and dental treatment, in Sarnat B.G. (ed.): *The Temporomandibular Joint.* Springfield, Ill., Charles C Thomas, Publisher, 1951, pp. 122–144.

20. Fox C.W. Jr., Abrams B.L., Doukoudakis A.A., et al.: A centric relation occlusal splint as an aid in diagnosis. *The Compendium of Continuing Education,* 3(2):142–150, 1982.

21. Wagner E.P., Crandall S.K., Oliver R.B.: Splints, in Morgan D.H., House L.R., Hall W.P., et al. (eds.): *Diseases of the Temporomandibular Apparatus,* ed. 2. St. Louis, C.V. Mosby Co., 1982, pp. 265–277.

22. Carraro J.J., Caffesse R.G.: Effect of occlusal splints on TMJ symptomatology. *J. Prosthet. Dent.* 40:563, 1978.

23. Clark G.T.: A critical evaluation of orthopedic interocclusal appliance therapy: Design, theory, and overall effectiveness. *J. Am. Dent. Assoc.* 108:359, 1984.

24. Clark G.T.: A critical evaluation of orthopedic interocclusal appliance therapy: Effectiveness for specific symptoms. *J. Am. Dent. Assoc.* 108:364, 1984.

25. Lerman M.D.: The hydrostatic appliance: A new approach to treatment of the TMJ pain-dysfunction syndrome. *J. Am. Dent. Assoc.* 89:1343, 1974.

26. Lerman M.D.: A complete hydrostatically derived treatment procedure for the TMJ pain-dysfunction syndrome. *J. Am. Dent. Assoc.* 89:1351, 1974.

27. Gale E.N.: Behavioral management of MPD, in *The President's Conference on the Examination, Diagnosis, and Management of Temporomandibular Disorders.* Chicago, American Dental Association, 1983, pp. 161–166.

28. Carlsson S.G., Gale E.N., Ohman A.: Treatment of temporomandibular joint syndrome with biofeedback training. *J. Am. Dent. Assoc.* 91:602, 1975.

29. Dohrmann R.J., Laskin D.M.: An evaluation of electromyographic biofeedback in the treatment of myofascial pain-dysfunction syndrome. *J. Am. Dent. Assoc.* 96:656, 1978.

30. Ayer W.A., Gale E.N.: Extinction of bruxism by massed practice therapy. *J. Can. Dent. Assoc.* 35:492, 1969.

31. Schwartz L.: Therapeutic exercises, in Schwartz L. (ed.): *Disorders of the Temporomandibular Joint.* Philadelphia, W.B. Saunders Co., 1959, pp. 223–231.

32. Rocabado M.: Joint distraction with a functional maxillomandibular orthopedic appliance. *J. Craniomand. Pract.* 2:358, 1984.

33. Danzig W.N., Van Dyke A.R.: Physical therapy as an adjunct to temporomandibular joint therapy. *J. Prosthet. Dent.* 49:96, 1983.

34. Murphy G.J.: Electrical physical therapy in treating TMJ patients. *J. Craniomand. Pract.* 1(2):67, 1983.

35. Esposito C.J., Veal S.J., Farman A.G.: Alleviation of myofascial pain with ultrasonic therapy. *J. Prosthet. Dent.* 51:106, 1984.

36. Travell J.G., Simons D.G.: *Myofascial Pain and Dysfunction.* Baltimore, Williams & Wilkins Co., 1983.

37. Greene C.S., Laskin D.M.: Meprobamate therapy for the myofascial pain-dysfunction (MPD) syndrome: A double-blind evaluation. *J. Am. Dent. Assoc.* 82:587, 1971.

38. Lupton D.E.: Psychological aspects of temporomandibular joint dysfunction. *J. Am. Dent. Assoc.* 79:131, 1969.

39. Marbach J.J., Dworkin S.F.: Chronic MPD: Group therapy and psychodynamics. *J. Am. Dent. Assoc.* 90:827, 1975.

40. Scott D.S.: Treatment of the myofascial pain-dysfunction syndrome: Psychological aspects. *J. Am. Dent. Assoc.* 101:611, 1980.

41. Fox C.W., Abrams B.L., Doukoudakis A.: Principles of anterior guid-

ance: Development and clinical applications. *J. Craniomand. Pract.* 2:23, 1983.

42. Williamson E.H., Lundquist D.O.: Anterior guidance: Its effect on electromyographic activity of the temporal and masseter muscles. *J. Prosthet. Dent.* 49:816, 1983.

43. DeBrul E.L.: The biomechanics of the oral apparatus. Chapter 3. Structural analysis, in DeBrul E.L., Menekratis A.: *The Physiology of Oral Reconstruction.* Chicago, Quintessence Publishing Company, 1981, pp. 21–38.

44. Carlsson G.E., Droukas B.C.: Dental occlusion and the health of the masticatory system. *J. Craniomand. Pract.* 2:141, 1984.

45. Ramfjord S.P.: Goals for an ideal occlusion and mandibular position, in Solberg W.K., Clark G.T. (eds.): *Abnormal Jaw Mechanics.* Chicago, Quintessence Publishing Company, 1984, pp. 77–95.

46. Okeson J.P.: *Fundamentals of Occlusion and Temporomandibular Disorders.* St. Louis, C.V. Mosby Co., 1985.

47. Weinberg L.A.: Definitive prosthodontic therapy for TMJ patients. Part I. Anterior and posterior condylar displacement. *J. Prosthet. Dent.* 50:544, 1983.

48. Annandale T.: On displacement of the interarticular cartilage of the lower jaw and its treatment by operation. *Lancet* 1:411, 1887.

49. Pringle J.: Displacement of the mandibular meniscus and its treatment. *Br. J. Surg.* 6:385, 1918.

50. Wakeley C.: The causation and treatment of displaced mandibular cartilage. *Lancet* 2:543, 1929.

51. Burman M., Sinberg S.E.: Condylar movement in the study of internal derangement of the temporomandibular joint. *J. Bone Joint Surg.* 28:352, 1946.

52. Dingman R.O., Moorman W.C.: Meniscectomy in treatment of lesions of temporomandibular joint. *J. Oral Surg.* 9:214, 1951.

53. Kiehn C.L.: Meniscectomy for internal derangement of temporomandibular joint. *Am. J. Surg.* 83:364, 1952.

54. Christie H.K.: Internal derangements of the temporomandibular joint. *J. Int. Coll. Surg.* 19:704, 1953.

55. Silver D.M., Simon S.D., Savastano A.: Meniscus injuries of the temporomandibular joint. *J. Bone Joint Surg.* 38:541, 1956.

56. Ireland V.E.: The problem of the clicking jaw. *Proc. Roy. Soc. Lond.* 44:363, 1951.

57. Farrar W.B.: Diagnosis and treatment of anterior dislocation of the articular disc. *N.Y. J. Dent.* 41:348, 1971.

58. Farrar W.B.: Differentiation of temporomandibular joint dysfunction to simplify treatment. *J. Prosthet. Dent.* 28:629, 1972.

59. McCarty W.L., Farrar W.B.: Surgery for internal derangements of the temporomandibular joint. *J. Prosthet. Dent.* 42:191, 1979.

60. Schultz L.W.: A curative treatment for subluxation of the temporomandibular joint or any joint. *J. Am. Dent. Assoc.* 24:1947, 1937.

61. Garcia R.: Radiofrequency lesioning of the posterior disk ligament: A new frontier. *Joint Effort* 1(2):1, 1984.
62. McNeill C.: Nonsurgical management, in Helms C.A., Katzberg R.W., Dolwick M.F. (eds.): *Internal Derangements of the Temporomandibular Joint.* San Francisco, Radiology Research and Education Foundation, 1983, pp. 193–227.
63. Gilboe D.B.: Posterior condylar displacement: Prosthetic therapy. *J. Prosthet. Dent.* 49:549, 1983.
64. Caswell C.W.: Treatment of anterior displaced meniscus with a flat occlusal splint. *J. Dent. Res.* 63 (special issue), Abstract No. 17, 1984.
65. Clark G.T.: Treatment of jaw clicking with temporomandibular repositioning: Analysis of 25 cases. *J. Craniomand. Pract.* 2:263, 1984.
66. Anderson G.C., Schulte J.K., Goodkind R.J.: Comparative study of two treatment methods for internal derangement of the temporomandibular joint. *J. Prosthet. Dent.* 53:392–396, 1985.
67. Niemann W.W.: The bicuspid buildup as a diagnostic aid in TMJ and muscular dysfunction. *J. Craniomand. Pract.* 2:369, 1984.
68. Bellavia W.D., Missert W.: Repositioning the mandible anteriorly with fixed composite overlays. *J. Craniomand. Pract.* 3:173–178, 1985.
69. Okeson J.P., Kemper J.T., Moody P.M.: A study of the use of occlusion splints in the treatment of acute and chronic patients with craniomandibular disorders. *J. Prosthet. Dent.* 48:708, 1982.
70. Goharian R.K., Neff P.A.: Effect of occlusal retainers on temporomandibular joint and facial pain. *J. Prosthet. Dent.* 44:206, 1980.
71. Manzione J.V., Tallents R., Katzberg R.W., et al.: Arthrographically guided splint therapy for recapturing the temporomandibular joint meniscus. *Oral Surg.* 57:235–240, 1984.
72. Dolwick M.F.; Surgical management, in Helms C.H., Katzberg R.W., Dolwick M.F. (eds.): *Internal Derangements of the Temporomandibular Joint.* San Francisco, Radiology Research and Education Foundation, 1983, pp. 167–191.
73. Eriksson L., Westesson P.: Long-term evaluation of meniscectomy of the temporomandibular joint. *J. Oral Maxillofac. Surg.* 43:263–269, 1985.
74. Hall M.B.: Meniscoplasty of the displaced temporomandibular joint meniscus without violating the inferior joint space. *J. Oral Maxillofac. Surg.* 42:788–792, 1984.
75. Bronstein S.L.: Closure of temporomandibular joint meniscoplasty with figure-of-eight vertical mattress suture. *J. Oral Maxillofac. Surg.* 40:248, 1982.
76. Zetz M.R., Irby W.B.: Repair of the adult temporomandibular joint meniscus with an autogenous dermal graft. *J. Oral Maxillofac. Surg.* 42:167, 1984.
77. *Criteria for TMJ Meniscus Surgery.* Chicago, American Association of Oral and Maxillofacial Surgeons, November 1984.
78. Howard J.: Questions and discussion, Session 2, in Moffett B.C. (ed.):

Diagnosis of Internal Derangements of the Temporomandibular Joint, Vol. 1. Seattle, University of Washington, 1984, pp. 51–57.

79. Bronstein S.L., Tomasetti B.J.: Temporomandibular joint surgery: Patient-based assessment and evaluation. *J. Am. Dent. Assoc.* 110:485–489, 1985.

80. Westesson P.: Clinical and arthrographic findings in patients with TMJ disorders, in Moffett B.C. (ed.): *Diagnosis of Internal Derangements of the Temporomandibular Joint*, Vol. 1. Seattle, University of Washington, 1984, pp. 59–71.

81. Hall M.B., Brown R.W., Sclar A.G.: Anatomy of the TMJ articular eminence before and after surgical reduction. *J. Craniomand. Pract.* 2:135, 1984.

82. Morgan D.H., House L.R., Hall W.P., et al.: Surgery of the temporomandibular joint, in Morgan D.H., House L.R., Hall W.P., et al. (eds.): *Diseases of the Temporomandibular Apparatus*, ed. 2. St. Louis, C.V. Mosby Co., 1982, pp. 355–442.

83. Irby W.B.: Surgical treatment of TMJ problems, in Irby W.B. (ed.): *Current Advances in Oral Surgery*, Vol. 3. St. Louis, C.V. Mosby Co., 1980, pp. 284–335.

84. Westwood R.M., Fox G.L., Tilson H.B.: Eminectomy for the treatment of recurrent temporomandibular joint dislocation. *J. Oral Surg.* 33:774, 1975.

85. Laskin D.M.: Myotomy for the management of recurrent and protracted mandibular dislocations. *Trans. Cong. Assoc. Oral Surg.* 4:264–268, 1967.

86. Hall W.P.: Pharmacological methods, in Morgan D.H., House L.R., Hall W.P., et al. (eds.): *Diseases of the Temporomandibular Apparatus*, ed. 2. St. Louis, C.V. Mosby Co., 1982, pp. 350–354.

87. Moffett B.: Histologic aspects of temporomandibular joint derangements, in Moffett B.C. (ed.): *Diagnosis of Internal Derangements of the Temporomandibular Joint*, Vol 1. Seattle, University of Washington, 1984, pp. 47–49.

88. Friedman M.H., Weisberg J., Agus B.: Emergency treatment of acute inflammation of the temporomandibular joint. *J. Prosthet. Dent.* 50:827, 1983.

89. Ward T.G., Smith D.G., Sommars M.: Condylotomy for mandibular joint arthrosis. *Br. Dent. J.* 103:147, 1957.

90. Henny F.A., Baldridge O.L.: Condylectomy for the persistently painful temporomandibular joint. *J. Oral Surg.* 15:24, 1957.

91. Morgan D.H.: Surgical correction of temporomandibular joint arthritis. *J. Oral Surg.* 33:766, 1975.

92. Sarnat B.G., Laskin D.M.: Surgical considerations, in Sarnat B.G., Laskin D.M. (eds.): *The Temporomandibular Joint*, ed. 3. Springfield, Ill., Charles C Thomas, Publisher, 1979, pp. 422–470.

93. Henny F.A.: Surgical treatment of the painful temporomandibular joint. *J. Am. Dent. Assoc.* 79:171, 1969.

94. Kent J.N., Misick D.J., Akin R.K., et al.: Temporomandibular joint con-

dylar prosthesis: A ten-year report. *J. Oral Maxillofac. Surg.* 41:245, 1983.

95. Hollander J.L.: *Arthritis and Allied Conditions.* Philadelphia, Lea & Febiger, 1966.

96. Poswillo D.E.: Experimental investigation of the effects of intra-articular hydrocortisone and high condylectomy on the mandibular condyle. *Oral Surg.* 30:161, 1970.

97. Hinds E.C., Pleasants J.E.: Reconstruction of the temporomandibular joint. *Am. J. Surg.* 90:931, 1955.

98. Walker R.V.: Arthroplasty of the ankylosed temporomandibular joint. *Am. Surg.* 24:474, 1958.

99. Caldwell J.B.: Surgical management of temporomandibular joint ankylosis in children. *Int. J. Oral Surg.* 7:334, 1978.

100. Hasse C.D., Morgan D.H.: Orthognathic surgery, in Morgan D.H., House L.R., Hall W.P., et al. (eds.): *Diseases of the Temporomandibular Apparatus,* ed. 2. St. Louis, C.V. Mosby Co., 1982, pp. 526–556.

101. Bell W.H. (ed.): *Surgical Correction of Dentofacial Deformities, Newer Concepts,* Vol. 3. Philadelphia, W.B. Saunders Co., 1985.

102. Okeson J.P., Moody P.M., Kemper J.T., et al.: Evaluation of occlusal splint therapy. *J. Craniomand. Pract.* 1(3):47, 1983.

103. Howard J.: A retrospective philosophy on treatment for internal derangements, in Moffett B.C. (ed.): *Diagnosis of Internal Derangements of the Temporomandibular Joint,* Vol. 1. Seattle, University of Washington, 1984, pp. 9–11.

104. Agerberg G., Carlsson G.E.: Late results of treatment of functional disorders of the masticatory system. *J. Oral Rehabil.* 1:309, 1974.

105. Greene C.S., Laskin D.M.: Long-term evaluation of conservative treatment for myofascial pain-dysfunction syndrome. *J. Am. Dent. Assoc.* 89:1365, 1974.

106. Magnusson T., Carlsson G.E.: Treatment of patients with functional disturbances in the masticatory system: A survey of 80 consecutive patients. *Swed. Dent. J.* 4:145, 1980.

107. Greene C.S., Turner C., Laskin D.M.: Long-term outcome of TMJ clicking in 100 MPD patients. *J. Dent. Res.* 61:218, 1982.

108. Bronstein S.L.: Postsurgical TMJ arthrography. *J. Craniomand. Pract.* 2(2):165, 1984.

109. Zinman E.J.: Legal aspects, in Morgan D.H., House L.R., Hall W.P., et al. (eds.): *Diseases of the Temporomandibular Apparatus,* ed. 2. St. Louis, C.V. Mosby Co., 1982, pp. 600–615.

Appendix | The Occlusal Splint

Temporary alteration of the occlusal relationship can be provided by utilizing interocclusal devices, known commonly as "occlusal splints." Occlusal splinting as a treatment method for different types of temporomandibular disorders is used to accomplish different objectives, namely: (1) occlusal disengagement; (2) temporary correction of occlusal disharmony; and (3) repositioning the mandible. Different splints accomplish different things.

Disengaging splints induce relaxation of the masticatory muscles. This is accomplished presumably by reducing, modifying, or more widely distributing the afferent neural input from the occluding teeth. *Occlusion-correcting splints* temporarily eliminate chronic (preexistent and possibly etiologic) malocclusion and acute (symptomatic) malocclusion. *Mandibular repositioning splints* are used to prevent the disc-condyle complexes from returning to the fully occluded position or to set the condyles more favorably in relationship to a displaced articular disc. The choice of the type of splint for a given case depends on the diagnosis of what is wrong and what is needed.

Several general principles should govern occlusal splinting as a treatment method:

1. If occlusal disengagement is to be used for only a few days, full coverage splinting is unnecessary. Such devices as anterior deprogramming jigs, anterior bite plates, flat plane occlusal splints, or conventional Thompson splints (covering the posterior teeth only) can be used. The danger of intrusion, extrusion, and drifting of teeth forbids the use of such devices for a longer period. *Full coverage of the teeth with*

306

an adequate occlusal matrix to securely hold them is mandatory for all long-term occlusal splinting. Damaging the occlusion is unnecessary and is much too high a price to pay for the benefits of splinting.

2. The splint should be constructed in such a manner as not to injure teeth, gingiva, or other oral structures.

3. The thickness of the splint should not exceed the interocclusal clearance (freeway space).

4. The device should be acceptable to the patient in stability, comfort, and appearance.

5. Short-term splinting should be simple, economical, and readily alterable. Long-term splinting should be more durable and satisfactory for mastication and other mouth functions.

6. Splints should be easily manageable by the patient so as not to interfere with normal oral hygiene.

The Thompson splint* modified to include the anterior teeth is a simple, easily constructed, economical device that is quite versatile in the management of many temporomandibular disorders. It can be used for disengagement and for temporarily correcting the occlusion. It also can serve as the base for making a mandibular repositioning splint. Its chief merit lies in the fact that it utilizes the patient's own masticatory structures without requiring transfer techniques, articulators, or occlusal adjustment, and it is easily alterable from day to day as normalization takes place. For long-term use, it can be converted into metal for durability. Although it can be used on either arch, usually the upper is preferred because of easier control of the mandibular anterior teeth. If it is to be used for only a few days for occlusal disengagement, coverage of the bicuspids and molars will suffice.

Making the Acrylic Splint. Take an impression of the arch and pour a cast. Adapt a single thickness of ordinary baseplate wax to cover the teeth (and palate, if the maxillary arch is used). Trim the wax to include the incisal edges of the anterior teeth and to a point slightly beyond the greatest contour of the posterior teeth, so that the finished splint will be retained by springing on. Process in transparent acrylic and fit to the mouth, being sure that it is securely retained and com-

*Thompson J.R.: Temporomandibular disorders: Diagnosis and dental treatment, in Sarnat B.G. (ed.): *The Temporomandibular Joint.* Springfield, Ill., Charles C Thomas, Publisher, 1951, pp. 122–144.

fortable (without pressure on the soft tissues). Remove the acrylic base from the mouth, and grind down the thickness in the occlusal matrix area until holes appear. This is done so that the finished splint will separate the teeth as little as possible. (Note: If the splint is for a measured occlusal stop, this step may not be needed.) Mix some self-curing acrylic material and place a thin layer over the occlusal matrix portion of the base. Place in the patient's mouth, and have him close by *gently resting the teeth together* against the splint. Do not use biting force. Do not guide him. *Let his own relaxed muscles establish the occlusal position.* After a few minutes, remove from the mouth and permit to cure completely. Trim excess material, and smooth any roughness, but leave most of the anchoring occlusal matrix intact.

Testing the Splint for Correctness.   The finished splint should meet the following criteria:

1. It should feel comfortable and secure in the mouth, with adequate retention.

2. When the teeth are occluded lightly against the splint, they should strike simultaneously.

3. When the teeth are clenched firmly against the splint, no movement should be sensed, and biting pressure should feel uniform bilaterally.

If any deficiency exists, grind away the added acrylic material, and repeat the step of adding self-curing material as outlined above. Several such trials may be required to achieve the objective of producing an occlusal matrix that will hold the mandible at the closed, unclenched position.

Conversion of the Acrylic Splint into Metal.   Take impressions of both arches, and pour casts. Mount the casts in an articulator, using the acrylic splint as a bite. Wax up for casting in metal. Use minimal bulk; include just the incisal edges of the anterior teeth and the occlusal contact area posteriorly. A palatal or lingual bar and clasps should be used for strength and retention. Cast, finish, and adapt to the mouth for comfort and retention. Equilibrate if needed. Mill in the finished splint with abrasive paste for a minute or so to eliminate minute discrepancies and to remove the surface glaze from the occlusal matrix area. Test for correctness as described above.

Note: With steeply inclined articular eminences, the full occlusal matrix as produced usually is quite comfortable and acceptable to the patient. Patients with relatively flat dentitions, however, may feel the occlusion as "too tight." In such cases, it should be eased a little by careful grinding to permit a little more freedom in the occluded position. This applies especially to the anterior teeth.

Mandibular Repositioning Splint. Make a narrow rapid-cure acrylic anterior jig in the new mandibular position that eliminates the opening symptoms of disc interference. Remove the jig and construct the splint base as described above. Cut out an anterior section of the splint so that both jig and splint can be placed in the mouth. Add rapid-cure acrylic to the splint in the posterior and cuspid areas to form the occlusal matrix (using the jig as a guide). Then, remove the jig and add acrylic to form the occlusal matrix anteriorly, being sure to include the incisal edges of the maxillary and mandibular teeth. Sufficient bulk should be left anteriorly to prevent retrusion of the mandible. Trim excess material, and smooth any roughness.

Periodically "stepping the mandible back" can be accomplished by grinding off the occlusal matrix, constructing a new jig, and replacing the matrix as before.

Index

A

Abduction, 17
Acromegaly, 160
Actin, 64
Actinomycosis, 131 f.
Activating factors, 267
Acupoints, 116
Acupuncture, 117
Adaptive changes, biomechanical, 32, 155
Adduction, 17
Adenocarcinoma, 129 f.
Adenosine triphosphatase, 64
Adhesions
  disc-condyle, 142, 189, 281
  intracapsular (see Ankylosis)
Age
  and incidence of articular disc displacement, 106
  and incidence of TM disorder, 105
Agonist muscles, 64
American Academy of Craniomandibular Disorders, 5, 173
American Association of Oral and Maxillofacial Surgeons, 285
American Dental Association, classification of TM disorders, 173–174
Amphiarthrosis, 17
Analgesics, 264
  balms, 116
  blocking, 120
    in confirmation of diagnosis, 250–252 f.

interruption of cycling myospastic activity and, 272–273
Anatomical concepts of TMJ, erroneous, 38–42
Ankylosis, 3, 18, 294
  and arthritic pain, 127
  fibrous, 177, 204, 208 f.
  of mandible, trauma and, 159
  osseous, 177, 206–207 f.
  radiographic confirmation, 244
  restriction of movement by, 134
  treatment, 294
Antagonist muscles, 64
Antigravity mechanism, muscle spindles as, 69
Anti-inflammatory medications, 290, 292, 294
Antinociceptive system, endogenous, 7
Athralgid, 219, 292
  classification, 114
  criteria for identification, 124–127 f.
Arthritis, inflammatory, 173, 177, 200–201
  deforming, 4
  degenerative, 141, 201–203 f., 292
    of articular hyaline cartilage, 31
    predisposing factors, 188, 189, 281
  gonorrheal, 204
  identification criteria, 236–237
  infectious, 203–204, 292–293
  intracapsular, 34, 134
  pain of, 114, 127